Revision Total Hip Arthroplasty

Revision Total Hip Arthroplasty

Edited by

Roderick H. Turner, M.D.

Clinical Professor of Orthopaedic Surgery
Tufts University School of Medicine

President, Medical Staff
New England Baptist Hospital

Senior Orthopaedic Physician
Lemuel Shattuck Hospital

Boston, Massachusetts

Arnold D. Scheller, Jr., M.D.

Assistant Professor of Orthopaedic Surgery
Tufts University School of Medicine

Director of Orthopaedic Implant Service
Boston Veterans Administration Medical Center

Staff Orthopaedic Surgeon
New England Baptist Hospital

Boston, Massachusetts

Editorial Consultant

Michael Joseph Carey

Medical Artwork

William T. Stillwell, M.D.
Daniel A. Williamson

Medical Photography

James F. Green

Grune & Stratton, Inc.

(Harcourt Brace Jovanovich, Publishers)
Orlando   San Diego   San Francisco
New York   London   Toronto   Montreal
Sydney   Tokyo   São Paulo

Library of Congress Cataloging in Publication Data
Main entry under title:

Revision total hip arthroplasty.

   Bibliography: p.
   Includes index.
     1. Hip joint—Surgery—Complications and sequelae.
2. Artificial hip joints—Complications and sequelae.
3. Arthroplasty—Complications and sequelae.
I. Turner, Roderick H.   II. Scheller, Arnold D.
[DNLM: 1. Hip joint—Surgery.   2. Hip prosthesis.
WE 860 R454]
RD549.R44   617'.5810592   82-6203
ISBN 0-8089-1466-9   AACR2

Grune & Stratton, Inc.
Orlando, Florida 32887

Distributed in the United Kingdom by
Grune & Stratton, Ltd.
24/28 Oval Road, London NW 1

Library of Congress Catalog Number 82-6203
International Standard Book Number 0-8089-1466-9
Printed in the United States of America

84 85 86 87   10 9 8 7 6 5 4 3

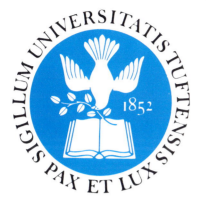

All of the authors of this book dedicate it to the New England Baptist Hospital and to the great men who have been responsible for the establishment of a strong Tufts University Orthopaedic Teaching Service at this institution:

Otto E. Aufranc, M.D.
Henry H. Banks, M.D.
Theodore A. Potter, M.D.
Morten Smith-Petersen, M.D.
Arthur A. Thibodeau, M.D.

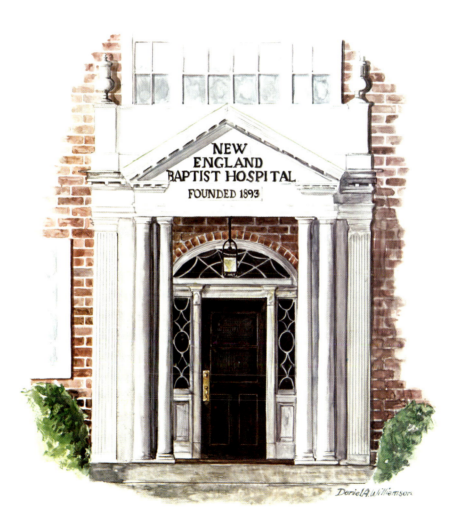

Contents

Color Plates I–IV follow page 92.
Color Plates V and VI follow page 316.

Acknowledgments

The authors would like to acknowledge those institutions and persons who contributed time, energy, loyalty, and support toward the completion of this book.

The project would not have been possible without the continuing support of the officers, administration, medical staff, nursing staff, and trustees of the New England Baptist Hospital. We would like particularly to thank Elinor Kirkby, R.N., who was administrator of the New England Baptist Hospital when the orthopedic surgical service was originally structured in conjunction with Tufts University School of Medicine. As acknowledged in the dedication, this service was made possible through the efforts of Drs. Otto E. Aufranc, Henry Banks, Morten Smith-Petersen, Arthur Thibodeau, and Theodore Potter. The continuing administrative cooperation of Mr. Raymond McAfoose has allowed this clinical and academic affiliation to flourish.

The editing and proofreading of several chapters of this book were greatly assisted by St. George Tucker Aufranc, M.D., and Sonya Scheller, R.N. Dr. Paul Woodard was tireless in his efforts to perfect and complete the references in each chapter. The reading and rereading of individual chapters were possible only because of the patient assistance of the following Aufranc fellows and postgraduate residents: Ron White, Richard Sweet, George Batten, Scott Oliver, Gregory Johnson, Steven Savonen, Bruce Leslie, Sheldon St. Clair, William McKenzie, Gary Peters, John Kazes, and Robert Randolph. Drs. Alan Robbins and Richard Pearl were most helpful in contributing to Chapter 2. Peter S. Walker, Ph.D., Peter Van Syckle, M.S., Victor Banko, Gerri Tavalaro, and Mark Phares were essential in the critical analysis and completion of Chapter 3.

We are deeply indebted to the following for extensive secretarial assistance: Christine Boly, Dorothy Bean, Margaret Leonard, Kaye Myers, Jacklyn Mayer, Denise Baffe, Betsy Turner, Kathy Thorsen, Mary Jane Downes, Donna Gilb, and Cynthia Turner. Individual chapters were greatly aided by the secretarial assistance of Christine Baranowski, Eleanor Busby, James Chambers, Tom DeJoie, Leonora Fisher, Patricia Flood, Jeannie Halligan, Mary Ellen Lyder, Kathryn McDonald, Dianne Mossey, and Josephine Wells.

The completion of Chapter 4 was possible only because of the assistance of Jan Woodbury, R.N., Elaine Marshall, R.N., and their excellent staff in the operating room at the New England Baptist Hospital. The contributions of Stacy Werner, R.N., Lester Borden, M.D., and Valarie Monnier immeasurably improved Chapter 5.

We are deeply indebted to William H. Harris, M.D., for suggestions and art work in reference to his careful work in the area of extraction of broken femoral stems. Richard Coup, E.Ed., and Espie Coup were extremely helpful in completing illustrations and text for this chapter. We are also indebted to William Jackson, M.D., and William Torgerson, M.D., for contributing their cases and critical evaluation of Chapter 7.

We would like to thank Stephen Wood, M.D., for his illustrations, which appear in Chapter 11. The illustrations and art work in Chapter 12 were made possible because of the contributions of Joanne Kineavy, Brad Milne, Susan Bright, Chuck Foltz, and Robert Benkovich of the medical art department at the Boston Veterans Administration Hospital. Chapter 13 was greatly aided by the contributions of Rodney Bond, M.D., Mary Delmar, R.N., Ann McNamara, R.N., and Charlotte McIntire. Editorial contributions were made to Chapter 14 by T. X. Kuriakose, M.D. The art work in Chapter 15 was done by Marilyn Lasek. Paula Collie, R.N., helped type and edit Chapter 15.

The authors would like to express their appreciation to the perfusionists and medical technologists in the New England Baptist Hospital Blood Bank for their contributions to Chapter 16. These people include Mary Crawford, James Kimbal, James Foley, Cheryl Bernard, Mark Cognata, Bruce Wacker, Carolyn Cardwell, Debbie Nelson, Hoda Sayed-Friel, Chris Werme, Cheryl Marson, Barbara Cross, Don Cartwright, and Leslie Lynch.

Dr. Lowell (Chapter 17) has asked us to thank his co-authors on the multi-center project: Gerald A. Finerman, M.D., Jack W. Bowerman, M.D., Richard H. Gold, M.D., Walter F. Krengel, M.D., William R. Murray, M.D., and Robert G. Volz, M.D., for their cooperation in this project.

Kathleen Driscoll, R.N., was inspirational in developing the thoughts and leadership necessary for completion of Chapter 18. The Physical Therapy Department at the New England Baptist Hospital contributed greatly to the formulation of the thinking that went into this chapter and its illustrations. We would like particularly to thank Dan Connelly, Shiela MacAllister, Arlene Colantuno, Debra Galinaro, Linda Cohen, Patty Healy, Margaret Francis, and Howard Pelkey.

Physicians other than contributors who contributed cases to this book are Alexander Wright, William Torgerson, Joseph Barr, Jr., William Shea, and William Dotter.

The medical art work and photography in this volume were made possible by grant assistance from the Boston Veterans Administration Hospital, Howmedica, Inc., Haemonetics, Inc., Davis & Geck, Inc., Midas Rex, Inc., and Proctor & Gamble, Inc.

We would like to thank specifically the Board of Trustees of the New England Baptist Hospital for creating an environment in which this project could be completed: President Allan R. White, Vice President Samuel Flemming, Treasurer Edward F. Brown, and Clerk Phillip R. White, Jr.

We would sincerely like to acknowledge the patience of our children: Jessica and Matthew Scheller and Rob, Cindy, and Betsy Turner, who were deprived of our time when we were working on this book.

All royalties paid to the authors will be contributed to the building fund of the New England Baptist Hospital.

Otto E. Aufranc, M.D.

Foreword

When facing a problem with the total hip arthroplasty, the surgeon should think first whether the problem can be managed without surgical intervention. As surgeons, we are always looking for a solution to a problem, but the problem is not solved well if the solution is merely a diversion—a need to have something different to offer. Results of such "solutions" are often far more difficult to manage than the original problem. If surgery is necessary, however, the patient must learn to manage his activities within the limits that may be imposed by even the best technical effort that we can offer by revision surgery.

The surgical problems in revision hip surgery are seldom solved fully unless they have limits that are easily defined, such as a loose or broken device, a poor or displaced portion of the implant, limited motion from new bone formation, etc. The patient's general health, bony and muscular "stock," cooperation, and desire to get well all come into play in achieving an end result.

It is very important to recognize that a complete solution may not exist so the efforts of both the surgeon and the patient can be directed toward the best *management* of the given situation, whether such management is supportive and nonsurgical in nature or a technical, well thought-out surgical plan.

The accumulated experience clearly shows the need to manage these problems in accordance with sound principles. If we are unable to translate these apparently complex problems into simple and easily understandable explanations, then we do not really understand the problems ourselves. In such situations I strongly advise seeking consultation and advice from associates.

As to the surgery itself, in order to have a firm feel for what to do and the confidence to carry it out, we must clearly have the following in mind: a thorough knowledge of the local anatomy; a capacity to visualize distortions of normal anatomy; the impact of congenital anomalies; changes introduced by injuries, dislocations, previous surgeries, or infections. If the previous surgeries have altered the battleground, then natural landmarks may be difficult to identify.

When operating on a patient who has had prior surgery, start the dissection in an area of known or normal anatomy and proceed toward the scarred area from above and below cautiously so that the unknown scarred area will yield its underlying hazards or innocence. In the surgical approach to any problem, the most direct route is usually the best. Sharp dissection is less damaging to the tissues, which will heal with less scar than those exposures produced by ripping and tearing (which may apear to be faster and more dramatic). While carrying out the surgical exposure, keep in mind the preservation of neurocirculatory life lines to the tissues left behind to insure their ability to repair themselves and regain function. Never dissect away viable tissue such as fat pads, gliding surfaces, fascia muscle, tendon, or bone unless you are sure that they will be an interference to repair or funcion. Gentleness to tissues is the hallmark of a mature and complete surgeon.

In implanting any device, a few basic principles must be remembered: (1) the simpler the device and the fewer parts, the fewer complications; (2) no matter how strong it is, it can be broken if overstressed; (3) no matter how securely it can be put in, it can loosen with the passage of time and with repetitive loading. Therefore, when implanting the device, visualize how it may later be removed or replaced with the least injury to the surrounding tissues.By developing a background of knowledge and incorporating the available experience, you can develop the confidence and the ability to do what needs to be done, keeping in mind that one should always be gentle to the tissues so that they will heal and return to their maximum potential or function. Patients should be made full participants in the process of recovery so that they understand their activities and limits and the reasons for them. They must be made aware of the need for their continued confidence, faith, and willingness to work with us so that they obtain the best available results.

Specificaly, patients who undergo revision hip surgery should accept the need for some external support for the remainder of their lives. Most revision patients will eventually be able to walk without the use of cane or crutch, at least for short distances. Even when revision patients have hips that are both strong and comfortable, they should be advised to walk with a cane anytime they go outside of the confines of their own homes. Patients with residual discomfort and patients with a Trendelenburg lurch in gait should use a cane at all times. The limitations of revision hip surgery must be impressed upon patients before, not after, the surgical procedure is performed.

Here the editors have produced a text that is the work of 34 contributing co-authors. I estimate that the collective experience of the orthopaedic contributors is drawn from well over 10,000 hip reconstructive operations and over 1000 revision total hip replacement procedures. The contributions from related specialties in Chapters 14 and 15 draw upon comparable wells of clinical and scientific expertise.

I have enjoyed working with Dr. Turner for over 20 years and have seen him evolve from an eager young resident to an innovative leader in the field of reconstructive hip surgery. There is no surgeon in my professional acquaintance more experienced or better qualified to address the highly complex subject material in this ambitious volume.

Dr. Scheller has joined Dr. Turner and me in our constant efforts to improve hip surgery by improved design, better materials, and meticulous surgical technique. In addition to being a brilliant graduate engineer, Dr. Scheller has had considerable surgical experience as Director of the Orthopaedic Implant Service at the Boston Veterans Administration Medical Center.

It is thrilling to me to know that such courageous and capable surgeons continue to review this type of pioneering work cautiously. It is only by such a permanent record and an ongoing observation plan that improvement in materials, design, surgical technique, and patient care comes about.

When working alone, one may accomplish much, but by working with others progress is accelerated geometrically. Individuals must be rewarded as virtue alone stands only as a statue, but virtue rewarded moves all obstacles.

I congratulate all of the coauthors of this impressive book for preparing a thorough and well organized treatise on these very challenging contemporary orthopaedic problems.

Preface

In the decade before January 1982 there were approximately 4000 reconstructive hip operations performed at the New England Baptist Hospital in Boston, Massachusetts. Approximately 760 (19 percent) of these operations were considered revision total hip arthroplasties. For the purposes of this volume and for the collection of our data base, the term "revision total hip arthroplasty" includes the following seven situations:

1. Failure of a total hip replacement
2. Failure of a hemiarthroplasty of the hip (stemmed proximal femoral endoprosthesis or cup arthroplasty)
3. Failure of a surface replacement system
4. Sepsis of the hip regardless of etiology
5. Femoral fracture adjacent to any prosthetic hip replacement system
6. Dislocation of any prosthetic hip replacement system
7. Failure of greater trochanteric fixation of sufficient severity to require major surgical intervention to restore abductor continuity

The 760 revision cases falling into the above-listed seven categories constitute the core subject material that has been analyzed in the preparation of this book.

Because the New England Baptist Hospital is a major referral center for hip problems developing in the northeastern sector of the country, it is reasonable to assume that we represent a microcosm of the national orthopedic experience.

A bar graph (Fig. 1) depicts the number of patients who came to revision total hip arthroplasty surgery in the lower segment of each vertical bar. The upper segment of the vertical bar shows the number of patients who were evaluated for failure of a prosthetic hip but who did not undergo revision arthroplasty. A number of patients undoubtedly appeared in the upper portion of the bar in one year in the chart and in a lower portion of the bar at a later year when their condition worsened.

The patients in the upper portion of the bar were involved in specific situations where the admission did not lead to major surgery, such as:

1. Arthrogram without surgery
2. Trochanteric wire removal for trochanteric bursitis (with trochanteric union)

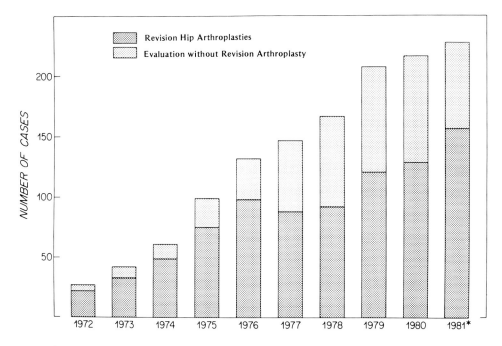

Figure 1.

3. Surgery canceled or delayed for some reason
4. Other surgical procedures performed (gallbladder, tooth extraction, hernia repair, etc.)
5. Other medical management (peptic ulcer, skin problems, digitalization, etc.)

The problem of failure of total hip replacements is real and is increasing steadily with the passage of time. This book is written to help orthopedic surgeons prepare to cope with the ever increasing hip revision decisions and operations. It has been our intention to make this volume a reference text such that each chapter can stand upon its own merit as a complete research source. Consequently, there is some inevitable duplication, both in the material presented and in the literature referenced in chapters dealing with closely related subjects. We apologize for this duplication, but we feel that it is necessary to achieve our ambitious overall goals for comprehensive coverage of the subject material.

Because our own clinical experience with surface replacement did not begin until the mid-1970s, we asked Professor Michael Freeman of the London Hospital to prepare a chapter discussing the management of failures included in group 3 as outlined above. Professor Freeman was a very early pioneer in resurfacing technology and his experience spans over a full decade. Furthermore, the London Hospital is a referral center for complex reconstructive hip problems and Professor Freeman has had wide experience with revision total hip arthroplasties of all types.

Dr. Jo Miller and his colleagues of Montreal, Canada, in discussing the critical subject of fixation, add additional international flavor to what we think is an outstanding list of contributing authors.

During the editing process some of the chapters of this book were reduced in scope and length. Consequently, some of the references are not cited in the body of the text, but we elected to leave all of the references so that the interested reader can pursue the literature in further detail.

Roderick H. Turner, M.D.
Arnold D. Scheller, M.D.

Contributors

Peter P. Anas, M.D.
Associate Professor of Orthopedics
University of Massachusetts Medical School
Staff Orthopaedic Surgeon
New England Baptist Hospital
Boston, Massachusetts

Otto E. Aufranc, M.D.
Clinical Professor Emeritus
Tufts University School of Medicine
Chairman Emeritus
Department of Orthopaedic Surgery
New England Baptist Hospital
Boston, Massachusetts

Forest C. Barber, M.D.
Honorary Member, American Academy of
    Neurological Orthopaedic Surgeons
Staff Physician
St. Joseph's Hospital
Forth Worth, Texas

Benjamin E. Bierbaum, M.D.
Orthopedic Surgeon-in-Chief
New England Baptist Hospital
Clinical Professor of Orthopaedic Surgery
Tufts University School of Medicine
Staff Surgeon
Childrens' Hospital Medical Center
Boston, Massachusetts

Gary W. Bradley, M.D.
Bone and Joint Research Unit
The London Hospital Medical College
Arthritis and Rheumatism Council Building
London, England

Stephan J. Camer, M.D.
Assistant Professor of Surgery
Tufts University School of Medicine
Clinical Instructor of Surgery
Harvard Medical School
Attending Surgeon
New England Baptist Hospital
Boston, Massachusetts

Joseph D'Errico, B.S., Eng.
Bradley University
Peoria, Illinois

Donna M. Dinardo, B.S., R.P.T.
Staff Physical Therapist
Student Clinical Supervisor
New England Baptist Hospital
Boston, Massachusetts

Roger H. Emerson, Jr., M.D.
Instructor in Orthopaedic Surgery
Harvard Medical School
Assistant in Orthopaedics
Massachusetts General Hospital
Chief of Orthopaedic Surgery
The Cambridge Hospital
Boston, Massachusetts

Michael A. R. Freeman, M.D.
Consultant Orthopaedic Surgeon
Bone and Joint Research Unit
The London Hospital Medical College
University of London, Whitechapel
London, England

Paul Fremont-Smith, M.D.
Physician-in-Chief
New England Baptist Hospital
Clinical Instructor, Harvard Medical School
Boston, Massachusetts

John McA. Harris, III, M.D.
Assistant Professor of Orthopaedic Surgery
Tufts University School of Medicine
Chief, Orthopaedic Section
Boston Veterans Administration Medical
    Center
Boston, Massachusetts

Michael Hume, M.D.
Professor of Surgery
Tufts University School of Medicine
Surgeon-in-Chief
New England Baptist Hospital
Chief of Surgical Services
Lemuel Shattuck Hospital
Boston, Massachusetts

Lydia C. Kalaby
Department of Orthopaedics
Montreal General Hospital
McGill University
Montreal, Canada

Klaus W. Korten, M.D.
Chairman, Department of Anaesthesia
New England Baptist Hospital
Boston, Massachusetts

William R. Krause, Ph.D.
Department of Orthopaedics
Montreal General Hospital
McGill University
Montreal, Canada

Walter G. Krengel, Jr., M.D.
Clinical Associate Professor
University of Washington
Swedish Hospital
Providence Hospital
Seattle, Washington

William N. Krug, B.S., Eng.
Department of Orthopaedics
Montreal General Hospital
McGill University
Montreal, Canada

J. Drennan Lowell, M.D.
Associate Professor of Orthopaedic Surgery
Harvard Medical School
Director of Clinical Services in Orthopaedic
    Surgery
Brigham and Womens' Hospital
Boston, Massachusetts

Sandra J. McKay, R. N.
Head Nurse, Orthopaedic Service
New England Baptist Hospital
Boston, Massachusetts

Joseph D. McKenzie
Biomedical Engineer
New England Baptist Hospital
Boston, Massachusetts

Gerald B. Miley, M.D.
Chairman, Infection Control Committee
Director, Rheumatology Clinic
New England Baptist Hospital
Boston, Massachusetts

Jo Miller, M.D.
Orthopedic Surgeon-in-Chief
Montreal General Hospital
Professor of Orthopaedics
McGill University
Montreal, Canada

Susan B. Mitchell, Ed. D.
Oklahoma State University
Stillwater, Oklahoma

Kenneth Moller, M.D.
Instructor in Orthopaedic Surgery
University of Vermont School of Medicine
Burlington, Vermont
Maine Medical Center
Portland, Maine

Arthur H. Newberg, M.D.
Assistant Professor of Radiology
Assistant Professor in Orthopaedics
Tufts University School of Medicine
New England Baptist Hospital
Boston, Massachusetts

Arnold D. Scheller, Jr., M.D.
Assistant Professor of Orthopaedic Surgery
Tufts University School of Medicine
Director of Orthopaedic Implant Service
Boston Veterans Administration Medical
    Center
Staff Orthopaedic Surgeon
New England Baptist Hospital
Boston, Massachusetts

James P. Schilz, M.D.
Otto E. Aufranc Fellow
New England Baptist Hospital
Boston, Massachusetts

Richard D. Scott, M.D.
Assistant Clinical Professor of Orthopaedic
    Surgery
Harvard Medical School
Staff Orthopaedic Surgeon
Brigham and Womens' Hospital
Staff Orthopaedic Surgeon
New England Baptist Hospital
Boston, Massachusetts

Kim. R. Sellergren, M.D.
Clinical Instructor in Orthopaedic Surgery
Tufts University School of Medicine
Assistant Chief, Orthopaedic Section
Boston Veterans Administration Medical
    Center
Boston, Massachusetts

Henry M. Steady, M.D.
Instructor in Pathology
Harvard Medical School
Adjunct Assistant Professor of
    Pathophysiology
Massachusetts College of Pharmacy and
    Allied Health Sciences
New England Deaconess Hospital
New England Baptist Hospital
Boston, Massachusetts

John T. Stinson, M.D.
Clinical Instructor in Orthopaedic Surgery
Tufts University School of Medicine
Staff Orthopaedic Surgeon
Lawrence Memorial Hospital
Bedford, Massachusetts
Staff Orthopaedic Surgeon
Winchester Hospital
Winchester, Massachusetts

Roderick H. Turner, M.D.
Clinical Professor of Orthopaedic Surgery
Tufts University School of Medicine
President, Medical Staff
New England Baptist Hospital
Senior Orthopaedic Surgeon
Lemuel Shattuck Hospital
Boston, Massachusetts

Steven M. Wetzner, M.D.
Assistant Professor of Radiology
Tufts University School of Medicine
Deputy Chairman, Department of Radiology
New England Baptist Hospital
Boston, Massachusets

John T. Stinson and
Arnold D. Scheller, Jr.

1

Clinical Evaluation of the Symptomatic Total Hip Replacement

There are myriad reasons for clinical failure of a hip arthroplasty. A growing list of complications and failure mechanisms is demonstrated in the literature. The relationship between the arthroplasty and its internal environment is exceedingly complex, with biological, mechanical, and structural factors contributing towards the integrity of the arthroplasty composite or to the failure thereof. A total hip arthroplasty, indeed, is a composite structure made up of bone, acrylic cement, metal, and high molecular-weight polyethylene. A mechanism of failure may occur in any one or a combination of these materials that form the composite. Failure mechanisms may occur at multiple levels, from the subatomic, as in component corrosion, to the macroscopic when the artificial components mechanically fail. Failure mechanisms in hip arthroplasty may occur at periarticular, articular, or extra-articular levels.

PERIARTICULAR MECHANISMS OF FAILURE

Soft-Tissue Contracture

Periarticular problems leading to suboptimal results are numerous and have a wide variety of clinical manifestations (Table 1-1). Soft-tissue contractures, usually flexion and occasionally adduction or abduction, can lead to gross gait disturbances, and functional limb length inequality.[1] The abnormal gait mechanism causes early fatigue of disproportionately stressed muscle groups, and continued muscle imbalance may place abnormal stresses on adjacent joints. Previously well-compensated arthritis in the lumbosacral spine, the contralateral hip, or the ipsilateral knee could then become prematurely symptomatic.

REVISION TOTAL HIP ARTHROPLASTY
ISBN 0-8089-1466-9

Table 1-1
Periarticular Problems Following Total Hip Replacement

1.	Soft-tissue contracture
2.	Neuropathy
3.	Vascular malfunction
4.	Trochanteric nonunion
5.	Heterotopic ossification
6.	Ectopic cement
7.	Limb length discrepancy
8.	Fatigue fracture

Neurologic Complications

Sciatic, femoral, and obturator neuropathies are well-documented complications of total hip replacement. Most nerve injuries are transient, rarely lasting beyond a year. The reported incidence has been approximately 1 percent.[4,7] Comparison of pre- and post-operative electromyographic studies, however, reveals a much higher incidence of subclinical nerve damage. The majority of nerve injuries consist of neuropraxias due to retraction, limb position or leg lengthening. Leg lengthening, especially when a result of reconstruction of long-standing dislocation, may produce a much more severe and lasting neuropraxia. So also may direct surgical trauma or cement entrapment and thermal injury cause more severe and lasting neurologic problems.[2,7] Hemorrhage and the resulting hematoma, whether operative or as a result of anticoagulant medication, produce a neuropathy of a more fleeting duration.[7,6]

Vascular Malfunction

The vascular system is an occasional source of reconstructive periarticular problems. Case reports of serious complications have been published in this regard. The femoral artery, separated from the hip by the capsule, the iliopsoas, and the pectinaeus muscles, was the site of pseudoaneurysm formation due to a protruding spike of methyl methacrylate.[8] Heralded by sciatic nerve palsy 9 months post-operatively, this complication ultimately resulted in hip disarticulation. Femoral artery damage, resulting in acute intraoperative bleeding or pseudoaneurysm,[10,13] has also been caused by over-zealous retraction. The iliac vessels have been injured by intrapelvic cement,[14] the heat of cement polymerization,[9] and by excessive reaming in patients with protrusio acetabuli.[11] The extensive debridement required to mobilize the hip or gain limb length may result in early or late limb ischemia, if the collateral circulation about the hip is comprised by arteriosclerosis or prior surgery.[12] With the expected increase in activity following successful total hip replacement, patients with borderline intra-arterial pressure often develop ischemia with exercise because of inadequate collateral circulation in the extremity.

Trochanteric Nonunion

The vast majority of osteotomized trochanters heal without incidence. Charnley evaluated trochanteric problems in his patients with a 9- to 10-year follow-up and noted a 2.7-percent incidence of nonunion.[17] However, avulsion, non- or fibrous union, wire breakage, and fragmentation, singularly or in combination, have led to a steady decrease in the use of this technique for uncomplicated hip reconstruction.[16,19,20] Trochanteric avulsion usually occurs within the first 4 weeks after arthroplasty, and is due to poor bone stock, improper wiring technique, rehabilitation in which flexion and extension of the hip is emphasized, or early abductor contraction. The incidence of trochanteric nonunion in dislocated total hips is approximately 10 to 18 percent.[18] While most of the trochanteric pseudarthroses are asymptomatic,[18] gluteal limp and pain may result. In trochanters with separation after hip replacement, significant abductor weakness occurs in about 50 percent of the cases; more weakness is evident if the fragment is widely gapped.[15] Persistent trochanteric pain has prompted wire removal in many patients, with inconsistent results. These unpredictable results are probably because most trochanteric pain is incisional with scarring of the iliotibial band and associated soft tissues. Late wire fatigue fracture is usually of minimal consequence.

Heterotopic Ossification

Ectopic bone formation following hip replacement has been reported incidences ranging from 5 to 30 percent.[22,23,32] In all series, male patients with osteoarthritis are by far the most vulnerable group, especially those patients with hypertrophic arthritic changes about the hip and spine. Heterotopic ossification was found in 8.1 percent of 501 Charnley-type replacements and correlated highly with the stiffer pre-operative hip and removal of osteophytes at surgery.[28] Patients undergoing revision hip replacement who formed ectopic bone following their initial procedure will, in all likelihood, have the same sequelae following the second procedure.[24] Bilateral disease is a strong predisposing factor, most likely due to the high percentage of patients with massive osteophytic osteoarthritis who have bilateral disease.[31] Other patients with a strong predilection for bone formation include those with Forestier's disease,[30] (DISH) syndrome,[25] and ankylosing spondylitis.[29] Those patients undergoing arthroplasty for congenital hip dysplasia (CDH), old Legg-Calvé-Perthes disease (LCP), and post-traumatic arthritis also appear to be at a higher risk,[24,26] presumably due to the greater amount of dissection required for successful reconstruction. The higher incidence following surface replacement and anterior surgical approaches to the hip is similarly explained, although the fundamental defect which transforms mesenchymal cells into osteoblastic precursors remains conjectural.

The clinical sequelae of heterotopic ossification are in large part benign,[23,31] however, the Harris hip rating scale is appreciably lower if significant amounts of new bone develop.[22] An association between ectopic ossification and femoral component loosening and fracture has been described.[27] It was believed that ectopic bone can magnify forces across the hip joint either by encouraging impingement or impeding subluxation of the prosthetic femoral head out of the socket. The onset of ectopic bone formation often produces signs and symptoms indicative of acute infection, a florid inflammatory response indicating a process of much more ominous nature.

Ectopic Cement

Another extra-articular source of problems is ectopic acrylic. The vascular and neurologic injuries associated with ectopic acrylic have been previously alluded to; its potential deleterious effects, by a local mass effect and thermal injury, are apparent. Ectopic cement has been the nidus of the problem in a number of locations about the hip. Cement-induced septic bladder fistula,[34] small bowel obstruction,[35] interference with musculotendinous units such as the quadriceps mechanism,[38] and an acrylic loose body in the ipsilateral knee following a long-stem hemiarthroplasty[33] have been reported in the literature. The more common ectopic cement villain relates to the articulating surfaces. As the prosthetic hip is reduced, a small amount of methacrylate may become interposed between the joint surfaces.[37] Ectopic cement may enter the articulating surfaces and impede concentric reduction of a dislocated total hip replacement.[39] In one instance, arthroscopic instrumentation and manipulation of the ectopic cement allowed reduction by manipulation of the fragment out of the joint.[36]

Limb-Length Discrepancy

Although leg-length discrepancy is a function of the accuracy of reconstruction of the joint per se, its manifestations are decidedly extra-articular. Moderate degrees of shortening are usually well tolerated, and patients rarely complain if a shoe lift of an inch or less is required.[42] Over-lengthening, however, is not as easily tolerated.[40] Patients take considerably more time in adjusting their gait pattern with a newly lengthened limb. Patients with chronic shortening from a congenital dislocation of the hip, however, have much less problem in adapting to their newly lengthened limb.[41] In many cases, limb lengthening cannot be avoided without placing the hip at risk for instability due to inadequate soft-tissue tension. Patients who do not have limb shortening prior to hip replacement are most likely to have some degree of over-lengthening post-operatively, and should be so warned.[43]

Fracture

Stress fractures following total joint replacement have been reported in the elderly,[44,45,49] and in congenital dislocations of the hip.[46] Relief of pain permits relatively vigorous activity on a previously unstressed pelvis or femur, as the bone yields to this unaccustomed stress. The pain from the fatigue fracture may point to an erroneous diagnosis of loosening or infection until a faint fracture line becomes visible on x-ray, establishing the proper diagnosis. A focal area of increased uptake on radionuclide scanning will precede the x-ray changes and in itself is often diagnostic.[47,48]

ARTICULAR MECHANISMS OF FAILURE

Problems directly involving the hip arthroplasty complex, ie, the bone-cement-metal-plastic composite, are categorized as articular problems (Table 1-2). These are of considerable complexity; most will be addressed in further detail elsewhere in this volume. In this chapter, emphasis will be placed on their clinical presentation.

Table 1-2
Articular Mechanisms of Failure

1. Loosening
2. Infection
3. Component failure
4. Instabililty
5. Osteolysis
6. Metal hypersensitivity and
   corrosion

Numerous questions must be answered when a patient with a painful total hip arthroplasty presents for evaluation and treatment. A complete history and physical evaluation are invaluable in distinguishing infection from aseptic loosening, and excluding other causes of pain and decreased motion. In spite of a complete pre-operative clinical evaluation, the etiology of component failure is not always clear until revision surgery; occasionally the mechanism of failure may never be explained.

Loosening

Femoral stem loosening is the major etiology for the mechanical failures in total hip arthroplasty that necessitate revision hip replacement. The magnitude of the loosening problem is significant; in 1974, there were approximately 100,000 primary total hip replacements performed in the United States. At a conservative revision rate of 8 percent, by 1984 there will be 8,000 patients who will need revision total hip replacement for loosening of their femoral components. Charnley and Cupic noted an 8.9-percent incidence of mechanical failure in a 9 to-10 year follow-up study.[54] Asymptomatic patients with x-ray evidence of fixation failure are much more frequently encountered, and their numbers appear to increase with time.[50,57]

Loosening of the femoral component was first mentioned in the literature in 1970.[70] Since that time, it has been variously reported as occurring in from 4 to 20 percent of patients.[50,58,61,67] Many causative mechanisms have been cited, including metal hypersensitivity,[52] calcar resorption,[62] and osteolysis.[59] More commonly cited reasons are varus position of the femoral stem and obesity.[53,61,64] Metal-to-metal prostheses increase torque and decrease the damping effect, which accentuates the mechanical stress on the supporting bone. In the case of McKee-Farrar prosthesis, it has been shown that neck-socket impingement was also an important cause for increased interface stress. A 16.2-percent incidence of loosening was observed in patients whose opposite hip was arthrodesed.[66,68,69] Other correlative factors are youthfulness,[63,72] increased height,[55] excellent initial surgical result and (in bilateral cases) a good result from a contralateral joint replacement.[53] Perhaps the single factor most generally accepted as contributory to femoral component loosening is poor cementing technique. An increased incidence of loosening has also been reported in cases with osteoporosis or osteopenia, and in as high as 24 percent of cases having had prior femoral replacement.[50,67,71] Certain metabolic bone diseases also predispose to loosening. Patients with Gaucher's disease are particularly prone, because the intramedullary infiltration of abnormal cells and the tendency for avascular necrosis can preclude adequate cement fixation.[60]

Acetabular component loosening has many factors in common with femoral loosening, ie, bone-cement-prosthesis structural fatigue secondary to stress of activity and poor fixation technique.[51] Interface radiolucency surrounding the socket-acrylic complex is frequently found in early post-operative x-rays, and has been seen in as high as 100 percent of cases.[56,65] Most of these radiolucent lines are noted within 1 year of surgery and subsequently do not progress.[65] It appears, however, that socket failure is a late clinical event which may be increasingly seen in the future,[56,58] Harris noted that socket radiolucencies are not appreciated in their malignancy beeause of this late failure, and that many patients with acetabular loosening continue to function well for considerable periods.[58] It wasn't until Charnley's follow-up study that a 9.2 percent acetabular loosening rate was apparent.[54] Most cases of socket loosening have been in females with broad pelves and wide midline-acetabular intervals.

Infection

Since the advent of prophylactic antibiotics, the infection rate has been between 1 and 2 percent, and about twice that for revision surgery. It has ranged from a low of .4 percent in primary arthroplasty,[81] to 17 percent in revision surgery for dislocation following the McKee-Farrar implantation.[78] While a disastrous complication, it may not be insurmountable.[75,85] About one third of the deep infections are diagnosed within the first 3 months after surgery; the remaining two thirds are diagnosed later.[82,90] While most infections are due to intra-operative contamination, an increasing number are metastatic from septic foci elsewhere.[77,79,89]

Although it has been generally recognized that obesity, advanced age, diabetes, and steroid therapy may influence the rate of post-operative deep sepsis, this may not be the case following total hip replacement.[82] Patients with prior hip surgery are at a greater risk for deep sepsis because of the limited healing ability of the dense scar tissue after incision, retraction, and suture.[80] Pre-existing infection and failure to aggressively evacuate post-operative hematomas are strong predisposing factors to deep sepsis.[82,86] While rheumatoid arthritis has been felt by many to be associated with a higher infection rate,[76,82,83] an equal incidence of infection between groups of osteoarthritics and rheumatoids was found in one series.[87] Gram-negative organisms have been increasingly encountered in deep sepsis of hip implants.[90]

The rheumatoid patient theoretically is more susceptible to infection because of the following factors: an increased incidence of spontaneous septic arthritis; steroid medication; a more sedentary life-style; an increased incidence of decubitis ulcer and pulmonary disease; and the chronic debilitating nature of the disease.[73,88] One group of rheumatoid patients is unusually susceptible to infections. These have hypocomplementemia and an elevated IgM.[84] Rheumatoid patients with impaired leukocyte chemotaxis are also at a higher risk.[74]

There is general agreement that the patient who has had a revision of a previous hip procedure is more susceptible to infection than a patient undergoing primary total hip replacement. Most investigators reproduce approximately the two-fold increase, noted by Charnley.[76] Despite refinements of surgical technique, the use of perioperative antibiotics, and the introduction of laminar flow systems, prosthetic infection remains a continual dire complication which may never be totally eliminated.

Component Failure

This topic is treated in considerable detail in Chapter 7 of this volume. Clinically, there is a distinct profile to patients most prone to this complication. It is usually seen in the active, overweight, tall individual whose mental image has not adequately addressed the limitations imposed by an artificial joint. Patients with prior femoral stem loosening are also at risk to develop component failure, but these problems may be mutually exclusive, metallurgical defects and design inadequacies being sometimes contributory.[91,93,97] If loosening occurs, the femoral component may subside to a relatively stable position, or may proceed to further loosening by one of four radiographic modes, depending on which portion of the supporting cement mantle is strongest.[101] Risk of stem fracture is highest with the cantilever mode of failure. Most authors feel that prior to component failure, cement failure occurs often or always,[92,94,100] and loosening of the prosthesis from the cement in varus inclination are clearly prejudicial to the survival of the prosthesis, because of the magnitude of the stresses developed.[98] Loss of calcar support is a constant finding in fractured stems.[96]

Technical and manufacturing conditions notwithstanding, several clinical factors which predispose to component failure have been noted in a number of reviews on fractured implants. Body weight and habitus, reduced motion of the hip, and the level of activity all may be contributory. In Charnley's series,[94] male patients weighing more than 88 kg had an incidence of fracture of 6 percent. When the rate of stem fracture was normalized to his entire series, however, the incidence was 0.23 percent. Taller patients with longer limbs acting as lever arms can be expected to have an increased vulnerability to component failure. In one series, patients taller than 1.8 meters and heavier than 91 kg had an incidence of stem fracture of 33 percent.[95] A relatively smaller range of motion of the hip both before and after surgery and diminished mobility in the contralateral hip and lumbar spine will also magnify stresses on the prosthesis and may result in fatigue failure. Ectopic bone-formers also are at increased risk of stem fracture, because normal cushioning of stresses may be diminished.[99] Stem fracture has also been seen in patients weighing less than 60 kg,[102] and it must be emphasized that there are a number of technical, manufacturing, and clinical factors that integrate an increasing fatigue on the stem.

Instability and Component Mismatch

Dislocation of the femoral from the acetabular component following total hip replacement ranges in incidence from about 1 to 8 percent of reported cases.[110] Subluxation is also known to occur, produce symptoms, and present a situation diagnostically more challenging.[113] Eftekhar classified this complication into three groups, according to the most probable cause: technical, mechanical, or anatomical.[106] He felt that often more than a single factor was responsible. Many believe, however, that the major cause is improper component alignment.[105,110,111] Other factors associated with instability are separation of the greater trochanter and previous hip surgery.[104,106,112] Patients who had previous surgery and patients with congenitally dislocated hips and acetabular dysplasia present more complex reconstructive problems and are associated with a higher incidence of dislocation.[108]

Stability is directly affected by prosthetic design, as a prosthesis with a greater neck recession allows greater freedom from impingement. A direct but inverse relationship has also been suggested between the femoral head diameter and the dislocation rate.[103,107,109] The cause of some dislocations of normally aligned prostheses remains enigmatic.[105,110] An accumulation of fluid in the closed periarticular space, due to infection or inflammatory reaction, may be responsible.[114] The recent trends of not performing trochanteric osteotomy and valgus positioning of the femoral component may be linked with a higher dislocation rate.[108]

Osteolysis or Diffuse Osteoporosis

Resorption of the supporting bone stock is another articular mechanism of total hip replacement failure. Its association with loosening of the prosthesis may be antecedent or secondary. Charnley, examining 5 necropsy specimens in 43 cemented endoprostheses at revision, noted resorption of the calcar but found no evidence of deterioration of the bone-cement bond up to 39 months post-operatively.[116] Progressive bone resorption following loosening is a well-recognized phenomenon; the etiology is unknown. Differential motion between cement and bone is a possible explanation,[121] but the reason why all loose prostheses do not show this phenomenon remains unexplained. Harris examined tissue from four patients undergoing revision surgery for extensive osteolysis following hip replacement.[117] His findings suggested that an adverse tissue response to fragmented acrylic might be the cause of bone resorption. The strong radiologic resemblance between this type of osteolysis and infection demands careful clinical evaluation. Resorption of the femoral neck following hip arthroplasty is a topic of continuing controversy; multiple explanations have been offered.[120] Resorption of bone from the calcar femorale can result from avascular changes in the region from the surgical preparation for the implant, diffuse osteoporosis because of inadequate stress to the calcar femorale or overload of the calcar femorale with microfracture and resorption. Loss of bone stock on the acetabular side resulting in intrapelvic protrusion of the socket is most commonly seen in rheumatoid arthritics, especially when metal-on-metal prostheses have been implanted.[118,119] Superior or medial socket migration may also be seen after reconstruction of the pagetoid hip.[115]

Metal Sensitivity and Corrosion

In determatologic practice, metals used in orthopedic implants are recognized as frequent causes of eczematous reaction. These reactions are attributed to a hypersensitivity to the elemental metals. Some cases of loosening of total joint prostheses have been attributed to the development of sensitivity to the metal component, and an especially high incidence of hypersensitivity to cobalt has been noted.[127,128] This has been especially implicated in failure of metal-to-metal implants.[124,125] It has been postulated that if elemental metal continues to be released into the tissues of the patient sensitized to that metal, a granulomatous reaction ensues, which leads to local small vessel occlusion and osteonecrosis. The infected bone may be resorbed, may be replaced by fibrous tissue, or may fatigue with failure of the implant.

An association between metal sensitivity and late prosthetic loosening was first demonstrated in 9 patients, from a total of 14 with loosened prostheses, found to be metal-sensitive by epicutaneous patch testing. In 24 patients with an intact prosthesis, no sensitivity was found.[125] Elves, et al found an incidence of 73.7 percent metal sensitivity in patients with unexplained prosthetic loosening.[124] On the other hand, one carefully designed study, including rigorously standardized patch tests and in vitro lymphokine assays, failed to demonstrate metal sensitivity in 20 patients with sterile loosening of the metal-c n-metal prosthesis.[122]

If wear products are the most important factor in producing metal sensitivity, this should occur much less frequently with metal-to-plastic prostheses; reports of this, indeed, are scarce.[124,125] While a metal-to-plastic prosthesis can sensitize a patient,[123] a definite correlation between this and implant failure remains to be demonstrated. More research in this regard with standardization of the techniques will be required before routine pre-operative skin testing can be recommended.

Extra-Articular Modes of Failure

Occasionally, the results of a technically perfect reconstruction may be marred by pathology extrinsic to the hip joint. Pain in and about the hip may be a manifestation of many disease states not primarily musculoskeletal in nature. An occasional patient with hip pain after joint reconstruction may be erroneously diagnosed as having a suboptimal surgical result.

A brief review of the pathways of pain referred to the hip and thigh is germane. This area is innervated by: (1) obturator nerve, from ventral divisions of L2, L3, and L4, and an accessory obturatory nerve from L3 and L4 in about 25 percent of patients; (2) femoral nerve, from dorsal divisions of L2, L3, and L4 by way of branches to the rectus femoris; and (3) sciatic nerve, from ventral divisions of L5 and S1, by way of the branch to the quadratus femoris.[133,137,139]

Sciatic neuropathy in particular, be it primary or secondary, may present a confusing symptom complex. Metabolic neuropathies, due to alcohol, avitaminosis, diabetes, or heavy-metal poisoning may produce continual buttock and posterior thigh pain. Episacral lipomas or osteoid osteomas may induce reflex sciatic nerve pain.[130] Protruding fourth or fifth lumbar discs are more common causes of sciatica, as is lumbar spondylosis or sacroiliac arthritis. Manipulation of the extremity during dislocation for hip arthroplasty may create stress along the lumbosacral spine and contribute to disc herniation.[135] Obturator neuropathies are much less common. The obturator nerve may be injured by pelvic tumors, the fetal head in difficult labor, and obturator hernias.[136] Obturator hernia may present as groin and medial thigh pain.[138] This is often severe in nature, characterized by dull pain and an intermittent burning sensation. Hyperesthesia may be associated. Early recognition is important, as mortality is high when intestinal obstruction complicates obturator hernia.

Abdominal tumors, infiltrating masses, adhesions, or infections in and about the iliopsoas muscle and the femoral or obturator nerves can also produce severe hip pain. Cholecystitis, nephrolithiasis, and aortic or iliac aneurysm may also be causes of referred pain and flexion contracture.[129] Patients with chronic aortoiliac occlusion may have low back, buttock, and leg pain as well as pain in the region of the hip.[132,134] Such a patient will have many complaints recognized to be of vascular origin, but often will have no calf claudication due to collateral circulation through the cruciate anastomosis. The clinical picture of ischemic neuritis of the sciatic nerve will frequently be superimposed.[139]

A final extra-articular mode of surgical failure is seen in those patients with emotional problems, whose initial procedure might well have been ill-advised. Characteristically, these patients will have high scores on the first three scales of the Minnesota Multiphasic Personality Inventory (MMPI). These are indices of depression, hysteria, and hypochondriasis. A high point-pairing score in two of these often predicts a poor result from elective surgery. These individuals usually lack insight into their behavior and are reluctant to acknowledge that their problems might be supratentorial in nature. Irritability, rigidity, and depression are characteristic, and psychological distress may be expressed through somatic complaints. The MMPI can be very helpful in ascertaining the candidacy of certain patients for hip reconstruction.[131]

CLINICAL EVALUATION

The patient presenting with a possible failed hip arthroplasty thus poses a diagnostic and therapeutic problem of considerable potential complexity. Our need to objectively address the situation is often tempered by the temporal and emotional investment that both the patient and the surgeon have made in the failed procedure. Such a patient may be scornful and distrustful and, understandably, somewhat depressed. A special effort must be made in support and understanding of these patients. The initial interview of a referred patient is crucial in establishing a productive patient–surgeon relationship. This rapport has hopefully been longstanding when the primary surgeon and revision surgeon are one and the same. Dr. Aufranc's admonitions never rang more true:

> Allow the patient to tell his story in his own way. Listen patiently until he has finished what he has to say. Do not interrupt the story until it is evident that some encouragement and direction are needed. Do not talk or try to explain conditions until all the essential facts of the patient's story, the preliminary examination, and any auxiliary studies that seem necessary have been evaluated. Ask more questions which will give a logical sequence of events in the development of the condition and in the past treatment.[129]

What were the patient's expectations from surgery? Were they ever realized? What is his or her customary life-style? How has joint replacement and its failure affected it? Aspersions cast on prior treatment are counterproductive. The story of a patient with a poor result following hip reconstruction warrants full attention.

History

Once the principal story has been told, a thorough medical history is taken. Disorders which may predispose a patient to infection, ectopic ossification, or osteopenia may thus be disclosed. Systemic complaints are specifically sought. Unexplained weight loss may point to malignancy with referred pain, as hematuria may herald intrapelvic cement. While patients with indolent prosthetic infection often have no systemic complaints, a history of fever, night sweats, or drainage will expedite the analysis. A bizarre symptom complex of kidney stones, gastrointestinal complaints, lethargy, and a loosened implant may be explained by an unsuspected parathyroid adenoma.

A thorough surgical history is essential. All prior operative reports are reviewed, looking specifically for details of operative findings, amount of dissection, anesthesia time, and operative complications. The number of prior procedures is noted, and any history of remote or recent sepsis should also be noted. The medical records are thoroughly reviewed, looking for problems such as delayed wound healing, prolonged drainage, or instability. The patient's progress with physical therapy is also scrutinized.

The pain pattern in failed hip replacements, while often nonspecific, is important to analyze. Pain, being in part a subjective phenomenon, may be described quite differently in patients sharing the same disease. The character of the pain, its primary location and radiation, its progression, and its temporal relationship to prior surgery all should be topics of inquiry. Provocative and palliative factors must also be uncovered. Pain on weight-bearing and a painful, restricted, passive range of motions are consistent findings in patients with deep pyogenic infection. This may be of fulminant onset, but more characteristically progresses insidiously. Subacute sepsis, often long-silent, may at first be only suggested on x-ray. Progressive pain and decrease in range of motion within the first month post-operatively may be due to heterotopic ossification, which may mimic an inflammatory process quite difficult to clinically distinguish from infection. Acute, severe pain usually accompanies component failure, although an occasional exception has been seen. The pain of femoral component loosening is usually experienced around the anteromedial thigh, and is made worse by passive internal rotation. The loosened femoral component often is associated with pain on rising from a chair due to resultant torque forces, but may improve after the first few steps are taken. (This is presumably due to microsubsidence to a stable position.) Knee pain may be the only complaint. Anteromedial knee pain is more likely to be referred from the hip, lateral knee pain more likely being due to strain. Loosened acetabular components often cause groin pain. The pain of aseptic loosening is more likely to be relieved with rest than that which is secondary to infection. Finally, atypical distribution or character of pain should alert us to possible pathology unrelated to the arthroplasty composite.

Specific complaints will generate suspicion of particular problems and dictate an appropriate line of questioning. Subluxation or recurrent dislocation should be clarified by defining what activities and which position(s) of the limb prompted the instability. The direction of dislocation should be known. This knowledge, coupled with x-ray analysis, will help decide whether component malposition, bony impingement, or poor muscle control and inadequate soft-tissue tension were contributory. The patient with loosening may describe, in addition to pain, progressive shortening of the limb due to subsidence or protrusio, or both, in combination. A decreasing range of motion may be the primary complaint. This may be associated with ectopic bone formation, soft-tissue contracture, subsidence, protrusio, and/or infection. In suspected hematogenous infection, inquiry is made regarding possible sites of primary sepsis and the performance of antecedent dental or urological procedures.

Physical Examination

The patient's height and weight are recorded, and age, both chronologic and physiologic, is noted. Gait, with and without ambulatory aids, is observed, looking carefully for antalgia, limb-length discrepancy, and compensatory mechanisms needed for maintenance of a stable center of gravity. In a painful total hip, a shortened stance phase, a shortened length of stride, abnormal pelvic rotation, and weight-bearing through the metatarsals is frequently noted. The patient's stance is checked for pelvic obliquity, compensatory scoliosis, and contractures; a Trendelenberg test is done. A positive Trendelenberg test may indicate abductor weakness or trochanteric nonunion, adduction deformity, a varus position of the femoral component, or ankylosis. A patient with a loosened femoral component may also present with a medius limp and a positive Trendelenberg. The general impression of the magnitude of the patient's disability becomes clearer.

With the patient recumbent, an active and passive range of motion of the hip is performed and documented. Those positions eliciting pain or instability are recorded. The patient with a failing femoral component may have a good range of motion but will often develop weakened straight-leg raising and quadriceps atrophy on the affected side. Patients with subluxation may have a palpable or even audible "thud" or "click," usually on hyperflexion in adduction, with a "click" of return on extension. A palpable "click" may be from a loosened acetabular component. Range of motion under fluoroscopy (with anesthesia) may be required in cryptic instances of suspected subluxation. The range of motion is compared to those values obtained in the operating room and during convalescence, and the operative report is again reviewed, looking specifically for impingement and the position and range prompting instability. Gross loosening may be palpable on passive ranging of the joint.

The skin is examined for abnormal healing, suture granulomata, or excessive scar formation, and any sinuses are probed and cultured. Dermatitis in association with a loosened prosthesis may point to skin sensitization to the implant. Palpation of the periarticular soft tissues may reveal abnormal scarring, heterotopic ossification, or ectopic cement. Swelling and local warmth will be detected in infection as well as in early heterotopic ossification.

The true and apparent leg lengths are then measured. Some feel that scanograms are necessary for truly accurate assessment. Comparison is made with pre- and post-operative measurements. A thorough neurovascular and motor examination is essential, as may be abdominal and rectal examinations in complicated situations. Functional evaluation of the ipsilateral and contralateral supporting joints, the spine, and any involved upper extremities is performed, in order to assess their contribution to the overall problem and to anticipate problems in postrevision rehabilitation.

Laboratory Analysis

Laboratory analysis is an important part of our diagnostic armamentarium. Routine screening tests done at New England Baptist Hospital and the Boston Veterans Administration Medical Center include complete blood count (CBC) and differential, erythrocyte sedimentation rate, a complete chemistry profile, urinalysis and culture, and bacterologic analysis of joint fluid aspirate. Additional tests done when appropriate are parathyroid hormone radioimmunoassay, EMG and nerve conduction studies, noninvasive vascular studies, serum electrophoresis, and determination of C-reactive protein. The radiologic evaluation of failed arthroplasty is covered in Chapter 2.

In many cases, the major decision to be made is whether or not the joint is infected. Often the history and physical examination is inconclusive in this regard; reliance must then be placed on x-rays and laboratory findings. Sometimes the diagnosis remains apocryphal, even to the pathologist, postoperatively. As a rule, it is impossible to definitely differentiate between infectious and noninfectious loosening by means of clinical, roentgenologic, and scintimetric examination.[149, 150] Infection after hip replacement generally does not present in the usual manner of temperature elevation, drainage, or leukocytosis. In one series, only 19 of 41 patients with deep sepsis had a fever of greater than 37.8°C.[143] The difficulties of defining deep sepsis after hip arthroplasty are compounded because of the long post-operative period during which the patient cannot be considered free from latent infection. Commonly the infection is indolent, and the patient appears with pain and some degree of osteolysis. Laboratory analysis may help us differentiate this from sterile loosening.

Generally speaking, the CBC has not been very helpful in cases of infected total hip replacement, as leukocytosis is not a common manifestation of this complication. In one series, a mean white blood cell count of 7,850 was found in 18 cases of documented deep sepsis; only 2 patients had elevations greater than 10,500.[147] In 41 cases of deep sepsis, the mean white blood cell count was 9,700, with an even lower white blood cell count with sepsis occurring in the immediate post-operative period.[143] We are aware of no series of infected implants where neutrophilia was a typical finding. Despite the lack of absolute white blood cell count elevation, however, a shift to the left may frequently be seen, and a differential should be ordered in all cases of suspected infection.

The erythrocyte sedimentation rate (ESR) is a rough indicator of serum fibrinogen and immunoglobulin concentration and, thereby, a barometer of inflammation. Although the precise mechanism remains elusive, it is thought that an accelerted rate points to a change in distribution and quantitation of plasma proteins, which leads to agglutination and rouleaux formation.[142] The sedimentation rate is commonly elevated physiologically in the post-operative period, returning to just above baseline at about 3 months.[140] Most reconstructive surgeons would agree that a persistently elevated sedimentation rate and pain in the operated hip are strong indicators of infection. Most patients with deep sepsis in whom this test is done by the Westergren method will have ESRs of about 40 mm/hour. The normal sedimentation rate, however, does not exclude sepsis, as was found in 3 of 19 patients with subacute infection who had readings less than 20 mm/hour.[153] The

42.9 mm/hour mean sedimentation rate found in 18 patients with pyogenic sepsis is more typical.[147] However, normal readings are not necessarily cause for complacency. The sedimentation rate is not necessarily a good indication of the activity of the infection and may even be markedly elevated without infection. Despite these shortcomings, it is our most valuable and reliable laboratory indicator of an infected prosthesis.

A valuable alternative to the erythrocyte sedimentation rate is determination of C-reactive protein. It is an abnormal protein that appears in blood in the acute stages of various inflammatory disorders, but is undetectable in the blood of healthy persons.[152] The ESR may be elevated in many conditions without inflammation, such as anemia, pregnancy, nephrotic syndrome, and hyperglobulinemia; it may be normal if an inflammatory process is associated with congestive heart failure, polycythemia, or a variety of other hematologic abnormalities. For the occasional patient in whom the ESR would be unrevealing, a latex fixation test for C-reactive protein may be helpful. A serum protein electrophoresis may also be helpful in the problem case. An elevated globulin fraction, with specific increases in the alpha and beta fractions point strongly towards infection. In patients with rheumatoid arthritis with elevated IgM, hypocomplementemia should also be ruled out through determination of serum levels. Abnormally low readings indicate a special susceptibility to infection.

The chemistry profile as a screening procedure is occasionally helpful in uncovering a metabolic cause of composite failure. Primary hyperparathyroidism may first be suspected through persistently elevated calcium levels. In an otherwise-unexplained case of aseptic loosening, parathyroid hormone radioimmunoassay should be considered. Calcium and phosphorus metabolism, as measured in the serum and also by 24-hour urinary excretion assays, may be abnormal in a variety of other, more occult causes of osteopenia and secondary loosening. The alkaline phosphatase will be mildly elevated in cases of sterile loosening and, of course, markedly elevated in instances of active heterotopic ossification.

A routine urinalysis may reveal hematuria due to bladder irritation by intrapelvic cement. Routine culture may help us in planning antibiotic prophylaxis for revision although a correlation between urinary tract infection and subsequent hip sepsis is questionable.[151]

Aspiration

When as much information as possible has been obtained through appropriate noninvasive means, aspiration is then considered. We feel this to be absolutely the single most revealing study in evaluating the painful hip arthroplasty. It is performed by us almost as a matter of course when hip pain cannot be easily ascribed to a periarticular or extra-articular mechanism. Through aspiration, we can obtain material for bacterologic analysis; inject contrast material to demonstrate occult loosening, abscesses, or sinuses; and inject local anesthetic to help exclude referred pain. When the question arises as to whether an infection is superficial or deep, aspiration, of course, is deferred until that question is resolved beyond all reasonable doubt. Acute suprafascial infection is clinically manifested by inflammation, incisional pain, and (occasionally) drainage, associated (but not invariably so) with fever and elevated white blood cell count. It usually manifests early within a 2-week post-operative period, and it is particularly likely to occur in patients with thick subcutaneous tissue. While bacterologically false-positive aspirates have been obtained, their infrequency makes a positive culture strongly indicative of deep infection. Conversely, a negative culture from aspirate should not be accepted as conclusive if other findings strongly suggest infection. In such cases, reoperation is indicated. Our approach to the patient with an infected prosthesis is covered in detail in Chapter 10.

We use a standard technique for hip joint aspiration. The patient is sedated and placed on the fluoroscopy table, and the hip is aseptically prepared and draped. We have found topical anesthesia to be adequate in most cases, but do not hesitate to give general anesthesia if pain or anxiety are considerable. An 18-gauge spinal needle is inserted 1 inch below and 1 inch lateral to the femoral artery on the line from the anterior/inferior iliac spine to the symphysis pubis. Under fluoroscopy, the needle is advanced until metal or bone is encountered, and an attempt is then made at aspiration. Repeated maneuvers may be necessary if considerable scar formation is present. If no fluid is obtained, several ccs of sterile saline are injected. This is then withdrawn and submitted for bacterologic analysis. Local anesthetic may be injected if referred pain is a consideration. An arthrogram may be performed. Specimens are then hand-carried to the laboratory, Gram-stained, and plated out on thioglycollate broth, sheep blood agar, MacConkey's media, and chocolate agar. Anaerobic specimens are incubated on colistin-nalidixic acid and kanamycin-vancomycin media, and plated out on laked blood agar. Further isolation can then be done, if necessary. If sufficient fluid is obtained, determinations of cell count, protein, and glucose are done. With this information in hand, combined with our clinical evaluation and other laboratory data, definitive therapy can then be planned.

PROPHYLACTIC ANTIBIOTICS
IN TOTAL HIP REPLACEMENT

After detailed and repeated reviews of the literature on prophylactic antibiotics in hip surgery, we strongly endorse their routine use in all cases of total hip replacement, both primary and revision.

Much has been written about prophylactic antibiotics in surgery; even a brief review of the literature would be impossible. The reader is referred to the writings of Sandusky, et al,[169] Di Piso, et al,[159,160] Chodak and Plaut,[158] and Medical Letter[165] for recent comprehensive reviews. Special attention is given to prophylactic antibiotics in orthopedic surgery by Boyd, et al,[155] Ericson, et al,[161] Burnett, et al,[156] Fogelberg, et al,[163] and Nelson and Schurman.[166]

The overwhelming majority of studies conducted to evaluate antibiotics in total hip replacement support the beneficial effects of prophylactic antibiotics immediately before, during, and immediately following total hip replacement.[157,160,164,167] Recommendations regarding the duration of antibiotic therapy after surgery vary, but there seems to be no proven value for continuing antibiotic therapy beyond 48 hours following uncomplicated surgery.[168]

The cephalosporin group of antibiotics had been very widely used for prophylaxis in total hip replacement surgery since the introduction of cepholothin in 1964.

Cefamandole nafate was introduced, as were other second-generation cephalosporin antibiotics, in 1978. Schurman, et al pointed out that cefamandole has a much broader antimicrobial spectrum than cephalothin, especially for Gram-negative organisms.[170] Cefamandole is resistant to degradation by beta-lactamase enzymes synthesized in Gram-negative organisms, thus resulting in the enhanced antimicrobial activity observed.

Schurman, et al have demonstrated that cefamandole is concentrated in bone and hematoma fluids at three times higher concentrations than cephalothin.[170] They further concluded that antibiotic bone concentration occurs so rapidly that antibiotics need not be administered to the patient prior to entering the operating room in routine total hip replacement cases.

Our habit in the uncomplicated total hip replacement case where there is no suspicion of sepsis (and or prior surgery) is to initiate intravenous (IV) cefamandole (1 gram) pre-operatively in the operating room, and to continue 1-gram doses every 4 hours for 48 hours. If there has been any previous surgery, or if there is any suspicion of sepsis, IV cefamandole is given immediately after intracapsular cultures of joint fluid, hip capsule, and bone have been harvested at surgery. If sepsis seems likely or probable, the dosage level is increased to 2 grams every 4 hours for 48 to 72 hours.

Cross-sensitivity between cefamandole and penicillin is now thought to be less than 5 percent; we use the former antibiotic even in patients with a vague history of penicillin allergy. If the patient has a history of cefamandole allergy, or if there is a documented history of severe penicillin allergy, we will change either the vancomycin or clindamycin. Antibiotic prophylaxis is continued for 72 hours following revision total hip arthroplasty, to be certain that all cultures and subcultures are negative. The management of antibiotic therapy in the proven septic hip is much more complex; it will be discussed in detail in Chapter 13.

REFERENCES

Soft-Tissue Contracture

1. Ireland J, and Kessel L: Hip adduction/abduction deformity and apparent leg-length inequality. *Clin Orthop* 153:156–157, 1980.

Neurologic Complications

2. Casagrande PA, Danahy PR: Delayed sciatic-nerve entrapment following the use of self-curing acrylic. *Bone and Joint Surg* 53(A):167–169, 1971.
3. Dunn HK, Hess WE: Total hip reconstruction in chronically dislocated hips. *Bone and Joint Surg* 58(A):838–845, 1976.
4. Eftekhar NS, Stinchfield F: Total replacement of the hip joint by low-friction arthroplasty. *Orthop Clin North Amer* 4 (2):483–501, 1973.
5. Fleming RE, Michelsen CB, Stinchfield FE: Sciatic paralysis. A complication of bleeding following hip surgery. *Bone and Joint Surg* 61(A):37–39, 1979.
6. Stern MB, Spiegel P: Femoral neuropathy as a complication of heparin anticoagulation therapy. *Clin Orthop* 106:140, 1975.
7. Weber ER, Daube JR, Coventry MB: Peripheral neuropathies associated with total hip arthroplasty. *Bone and Joint Surg* 58(A):66–69, 1976.

Vascular Malfunction

8. Dorr LD, Conaty JP, Kohl R, et al: False aneurysm of the femoral artery following total hip surgery. *Bone and Joint Surg* 56(A):1059–1062, 1974.
9. Hirsch SA, Robertson H, Gorniosky M: Arterial occlusion secondary to methyl methacrylate use. *Arch Surgery* III:204, 1976.
10. Kroese A, Mollerud A: Traumatic aneurysm of the common femoral artery after hip endoprosthesis. *Acta orthop Scand* 46:119–122, 1975.
11. Mallory TH: Rupture of the iliac vein from reaming the acetabulum during total hip replacement. *Bone and Joint Surg* 54(A):276–277, 1972.
12. Matos MH, Amstutz H, Machleder HI: Ischemia of the lower extremity after total hip replacement. *Bone and Joint Surg* 61(A):24–27, 1979.
13. Salama R, Stavorovsky MM, Iellin A, et al: Femoral artery injury complicating total hip replacement. *Clin Orthop* 89:143–144, 1972.
14. Scullin JP, Nelson CL, Beven EG: False aneurysm of the left external iliac artery following total hip arthroplasty. *Clin Orthop* 113:145–149, 1975.

Trochanteric Nonunion

15. Amstutz HC, Maki S: Complications of trochanteric osteotomy in total hip replacement. *Bone and Joint Surg* 60(A):214–216, 1978.
16. Charnley J: Transplantation of the greater trochanter in arthroplasty of the hip. *Bone and Joint Surg* 46(B):191–197, 1964.
17. Charnley J, Cupic Z: The nine and ten year results of the low–friction arthroplasty of the hip. *Clin Orthop* 95:9–25, 1973.
18. No lan DR, Fitzgerald RH, Beckenbaugh RD, et al: Complications of total hip arthroplasty treated by reoperation. *Bone and Joint Surg* 57(A):977–981, 1975.
19. Parker HG, Weisman HG, Ewald FC, et al: Comparison of preoperative, intraoperative and early post-operative total hip replacement with and without trochanteric osteotomy. *Clin Orthop* 121:44–49, 1976.
20. Thompson RC Jr, Culver JE: The role of trochanteric osteotomy in total hip replacement. *Clin Orthop* 106:102–106, 1975.

Heterotopic Ossification

21. Bisla RS, Ranwat CS, Inglis AE: Total hip replacement in patients with ankylosing spondylitis with involvement of the hip. *Bone and Joint Surg* 58(A):233–238, 1976.
22. Brooker AF, Bowerman JW, Robinson RA, et al: Ectopic ossification following total hip replacement. Incidence and a method of classification. *Bone and Joint Surg* 55(A):1629–1632, 1973.
23. Charnley, J: The long-term results of low-friction arthroplasty of the hip performed as a primary intervention. *Bone and Joint Surg* 54(B):61–76, 1972.
24. DeLee J, Ferrari A, Charnley J: Ectopic bone formation following low-friction arthroplasty of the hip. *Clin Orthop* 121:53–59, 1976.
25. Halpern AA, Rinsky L: Massive ankylosis following total hip arthroplasty. *Clin Orthop* 137:51–54, 1978.
26. Harris WH: Traumatic arthritis of the hip after dislocation and acetabular fractures: Treatment by mold arthroplasty. *Bone and Joint Surg* 51(A):737–755, 1969.
27. Langan P, Weiss CA: Femoral stem failure and ectopic bone formation in total hip arthroplasty. *Clin Orthop* 146:205–208, 1980.
28. Lazansky MG: Complications revisited. The debit side of total hip replacement. *Clin Orthop* 95:96–103, 1973.
29. Resnick D, Dwosh IL, Goergen TG, et al: Clinical and radiographic "reankylosis" following hip surgery in ankylosing spondylitis. *Amer J Roentgenol* 126:1181, 1976.

30. Resnick D, Linovitz RJ, Feingold MC: Post-operative heterotopic ossification in patients with ankylosing hyperostosis of the spine (Forestier's disease). *J Rheum* 3:3, 1976

31. Ritter MA, Vaughan RB: Ectopic ossification after total hip arthroplasty. *Bone and Joint Surg* 59(A):345–351, 1977.

32. Salvati E, Im VC, Aglietti P, et al: Radiology of total hip replacements. *Clin Orthop* 121:74–82, 1976.

Ectopic Cement

33. Hallel T, Salvati, EA, Botero PM: Polymethyl methacrylate in the knee. A complication of total hip replacement. *Bone and Joint Surg* 58a:556–557, 1976.

34. Lowell JD, Davies JA, Bennet AH: Bladder fistula following total hip replacement using self-curing acrylic. *Clin Orthop* 111:131–133, 1975.

35. Michel AG, Haskell J: Small bowel obstruction after total hip replacement. *J Bone and Joint Surg* 59(A):1115, 1977.

36. Shifrin LZ, Reis ND: Arthroscopy of a dislocated hip replacement. *Clin Orthop* 146:213–214, 1980.

37. Tailor CC, Murphy WA, Smith EL: Intra-articular methyl methacrylate: Complication of hip surgery. *Amer J Roentgenol* 131:1055–1057, 1978.

38. Turner RH: Personal communication.

39. Vakili F, Salvati EA, Warren RF: Entrapped foreign body within the acetabular cup in total hip replacement. *Clin Orthop* 150:159–162, 1980.

Limb-Length Discrepancy

40. Dunn HK, Hess, WE: Total hip reconstruction in chronically dislocated hips. *J Bone and Joint Surg* 58(A):838–845, 1976.

41. Green WT, Wyatt GM, Anderson M: Orthoroentgenography as a method of measuring the bones of the lower extremity. *Clin Orthop* 61:10, 1968.

42. Lowell JD: Complications of arthroplasty and total joint replacement in the hip, *in* Epps CH (ed.): *Complications in Orthopaedic Surgery.* Philadelphia, Lippincott, 1978, pp 928–929.

43. Williamson JA, Reckling FW: Limb length discrepancy and related problems following total hip replacement. *Clin Orthop* 134:135–138, 1978.

Fracture

44. Marmor L: Stress fracture of the public ramus simulating a loose total hip replacement. *Clin Orthop* 121:103–104, 1976.

45. McElfresh EC, Coventry MB: Femoral and pelvic fractures after total hip arthroplasty. *J Bone and Joint Surgery* 56(A):483–493, 1974.

46. Oh I, Hardacre JA: Fatigue fracture of the inferior public ramus following total hip replacement for congenital hip dislocation. *Clin Orthop* 147:154–156, 1980.

47. Prather JL, Nvsynowitz ML, Snowdy HA, et al: Scintigraphic findings in stress fractures. *J Bone and Joint Surg* 59(A):869–874, 1977.

48. Savoca CJ: Stress fractures. *Radiology* 100:519–524, 1971.

49. Torisu T: Fatigue fracture of the pelvis after total knee replacement. *Clin Orthop* 149:216–219, 1980.

Loosening

50. Amstutz HC, Markolf KL, McNeice GM, et al: Loosening of total hip components: Cause and prevention, *in The Hip Society:* The Hip. Proceedings of the Fourth Open Scientific Meeting of the Hip Society. St. Louis, CV Mosby, 1976, pp 102–116.

51. Andersson GB, Freeman MAR, Swanson SAV: Loosening of the cemented acetabular cup in total hip replacement. *J Bone and Joint Surgery* 54(B):590–599, 1972.

52. Brown GC, Lockshin MD, Salvati EA, et al: Sensitivity to metal as a possible cause of sterile loosening after cobalt-chromium total hip replacement arthroplasty. *J Bone and Joint Surg* 59(A):164–168, 1977.

53. Charnley J: Fatigue fracture of femoral prosthesis in total hip replacement—A clinical study. *Clin Orthop* 111:105–109, 1975.

54. Charnley J, Cupic Z: The nine and ten year results of the low-friction arthroplasty of the hip. *Clin Orthop* 95:9–25, 1973.

55. Collis DK: Femoral stem failure in total hip replacement. *J Bone and Joint Surg* 59(A): 1033–1041, 1977.

56. DeLee JG, Charnley, J: Radiological demarcation of cemented sockets in total hip replacement. *Clin Orthop* 121:20–32, 1976.

57. Dietschi C, Huggler A, Suezawa Y: Problems of loosening, *in* Geschwerd N, Debrunner HU (eds): *Total Hip Prostheses.* Baltimore, Williams and Wilkins, 1976, pp 144–152.

58. Harris WH: Loosening. *In* The Hip Society: *The Hip.* Proceedings of the Sixth Open Scientific Meeting of the Hip Society. St Louis, CV Mosby, 1978, pp 162–175.

59. Harris WH, Schiller AL, Scholler JM, et al: Extensive localized bone resorption in the femur following total hip replacement. *J Bone and Joint Surg* 58(A): 612–618, 1976.

60. Lau MM, Lichtman DM, Hamati YI, et al: Hip arthroplasties in Gaucher's disease. *J Bone and Joint Surgery,* 63(A): 591–601, 1981.

61. Marmor, L: Femoral loosening in total hip replacement. *Clin Orthop* 121:116–119, 1976.

62. McNeice, GM, Amstutz HC: Stresses in prosthesis stems and supporting acrylic—A finite element study of hip replacement, *in Transactions of the 22nd Annual Meeting,* Orthop Res Soc, p 172, 1976.

63. Debrunner N, Muller ME: Complications of total hip replacement, in Geschwend N, Debrunner HU (eds): *Total Hip Prosthesis.* Baltimore, Williams and Wilkins, 1976, pp 57–64.

64. Pellici PM, Salvati EA, Robinson HJ: Mechanical failures in total hip replacement requiring reoperation. *J Bone and Joint Surg* 61(A):28–36, 1979.

65. Salvati EA, Im VC, Aglietti P, et al: Radiology of total hip replacement. *Clin Orthop* 121:74–82, 1976.

66. Simon SR, Paul IL, Rose RM, et al: "Stiction-friction" of total hip prostheses and its relationship to loosening. *J Bone and Joint Surg* 57(A):226–230, 1975.

67. Stuhmer G: Loosening of prostheses. *in* N. Gesclhwend N, Debrunner HU (eds): *Total Hip Prosthesis.* Baltimore, Williams and Wilkins, 1976, pp 125–131.

68. Walker PS, Salvati EA: The measurement and effects of friction and wear in artificial hip joints. *JL Biomed Mat Res Symposium,* 4:327–342, 1973.

69. Walker PS, Salvati EA, Hotzler RK: The wear on removed McKee-Farrar total hip prostheses. *J Bone and Joint Surg* 56(A):92–100, 1974.

70. Wilson JN, Scales JT: Loosening of total hip replacements with cement fixation. *Clin Orthop* 72:145–160, 1970.

71. Wilson PD Jr, Amstutz HC, Czeniedci A, et al: Total hip replacement with fixation by acrylic cement. *J Bone and Joint Surg* 54(A):207–235, 1972.

72. Wilson PD Jr, Salvati EA, Hughes PW, et al: Total prosthetic replacement of the Hip-1977, *in Total Joint Replacement.* Proceedings of a workshop held at Northwestern University, Chicago, 1977, pp 38–61.

Infection

73. Baum J: Infection in rheumatoid arthritis. *Arthritis Rheumatol* 14:135–137, 1971.

74. Bodel PT, Hollingsworth JW: Comparative morphology, respiration and phagocytic

function of leukocytes from blood and joint fluid in rheumatoid arthritis. *J Clin Invest* 45:580–589, 1966.

75. Bucholz HW: Clinical experiences in the use of gentamycin-polymethyl methacrylate for prophylaxis against infection in hip surgery and in the treatment of deep infections in cases of total prosthetic replacement, *in Proceedings of the First International Congress on Prosthetic Techniques and Functional Rehabilitation.* Vienna, 1973, pp 119–135.

76. Charnley J: Post-operative infection after total hip replacement with special reference to air contamination in the operating room. *Clin Orthop* 87:167–187, 1972.

77. Cruess RL, Bickel WS, von Kessler KL: Infections in total hips secondary to a primary source elsewhere. *Clin Orthop* 106:99–101, 1975.

78. Dandy DJ, Theodorou BC: The management of local complications of total hip replacement by the McKee-Farrar technique. *Bone and Joint Surg* 57(B):30–35, 1975.

79. D'Ambrosia R, Shoji H, Heater R: Secondarily infected total joint replacements by hematogenous spread. *J Bone and Joint Surg* 58(A):450–453, 1976.

80. Dupont JA, Charnley J: Low-friction arthroplasty of the hip for the failures of previous operations. *J Bone and Joint Surg* 54(B):77–87, 1972.

81. Eftekhar NS, Stinchfield FE: Experience with low-friction arthroplasty. A statistical review of early results and complications. *Clin Orthop* 95:60–68, 1973.

82. Fitzgerald RH Jr, Nolan DR, Ilstrup DM, et al: Deep wound sepsis following total hip arthroplasty. *J Bone and Joint Surg* 59(A):847, 1977.

83. Harris J, Lighttowler CD, Todd RC: Total hip replacement in inflammatory hip disease using the Charnley prosthesis. *Brit Med J* 2:750–752, 1972.

84. Hunder GG, McDuffie FC: Hypocomplemintemia in rheumatoid arthritis. *Amer J Med* 54:461–472, 1973.

85. Jupiter JB, Karchmer AW, Lowell JD, et al: Total hip arthroplasty in the treatment of adult hips with current or quiescent sepsis. *J Bone and Joint Surg* 63(A):194–200, 1981.

86. Nelson JP: Deep infection following total hip arthroplasty. *J Bone and Joint Surg* 59(A):1042–1044, 1977.

87. Poss R, Ewald FC, Thomas WH, et al: Complications of total hip replacement arthroplasty in patients with rheumatoid arthritis. *J Bone and Joint Surg* 58(A):1130–1133, 1976.

88. Rimoin DL, Wennberg JE: Acute septic arthritis complicating chronic rheumatoid arthritis. *JAMA* 196:617–621, 1966.

89. Wigren A, Karlstrom G, Kaufer H: Hematogenous infection of total joint implants. A report of multiple joint infections in three patients. *Clin Orthop* 152:288–291, 1980.

90. Wilson PD, Salvati EA, Hughes PW, et al: Total prosthetic replacement of the hip-1977, *in Total Joint Replacement.* Proceedings of a workshop held at Northwestern University, Chicago, 1977, pp 38–61.

Component Failure

91. Amstutz HC, Markolf KL: Design features in total hip replacement, *in The Hip Society:* The Hip. Proceedings of the Second Open Scientific Meeting of the Hip Society. St Louis, CV Mosby, 1974, pp 111–124.

92. Amstutz HC, Markolf KL, McNeice GM, et al: Loosening of total hip components: cause and prevention, *in The Hip Society:* The Hip. Proceedings of the Fourth Open Scientific Meeting of the Hip Society. St Louis, CV Mosby, 1976, pp 102–116.

93. Cahoon JR, Paxton HW: Metallurgical analysis of failed orthopedic implants. *J Biomed Mat Res* 2:1–22, 1968.

94. Charnley J: Fatigue fracture of femoral prosthesis in total hip replacement—A clinical study. *Clin Orthop* 111:105–109, 1975.

95. Collis DK: Femoral stem failure in total hip replacement. *J Bone and Joint Surg* 59(A):1033–1041, 1977.

96. Galante JO: Causes of fractures of the femoral component in total hip replacement. *J Bone and Joint Surg* 62(A):670–673, 1980.

97. Galante JO, Andriacchi T, Rostoker W, et al: Femoral stem failures in total hip replacement, *in The Hip Society:* The Hip. Proceedings of the Third Open Scientific Meeting of the Hip Society. St Louis,CV Mosby, 1975, pp 231–239.

98. Galante JO, Rostoker W, Doyle JM: Failed femoral stems in total hip prostheses. A report of six cases. *J Bone and Joint Surg* 57(A):230–236, 1975.

99. Langan P, Weiss CA: Femoral stem failure and ectopic bone formation in total hip arthroplasty. *Clin Orthop* 146:205–208, 1980.

100. Martens M, Aernoudt E, DeMeester P, et al: Factors in the mechanical failure of the femoral component in total hip prosthesis. *Acta Orthop Scand* 45:693–710, 1974.

101. McNeice GM, Gruen TA: Mechanical failure modes of femoral components. *Trans Orthop Res Soc* 1:6, 1976

102. Rostoker W, Chao EY, Galante JO: Defects in failed stems of hip prostheses. *J Biomed Mat Res* 12:635–651, 1978.

Instability

103. Amstutz HC, Markolf KL: Design features in total hip replacements, *in The Hip Society:* The Hip. Proceedings of the Second Open Scientific Meeting of the Hip Society. St Louis, CV Mosby, 1974, pp 111–124.

104. Charnley J, Cupic Z: Etiology and incidence of dislocation in Charnley low-friction arthroplasty. Internal Publication, Centre for Hip Surgery, Wrightington Hospital, Wigar, England, No 46, 1974.

105. Coventry MB, Beckenbaugh RD, Nolan DR, et al: 2,012 total hip arthroplasties. A study of post-operative course and early complications. *J Bone and Joint Surg* 56(A):273, 1974.

106. Eftekhar NS: Dislocation and instability complicating low-friction arthroplasty of the hip joint. *Clin Orthop* 121:120–125, 1976.

107. Evanski PM, Waugh TR, Orofino CF: Total hip replacement with the Charnley prosthesis. *Clin Orthop* 95:69–72, 1973.

108. Fackler CD, Poss R: Dislocation in total hip arthroplasties. *Clin Orthop* 151:169–178, 1980.

109. Harris WH: A new total hip implant. *Clin Orthop* 81:105–113, 1971.

110. Lewinnek GE, Lewis JL, Tarr R, et al: Dislocations after total hip replacement arthroplasties. *J Bone and Joint Surg* 60(A):217–220, 1978.

111. Nolan DR, Fitzgerald RH, Beckenbaugh RD: Complications of total hip arthroplasty treated by re-operation. *J Bone and Joint Surg* 57(A):977–981, 1975.

112. Pellici PM, Salvati EA, Robinson AJ: Mechanical failures in total hip replacement requiring re-operation. *J Bone and Joint Surg* 61(A):28–36, 1979.

113. Ritter MA: Dislocation and subluxation of the total hip replacement. *Clin Orthop* 121:92–94, 1976.

114. Ritter MA: A treatment plan for the dislocated total hip arthroplasty. *Clin Orthop* 153:153–155, 1980.

Osteolysis

115. Calandruccio RA: Anthroplasty, *in* Edmonson AS, Crenshaw AH (eds): *Campbell's Operative Orthopedics (ed 6),* St Louis, CV Mosby, 1980, pp 2301–2303.

116. Charnley, J: The bonding of prostheses to bone by cement. *J Bone and Joint Surg* 46(B):518–529, 1964.

117. Harris WH, Schiller AL, Scholler JM, et al: Extensive localized bone Resorption in the femur following total hip replacement. *J Bone and Joint Surg* 58(A):612–618, 1976.
118. Hastings DE, Parker SM: Protrusio acetabuli in rheumatoid arthritis. *Clin Orthop* 108:76–83, 1975.
119. Salvati EA, Bullough P, Wilson PD Jr: Intrapelvic protrusion of the acetabular component following total hip replacement. *Clin Orthop* 111:212–227, 1975.
120. Sarmiento A, Turner TM, Latta LL, et al: Factors contributing to lysis of the femoral neck in total hip arthroplasty. *Clin Orthop* 145:208–212, 1979.
121. Scales JT: Acrylic bone cement—bone or plug? *J Bone and Joint surg* 50(B):698–700, 1968.

Metal Sensitivity

122. Brown GC, Lockshin MD, Salvati EA, et al: Sensitivity to metal as a possible cause of sterile loosening after cobalt-chromium total hip replacement arthroplasty. *J Bone and Joint Surg* 59(A):164–168. 1977.
123. Deutman R, Mulder TJ, Brian R, et al: Metal sensitivity before and after total hip arthroplasty. *J Bone and Joint Surg* 59(A):862–865, 1977.
124. Elves MW, Wilson JN, Scales JT, et al: Incidence of metal sensitivity in patients with total joint replacements. *Brit Med J* 4:376–378, 1975.
125. Evans EM, Freeman MAR, Vernon-Roberts B: Metal sensitivity as a cause of bone necrosis and loosening of the prosthesis in total joint replacement. *J Bone and Joint Surg* 56(B):626–642, 1974.
126. Ferguson AB Jr, Laing PG, Hodge ES: The ionization of metal implants in living tissues. *J Bone and Joint Surg* 42(A): 77–90, 1960.
127. Jones DA, Lucas HK, O'Driscoll M, et al: Cobalt toxicity after McKee hip arthroplasty. *J Bone and Joint Surg* 57(B):289–296, 1975.
128. Munro-Ashman D, Miller AJ: Rejection of metal-to-metal prostheses and skin sensitivity to cobalt contact. *Dermat* 2:65–67, 1976.

Extra-Articular Modes of Failure

129. Aufranc OE: *Constructive Surgery of the Hip.* St Louis, CV Mosby, 1962, p 18.
130. Copeman WS: Fibrofatty tissue and its relation to rheumatic syndromes. *Brit Med J* 2:191–197, 1949.
131. Dennis MD, Greene RL, Farr SP, et al: The Minnesota Multiphasic Personality Inventory: General guidelines to its use and interpretation in orthopedics. *Clin Orthop* 150:125–130, 1980.
132. DeWolfe VG et al; Intermittent claudication of the hip and the syndrome of chronic aortoiliac thrombosis. *Circulation* 9:1–16, 1954.
133. Kaiser RA: Obturator neurectomy for causalgia. *J Bone and Joint Surg* 31(A):815–819, 1949.
134. Leriche R, Morel A: The syndrome of thrombotic obliteration of the aortic bifurcation. *Ann Surg* 127:193–206, 1948.
135. Mallory TH, Halley D: Posterior buttock pain following total hip replacement. *Clin Orthop* 90:104–106, 1973.
136. Merritt HH: *A textbook of Neurology* (ed 3). Philadelphia, Lea and Febiger, 1973, p 391.
137. Obletz BE, Lockie, LM, Milch E et al: Chronic arthritis of the hip: Effects of partial denervation. *J Bone and Joint Surg* 31(A):805–814, 1949.
138. Sumell A, Ljungdahl I, Spangen L: Thigh neuralgia as symptom of obturator hernia. *Acta Chir Scand* 142:457–459, 1976.
139. Turek SL: *Orthopaedics. Principles and Their Application (ed 3)* Philadelphia, Lippincott, 1977, p 106.

Laboratory Analysis

140. Carlsson AS: Erythrocyte sedimentation rate in infected and non-infected total hip arthroplasties. *Acta Orthop Scand* 49:287–290, 1978.

141. Carlsson AS, Josefsson G, Lindberg L: Revision with gentamicin-impregnated cement for deep infections in total hip arthroplasties. *J Bone and Joint Surg* 60(A):1059–1064, 1978.

142. Davidsohn I, Nelson DA: Chapter 5, *in* Davidsohn I, Henny JB (eds): *Clinical Diagnosis by Laboratory Methods* (ed 14). Philadelphia, WB Saunders, 1969, pp 152–153.

143. Fitzgerald RH, Nolan DC, Illstrup DM, et al: Deep wound sepsis following total hip arthroplasty. *J Bone and Joint Surg* 59(A):847–856, 1977.

144. Fitzgerald R, Peterson L, Washington J II, et al: Bacterial colonization of wounds and sepsis in total hip arthroplasty. *J Bone and Joint Surg* 55(A):1242–1250, 1973.

145. Fitzgerald RH, Washington J II: Contamination of the operative wound. *Orthop Clin North Am* 6:1105–1114, 1975.

146. Hunder GG, McDuffie FC: Hypocomplementemia in rheumatoid arthritis. *Am J Med* 54:461–472, 1973.

147. Jupiter JB, Karchmer AW, Lowell JD, et al: Total hip arthroplasty in the treatment of adult hips with current or quiescent sepsis. *Bone and Joint Surg* 63(A):194–200, 1981.

148. Kamme C, Lindberg L: Aerobic and anaerobic bacteria in deep infections after total hip arthroplasty. *Clin Orthop* 154:201–207, 1981.

149. Lindberg L: Diagnosis of infection in total hips, in *Revision Arthroplasty*. Oxford, Oxford Medical Education Services, 1979.

150. Lindberg L, Sjostrand LO, Mortenson W: Assessment of the painful total hip arthroplasty with arthrography and bone scanning, *in* St Louis, CV Mosby, 1977, p 197.

151. Nelson JP: Deep infection following total hip Arthroplasty. *J Bone and Joint Surg* 59(A):1042–1044, 1977.

152. Sonnenwirth AC: Miscellanbeous Serologic Tests, *In* Frankel S, Reitman S, Sonnenwirth AC (eds): *Gradwohl's Clinical Laboratory Methods and Diagnosis (ed 7)* Saint Louis, CV Mosby, 1970, pp 1563–1564.

153. Wilson PD Jr, Aglietti P, Salvati EA: Subacute sepsis of the hip treated by antibiotics and cemented prosthesis. *J Bone and Joint Surg* 56(A):879–898, 1974.

154. Wilson PD Jr, Salvati EA, Aglietti P, et al:The problem of infection in endoprosthetic replacement of the hip joint. *Clin Orthop* 96:213–221, 1973.

Prophylactic Antibiotics

155. Boyd RJ, Burke JF, Colton T. A double-blind clinical trial of prophylactic antibiotics in hip fractures. *J Bone and Joint Surg* 55(A): 1251–1258, 1973.

156. Burnett JW, Gustilo RB, Williams DN, et al: Prophylactic antibiotics in hip fractures. *J Bone and Joint Surg* 62(A):457–462, 1980.

157. Carlsson AS, Lidgren L, Lindberg L: Prophylactic antibiotics against early and late deep infections after total hip replacements. *Acta Orth Scand* 48: 405–410, 1977.

158. Chodak GW, Plaut ME; Use of systemic antibiotics for prophylaxis in surgery. *Arch Surg* 112:326–334, 1977.

159. DiPiro JT, Record KE, Schanzenbach KS, et al: Antimicrobial prophylaxis in surgery: Part 1. *Amer J of Hosp Pharmacy* 38:320–334, 1981.

160. DiPiro JT, Record KE, Schanzenbach KS, et al: Antimicrobial prophylaxis in surgery: Part 2. *Amer J of Hosp Pharmacy* 38:487–494, 1981.

161. Ericson C, Lidgreen L, Lindberg L: Cloxacillin in the prophylaxis of post-operative infections of the hip. *J Bone and Joint Surg* 55(A):808–813, 1973.

162. Fitzgerald RH Jr, Kelly PJ, Snyder RJ, et al: Penetration of methicillin,oxacillin and cephalothin into bone and synovial tissues. *Antimicrob Chemother* 14:723–726, 1978.

163. Fogelberg EV, Zitzmann EK, Stinchfield FE: Prophylactic penicillin in orthopaedic surgery. *J Bone and Joint Surg* 52(A):95–98, 1970.

164. Hill C, Mazas F, Flamant R, et al: Prophylactic cefazolin versus placebo in total hip replacement. *Lancet* 1:795–797, 1981.

165. Medical letter on drugs and therapeutics. Antimicrobial prophylaxis for surgery. *Medcial Letter* 23:77–80, 1981.

166. Nelson CL, Schurman DJ: *Preventive Antibiotics, Instructional Course Lectures of AAOS,* Vol 30. St Louis, CV Mosby and Co, 1981.

167. Pavel A, Smith RK, Ballard A, et al: Prophylactic antibiotics in clean orthopaedic surgery. *J Bone and Joint Surg* 56(A):777–782, 1974.

168. Pollard JP, Hughes SPF, Scott JE, et al: Antibiotic prophylaxis in total hip replacement. *Brit Med J* 1:707–709, 1979.

169. Sandusky WR: Use of prophylactic antibiotics in surgical patients. *Surg Clin No Amer* 60:83–92, 1980.

170. Schurman DJ, Hirshman HP, Burton DP: Cephalothin and cefamandole penetration into bone, synovial fluid and wound drainage fluid. *J Bone and Joint Surg* 62(A): 981–985, 1980.

Steven M. Wetzner,
Arthur H. Newberg, and
Joseph D. McKenzie

2

Radiographic Evaluation of the Symptomatic Hip Replacement

The successful development of reliable total hip arthroplasties for the treatment of severely diseased hips has led to its increasing application in this country (greater than 75,000 such operations annually).[22] As with any mode of therapy, the more frequent its use, the greater the chance of complication or failure. Component failure involving the total hip arthroplasty is a complex mechanism, involving mechanical, biological, and structural factors that affect the integrity of the component as a whole. The most frequent of these complications are infection and component loosening.[1] The presenting clinical symptom in such cases is almost always a painful joint. The clinician must utilize information derived from plain radiographic, radionuclide, and arthrographic examinations to determine the cause of the symptoms. In the end, however methodical the work-up, clinical judgment may be the deciding factor in dictating a treatment course. The following discussion of the plain radiographic as well as complementary arthrographic and radionuclide findings will make the evaluation of the symptomatic patient less susceptible to an inconclusive result.

RADIOGRAPHY OF THE TOTAL HIP JOINT REPLACEMENT

The total hip prosthesis may consist of a metal-to-metal articulation, such as the McKee-Farrar or Ring prosthesis. More commonly, it consists of a low-friction metal femoral component and a high molecular-weight polyethylene acetabular

25

REVISION TOTAL HIP ARTHROPLASTY
ISBN 0-8089-1466-9

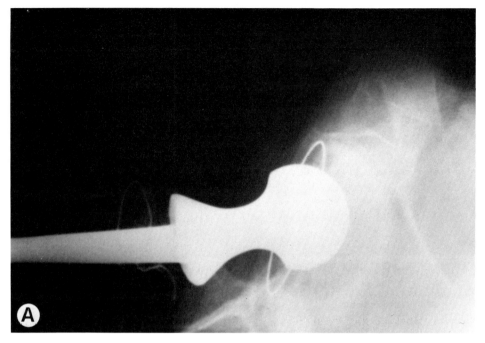

Fig. 2-1A.   An example of 15° of anteversion of the acetabular component.

component, such as in the Charnley,* Aufranc-Turner,† and the newer ATS†
prostheses. The initial priority that must be established in the plain film assessment
of the prosthesis is the accurate determination of the position of the femoral and
acetabular components.[6] Anteroposterior (AP) pelvis and true lateral radiographs
centered on the acetabulum are required for adequate evaluation. In each prosthesis,
the acetabular component is placed so that the acetabular cup is at a particular
angle to the base of the pelvis (30° for the Aufranc-Turner prosthesis and 45° for
the Charnley), in an effort to provide as much motion as possible without
dislocation.[6] The acetabular component ideally is placed in slight anteversion. The
actual degree of acetabular anteversion can only be measured in the true lateral
film. On the frontal view, the acetabular equatorial marker wire should form a thin
ellipse if the cup is properly positioned in slight anteversion. If the equatorial
marker wires begin to assume a more circular configuration, increasing anteversion
may be inferred.[20] Without the true lateral film, retroversion cannot be ruled out,
even though the cup appears to be in anteversion (Fig. 2-1).. The degree of apparent
anteversion seems to vary considerably with the accuracy in centering the film over
the acetabulum.[20]

The femoral component should be centered in the medullary canal or placed
in slight valgus.[27,35] The prosthesis should be positioned so that the lesser trochanters
are at symmetrical levels, thus minimizing the possibility of leg length discrepancy.
A horizontal line, drawn through the inferior margin of the ischium, provides a
reference point for evaluating these discrepancies. The radiographic evaluation of

*Chas. F. Thackray, Ltd.
†Howmedica Inc.

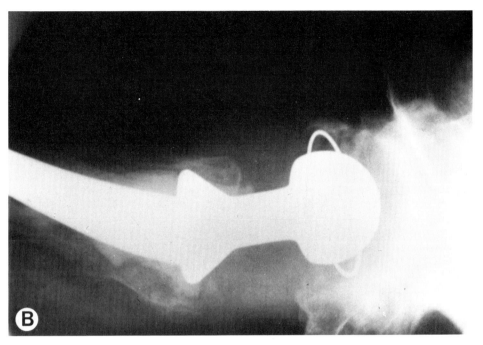

Fig. 2-1B. An example of a retroverted acetabular cup which might predispose to posterior dislocation.

the total hip arthroplasty allows analysis of the components' interactive environment between the bone, acrylic cement, metal, and high density polyethylene. The use of barium-impregnated cement allows easier evaluation of the cement-bone, as well as cement-metal, interface. The acrylic must be thought of as a space-filler within the bony matrix, rather than as an adhesive.[23] It allows interdigitation within the surrounding bone and serves as a mechanism of absorbing and uniformly transmitting forces to the bone. The effectiveness of the methacrylate relies upon its symmetrical distribution of even thickness around the prosthesis with meticulous detail to the absence of voids. Chou and Coventry have developed a criteria of risk factors predisposing to prosthesis failure, especially stem fracture.[10] These include uneven distribution of cement; inadequate cement beyond the tip; voids greater than 4 mm; and bone-cement interface gaps greater than 2 mm (Fig. 2-2).[10] Beckenbaugh and Ilstrup found loosening of the femoral component to be inversely related to the degree of extension of cement past the prosthesis tip.[7] Extension of cement past the tip by a distance of at least 2 cm is optimal.[7] The use of a silastic intramedullary plug distal to the tip of the prosthesis ensures adequate filling with cement. This plug limits the distal spread of cement, as well as increases filling pressure, thus effecting a more even cement distribution around the prosthesis.

The diagnosis of "loosening of prosthetic components" has been radiographically defined by the presence of a radiolucent line at the cement-bone interface. However, the presence of a 1-mm radiolucent zone at the cement-bone interface is a frequent occurrence noted in the acetabular region in as many as 100 percent of the patients in Salvati's series,[27] and in 99 percent of patients in a series by

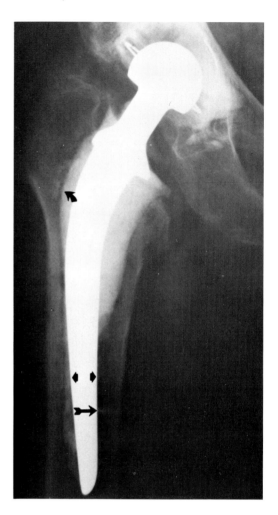

Fig. 2-2. Plain radiograph of a right total hip prosthesis demonstrates several factors which predispose to component failure. These include inadequate cement (arrow), unequal cement distribution (arrowheads), and cement-bone lucency greater than 2 mm (curved arrow).

Beckenbaugh and Ilstrup.[7] It is less frequently seen in the femoral region, at a rate of approximately 50 percent.[15] The radiolucent zone can be seen in the immediate post-operative period, or may develop post-operatively, in the first 6 months.[2] Only when the zone progresses to a width greater than 2 mm is there evidence of mechanical loosening (Fig. 2-3).[2,3,13,15,27] What the radiolucent zone represents is

Fig. 2-3A. Radiograph of the pelvis demonstrates bilateral total hip replacements. Note a 1-mm cement-bone lucency in the acetabular component of the right hip. This is considered normal.

Fig. 2-3B. Two years later, there is an increased lucency at the cement-bone interface of the acetabular component of the right hip suggestive of loosening (arrows).

Fig. 2-3C. The arthogram confirms the acetabular loosening. Contrast appears at the cement-bone interface (arrows). There is filling of a pseudobursa and early lymphatic opacification (arrowheads).

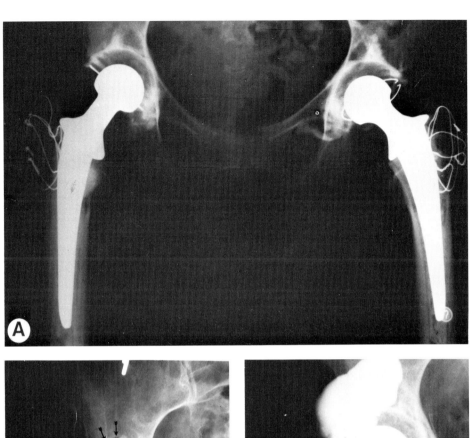

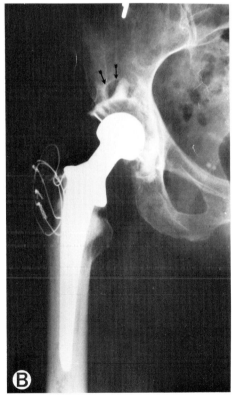

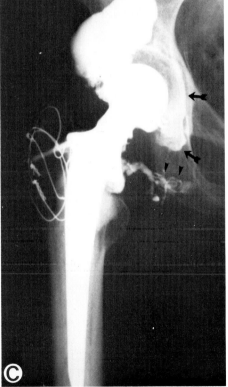

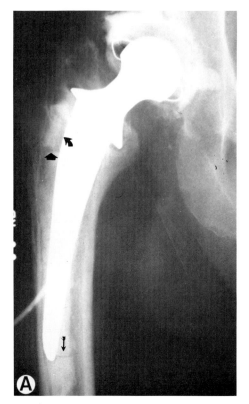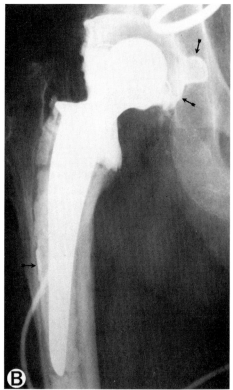

Fig. 2-4A. Anteroposterior radiograph of the right hip demonstrates a cement fracture adjacent to the femoral stem (arrow) and a second fracture lateral to the proximal stem (arrowhead). There has been settling and medial migration. There is an increased radiolucency between the prosthesis and cement consistent with loosening (curved arrow).

Fig. 2-4B. Arthrogram confirms both femoral and acetabular loosening (arrows).

speculative. The immediate post-operative appearance of the lucent line most probably represents residual cartilage, soft tissue, marrow, or blood trapped at the cement-bone interface.[8,15] Later changes may be secondary to necrosis and fibrosis, set up either by a thermal injury related to polymerization of methylmethacrylate, or to endosteal cortical necrosis caused by arterial damage during the reaming process during the insertion of the component.[32] If there is progression of the lucency in the radiographs after 6 months, this is more suggestive of loosening.[9]

A lucent zone occurring at the cement-metal interface is a less frequent event. This failure almost always occurs along the lateral aspect of the proximal third of the femoral stem, and usually occurs within the first post-operative year.[12] The etiology of cement-metal failure is similarly not well understood, but is thought to be either the result of prosthesic movement during the curing of the methyl-methacrylate, improper filling of the acrylic with subsequent void formation, or actual fractures of the cement.[12] Failure at the cement-metal interface often leads to eventual component loosening.

Loosening of one or both components of a total hip prosthesis is the most frequent cause of failure.[21] The acetabular component appears more frequently affected than the femoral component, and single component loosening occurs more frequently than the simultaneous involvement of both components.[2] The actual frequency of occurrence is reported to lie between 1 and 35 percent, depending on the series.[22] This discrepancy is probably due to varying criteria for the radiographic diagnosis of loosening. Carlsson and Gentz consider a width of the juxtaarticular radiolucent zone in excess of 1 mm to be evidence of loosening, while the majority of investigators define a radiolucent zone in excess of 2 mm width to be suggestive of loosening.[14]

As described earlier, various factors are thought to contribute to loosening, including insufficient cement or uneven distribution of cement; the presence of less than 1 cm of cement between the calcar and the stem; insufficient removal of cancellous bone lateral to the stem; insufficient cement beyond the stem tip; and positioning of the femoral component in alignment other than slight valgus.[7] Additional radiographic observations include migration of a component; cement fracture; widening of the lucent zone; or actual radiographic demonstration of motion on stress views (Fig. 2-4).

In addition to the radiographic observations relating to the integrity of the prosthesis-cement-bone interface, other radiographic observations regarding the configuration and position of the prosthesis are notable. Dislocation of the total hip prosthesis most commonly occurs in the immediate post-operative period, and relates either to improper positioning of the patient's leg during that time, or to improper positioning of components. When dislocation occurs later than 3 months post-operatively, it is usually indicative of malposition of the prosthetic components or due to over-zealous rehabilitation, with the development of a range of motion that exceeds the limits of the prosthesis.[31] The position of the greater trochanter relative to the lateral acetabular rim is of importance: a high trochanter at this level can act as a lever to facilitate dislocation, as it abuts the acetabular rim during abduction. In addition, excessive anteversion or retroversion potentiates dislocation (Fig. 2-5). The radiographic diagnosis of dislocation may be self-evident; however, AP and true lateral views are essential for the best definition of prosthesis position. Subtle dislocations may be diagnosed on the AP film by the use of the *Saturn ring sign.* This sign relates to the position of the femoral head within the acetabular cup, so that the measurement of the medial and lateral distances from the equatorial wires of the cup to the femoral head should be equal. An unequal measurement suggests dislocation in a concentric prosthesis, such as the Charnley; however, for the eccentric prostheses, such as the Aufranc-Turner, the lateral measurement should be approximately twice that of the medial aspect; in this case equality implies dislocation.[31]

In addition to dislocation, migration, or change in the position of the prosthetic component, should be noted. Amstutz describes four modes of failure that lead to medial migration of the proximal stem and lateral migration of the distal stem, thus leading to motion of the femoral component.[2] The presence of heterotopic bone formation (Fig. 2-6), as well as loose surgical wires in the area surrounding the joint space should also be noted. These potentiate pain and cause component failure. The progression of heterotopic bone can be followed by radionuclide bone scans (described in a later section). Pronounced heterotopic bone formation is seen in patients with ankylosing spondylosis or diffuse idiopathic skeletal hyperostosis (DISH) syndrome.

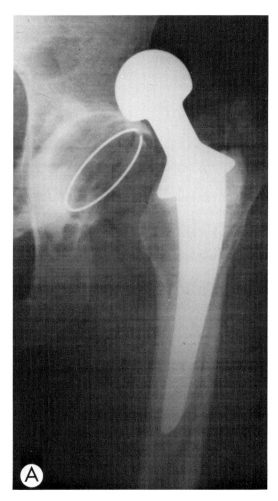

Fig. 2-5A and B. Two examples of dislocated total hip arthroplasties.

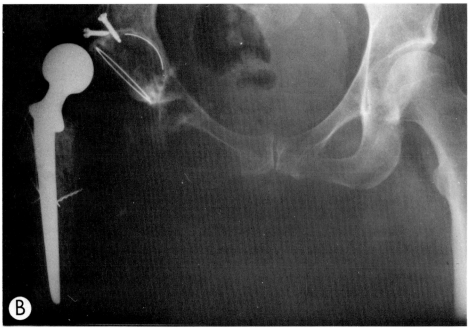

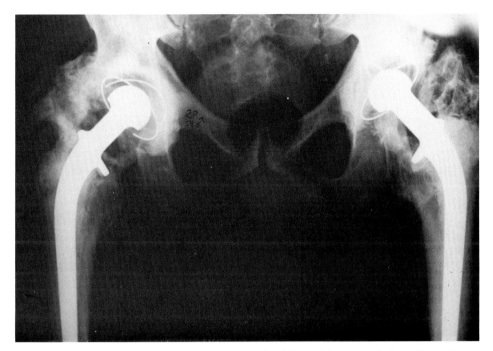

Fig. 2-6.   Pelvis radiograph demonstrates extensive bilateral heterotopic bone formation.

Ectopic distribution of cement must be noted. Rarely, cement in the pelvis has eroded the bladder and/or femoral vessels, with resultant sepsis, and hemorrhage or hematuria.[31] In addition, the extension of cement through breaks in the femoral shaft cortex should be noted. Such breaks may be potential sites of component failure. Examination of the AP pelvis film may yield information with regard to the post-operative presence of protrusio acetabuli, or stress fractures of the contralateral ischium. A summary of plain radiographic findings is provided in Table 2-1.

One final point must be emphasized. It is imperative that the entire prosthesis, including the tip, be included on the radiograph to ensure adequate evaluation of the entire arthroplasty. Position change, component fracture (Fig.2-7), motion, or infection can easily be missed if the information is not visible (Fig. 2-8).

Table 2-1
Radiographic observations involving the total hip prosthesis

Early	Late
1. Position of components	1. Dislocation
2. Presence of dislocation	2. Migration of components
3. Cement voids	3. Cement-bone radiolucent zone greater than 2 mm
4. Heterotopic bone	4. Rapid change in radiolucent zone width
5. Ectopic cement	5. Cement-metal radiolucent width
6. Broken wires	6. Periosteal reaction
7. Trochanteric separation	7. Bone destruction
	8. Cement fractures
	9. Motion on stress views
	10. CHANGE FROM PREVIOUS EXAM

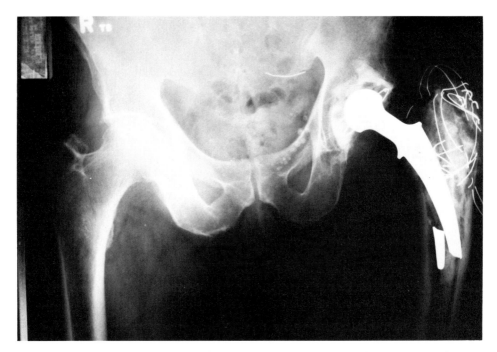

Fig. 2-7. An example of a fractured femoral component stem secondary to abnormal varus positioning of the prosthesis with accompanying settling. Note also fractured and migrating trochanteric wires.

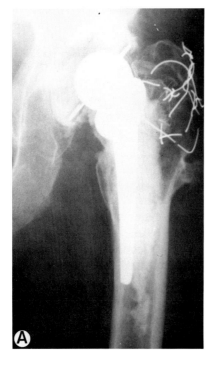

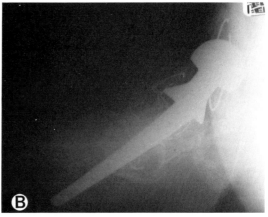

Fig. 2-8A. Anteroposterior radiograph of the left hip demonstrates that the stem of the arthroplasty appears foreshortened. The diagnosis of a malpositioned femoral component may be questioned.

Fig. 2-8B. The true lateral radiograph, however, confirms that the femoral stem has penetrated the posterior cortex of the femur.

34

Hip Arthrography

Hip arthrography is a valuable method of demonstrating component loosening. In symptomatic patients, the tracking of contrast material along the cement-bone or cement-prosthesis interface is useful in the overall evaluation and management of those patients. There are, however, subtle cases in which the contrast material cannot be clearly distinguished from the adjacent acrylic or metallic contours. A subtraction technique may enhance the diagnosis in these cases.[4] In 1936, Ziedes Des Pointes first described a method of subtraction of photographic images, whereby all picture elements common to a pair of radiographs could be subtracted, or cancelled, by superimposition of the images after one image had been converted to a densimetric diapositive.[17] If injected contrast has been added to a radiograph, it would stand out with increasing clarity on the subtracted radiograph.[28] If perfect subtraction were obtained, it would result in complete obliteration of the background. For this technique to be useful, it is necessary to reproduce the film in a darkroom; this adds additional time and expense to the procedure.

Subtraction of radiographic images by color addition overcomes many of these disadvantages.[14] The method also depends upon the superimposition of two radiographic images before and after the injection of a contrast agent. The method is rapid, inexpensive, and extremely accurate. It permits analysis of radiographs within seconds after processing, thus allowing immediate decisions to be made with respect to further diagnostic work-up.

The technique of subtraction by color addition depends on the principle of addition of primary colors to produce white light. Application of this technique has been described by Frey and Norman.[17] Drinker and co-workers have modified the technique to some degree.[14] Their technique utilizes two filters of opposite primary colors. A "scout" (preliminary radiograph of the symptomatic hip) is exposed, and compared to a second radiograph taken following the administration of contrast. They are identical, except that one contains added contrast material. After processing, one is placed behind each filter, optically superimposed and viewed through a split-beam mirror. Identical anatomical landmarks will appear in normal gray tones, while the added contrast material will appear in the color of its contiguous filter. If a permanent record is desired, one can photograph through the beam-splitting mirror. Examples of color subtraction arthrography are seen in Figures 2-9, 2-10, and Color Plate I.

Arthrographic Technique

Hip aspiration and arthrography is considered to be the "gold standard," when applied to the symptomatic prosthetic hip.[21] The technique is most easily performed in a radiographic room equipped with an image intensifier so that all phases of the exam can be carried out under precise radiographic control. The examination may be performed under local anesthesia, or, in the extremely symptomatic patient, under general anesthesia. The patient is positioned supine on the radiographic table, and the symptomatic leg is immobilized in a neutral position. The thigh and groin are prepared with both iodine scrub and solution and are draped with sterile towels. Local anesthesia with 1 percent lidocaine is then administered as indicated. An 18-gauge disposable short-beveled spinal needle is

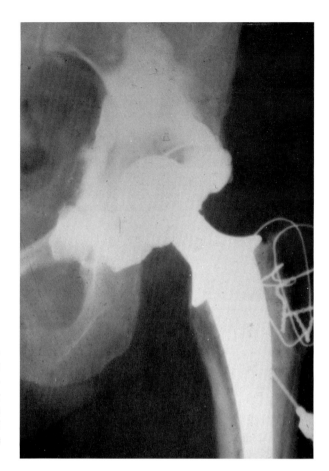

Fig. 2-9. A radiograph obtained during arthrography suggests faint tracking of contrast around the acetabular component consistent with loosening. (see Color Plate I for color subtraction technique demonstration of loosening.)

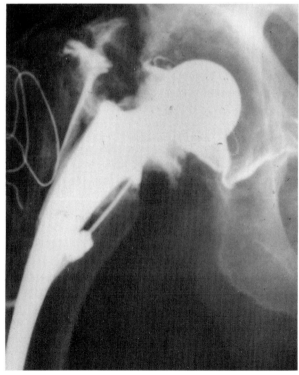

Fig. 2-10. A radiograph obtained during arthrography suggests femoral component loosening. (See Color Plate I for color subtraction technique demonstration of loosening.)

inserted at the level immediately cephalad to the greater trochanter, distal to the inguinal ligament, and lateral to the femoral neurovascular bundle. It is advanced angularly under fluoroscopic control until it strikes the medial femoral neck. After striking the metal of the neck, the needle is advanced medially along the neck. Penetration of the joint space in the post-operative hip may present some difficulty, as the fibrous pseudocapsule formed post-operatively can achieve significant thickness and thus offer substantial resistance to the progress of the needle. The advantage of the lateral approach is that the needle position is fluoroscopically discernable from the contour of the metallic prosthesis. If a direct anterior approach is utilized, the needle is obscured by the metallic prosthesis. In patients suspected of having tight, small capsules, the needle tip can be inserted medially, beneath the lip of the acetabular cup.

As the needle is advanced into position, a continuous, slow injection of lidocaine can confirm when the tip has entered the pseudocapsule: resistance to injection is felt as the tip passes through the wall of the capsule; this resistance is suddenly reduced upon entering into the joint space. When the needle tip is in position, if fluid can be aspirated, the intra-articular position of the needle is confirmed. The fluid is sent for aerobic and anerobic culture. If no fluid can be aspirated, sterile nonbacteriostatic saline is injected, aspirated, and sent for culture. A few drops of contrast are then slowly injected under fluoroscopic control. We recommend the use of meglumine diatrozoate for the radio-opaque contrast media, as its lower sodium content is less irritating to the synovial lining of the joint. If the needle is intra-articular, the contrast will flow freely away from the needle tip.[16] If it is extra-articular, the contrast will pool at the needle tip. In the latter case, the needle must be repositioned and its location determined again.[16] When appropriate position of the needle is confirmed, approximately 20 cc of contrast is injected under pressure and fluoroscopically observed. Sequential radiographs are taken for subsequent subtraction. After an initial "scout" film, three films are taken during the slow, forceful injection of contrast. Delayed films are then obtained, following compression and traction. We have found these delayed films extremely helpful in showing contrast tracking not previously seen on conventional views; delayed films are essential for a diagnostic examination (Fig. 2-11).

Arthrography of a well-seated prosthesis normally demonstrates contrast confined only to the region of the pseudocapsule. Extension of contrast media into the bone-cement or cement-metal interface implies loosening (Fig. 2-12). Freiberger accepts tracking of contrast up to 1 cm down the femoral stem as a "normal" appearance, and not representative of loosening.[16] Extension of contrast media throughout the entire bone-cement interface definitely indicates that the component is loose (Fig. 2-13). However, focal areas of contrast tracking do not necessarily indicate that the component is entirely loose.[20] The accuracy of an arthrographic diagnosis of loosening varies according to the series. Gelman and co-workers were accurate in correctly diagnosing loosening in 16 of 17 hips for a 94-percent correlation level.[18,19] However, Murray and Rodrigo found 58-percent accuracy for the diagnosis of loosening, noting three false-positives and two false-negatives.[25] In addition, they demonstrated loosening of the acetabular component in 22.6 percent of asymptomatic patients, leading to the impression that the demonstration of acetabular loosening on arthrography may be a less-accurate diagnostic finding.[25] Arthrographic findings are summarized in Table 2-2.

The divergence of views as to the accuracy of arthrography again most

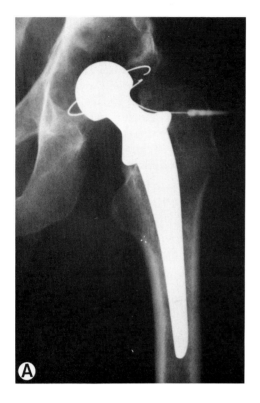

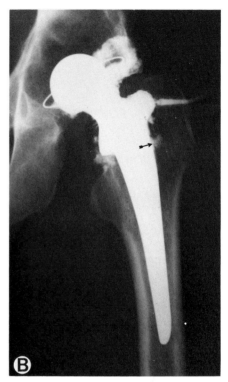

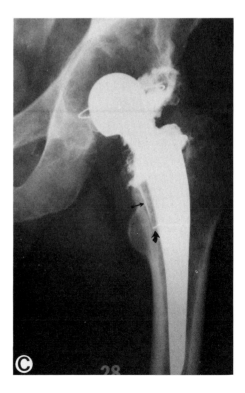

Fig. 2-11A. Plain radiograph demonstrates left total hip prosthesis utilizing nonbarium impregnated cement. No definite signs of loosening are noted.

Fig. 2-11 B. Early film obtained during an arthrogram shows no evidence of acetabular loosening and only minimal tracking laterally in the femoral component (arrow).

Fig. 2-11C. A delayed radiograph obtained during arthrography demonstrates medial tracking (arrow), as well as outlining a cement fracture (curved arrow). The value of the delayed film must be emphasized, as it frequently demonstrates previously nonvisualized abnormalities.

38

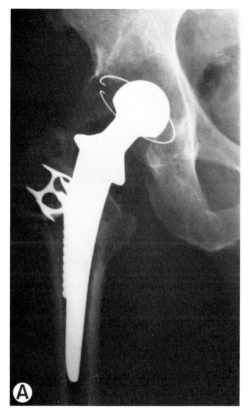
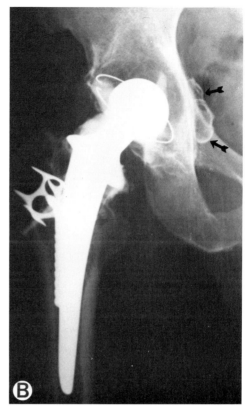

Fig. 2-12A. Anteroposterior radiograph of a right total hip arthroplasty with nonbarium impregnated cement. The diagnosis of loosening of acetabular component is impossible.

Fig. 2-12B. Arthrogram reveals contrast tracking around the lucent cement medially in the acetabulum (arrows). These findings suggest acetabular loosening.

probably relates to the ambiguity in the definition of loosening. Amstutz defined loosening in the following manner: (1) in the mechanical sense, the result of motion occurring when there is inadequate bonding between materials of different elasticity in a composite structure; (2) radiographically, by the presence of cracks or the occurrence of radiolucent zones at the bone-cement or cement-metal interface; and (3) visual demonstration of motion following the application of stress.[2] The tracking of contrast at the time of arthrography does in fact broadly represent loosening; however, the findings must be closely correlated with the patient's clinical symptoms to determine the true significance of the radiographic observations.[4, 25]

Table 2-2
Pertinent arthrographic findings

1. Extension of contrast media into cement-bone or cement-metal interface
2. Filling of fistulous tracts or abscess cavities
3. Lymphatic opacification
4. Bacteriologic results from fluid aspirate

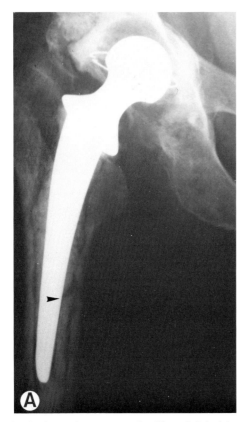

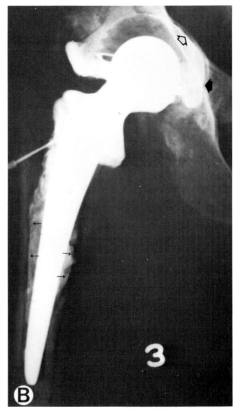

Fig. 2-13A. Anteroposterior film of right hip demonstrates a cement fracture (arrowhead) and varus migration of the femoral component.

Fig. 2-13B. An arthrogram demonstrates loosening with contrast appearing around the femoral component at the cement-bone interface (arrows), as well as the acetabular cement-bone interface (arrowheads).

Infection

There is no apparent time frame for the occurrence of post-operative infection in the hip arthroplasty.[22] The incidence of delayed sepsis appears to increase as the post-operative interval lengthens. Early infections tend to be fulminant in character, whereas late infections may either be fulminant or indolent.[23] Patients undergoing reoperations have an increased incidence of infection twice that of the virgin hip.[15] Prosthetic loosening is a severe complication of joint space infection, accounting for 7 to 56 percent of the total number of loose prostheses.[7,27] Delay in the treatment of an infected joint favors increased bone destruction with resultant loosening of components.

It is usually difficult to distinguish between loosening secondary to infection and that due to mechanical factors on the basis of either plain radiographs or arthrography. The diagnosis usually rests on the results of culture from the joint aspiration at the time of arthrography.[15] There are, however, some radiographic findings that indicate infection. Rapid bone resorption and widening of the radiolucent zone at the bone-cement interface greater than 2 mm both suggest the possibility of infection.[15] Similarly, the presence of periosteal bone adjacent to the joint space is indicative of infection. During an arthrogram, filling of adjacent abscess cavities or communication with periarticular cavities may suggest an infected joint (Fig. 2-14). Dussault found five patients in whom there was contrast filling of such communicating cavities who subsequently were proven to have infected hip replacements.[15]

Lymphatic opacification during arthrography may be minimally suggestive of infection; more likely, it represents synovial inflammation. Dussault[15] and Coren et al[11] describe a number of patients with lymphatic opacification demonstrated at arthrography, most of whom had no evidence of demonstrable infection. This finding must be considered nonspecific, and may relate to the volume of dye used during arthrography and the force of contrast injection. The application of [67] Ga scanning to the evaluation of the patient with an infected joint will be discussed in a later section. In spite of radiographic evaluation, in the end, surgical exploration alone may be the definitive method for diagnosing infection of prosthetic joints, because hips with negative culture aspiration/arthrography have confirmed infection at surgery. This is most probably due to the ability of obtaining specimens from the

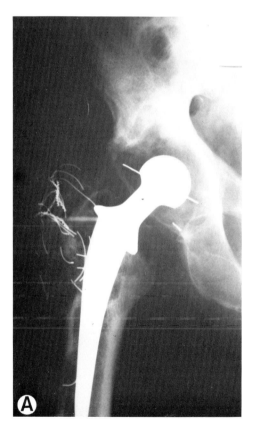

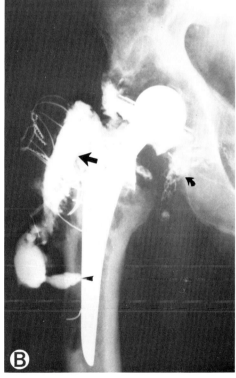

Fig. 2-14A. Radiograph of the right hip before the injection of contrast demonstrates fracture of wire sutures and a nonunion of the greater trochanter.

Fig. 2-14B. The arthrogram demonstrates contrast tracking between the greater trochanter and the femur (arrow). Filling of a sinus tract, suggests infection (arrowhead). Note the medial filling of lymphatic vessels (curved arrow).

actual joint space during surgery, as opposed to a potential peripheral location during arthrography.[15,25]

NUCLEAR MEDICINE: RADIONUCLIDE BONE SCANNING

Radionuclide bone scanning is an adjunct method for evaluating possible loosening or infection of a prosthetic joint. Where conventional radiography may provide equivocal information, Technetium-99m MDP (methylene diphosphonate) may add significant information that would substantiate a scintigraphic diagnosis of loosening or infection.

Three hours following the injection of 15 mCi of ^{99m}Tc, the patient is scanned with a gamma camera. The total hip arthroplasty patient will normally demonstrate increased isotopic activity in the region of the prosthesis for 3 to 6 months following surgery. By 6 months, the activity should begin to return to normal in both the femoral and acetabular components. Focal increased activity demonstrated greater than 6 months post-operatively is considered abnormal and consistent either with loosening or infection.[33,34] Campeau et al studied 36 patients undergoing total hip replacement via serial ^{99m}Tc pyrophosphate bone scans.[8] Sixteen patients demonstrated increased scan activity in either femoral or acetabular components greater than 6 months post-operatively; all 16 were symptomatic. While seven of the patients with abnormal scans showed no radiographic abnormality, no patient with a proven complication had a normal scan. Williamson et al utilized ^{99m}Tc MDP bone scanning to evaluate 20 symptomatic patients.[34] Their study indicated that bone imaging was capable of differentiating loosening from prosthesic infection. Loosened prostheses demonstrated discrete focal increased activity, primarily at the prosthesis stem tip and the trochanteric regions, whereas infection presented as a less-defined, diffuse uptake. They also described bone scanning as effective for the diagnosis of ectopic bone formation in the symptomatic hip replacement.

While technetium MDP bone imaging is extremely sensitive to localized areas of inflammation or bony erosion, its specificity is often in question. Weiss et al conducted a retrospective study of 35 symptomatic prostheses.[30] They found bone imaging to be 100-percent sensitive but only 77-percent specific with a diagnosis of loosening or infection. They describe increased uptake in the greater and lesser trochanters as normal variants in the post-operative hip. This is attributed to increased bone turnover in high-stress regions, and to heterotopic ossification that occurs following trochanteric osteotomy.[30] Focally increased uptake in the stem tip region is viewed as a specific sign of loosening.[30,34] Repeated impact loading of a loose prosthesis, as well as a toggle motion of the tip that occurs with loosening, acts to stimulate bone formation and blood flow in the tip region.[30] This results in increased activity visualized on scans.

The bone scan can also be utilized to follow the therapeutic progress of the treatment of symptomatic joints. McInerny and Hyde described six patients whose scans returned to normal as their symptoms resolved.[24] Gelman et al evaluated 10 patients with symptomatic joints,[19] and found radionuclide evaluation 85-percent accurate in determining the cause and site of symptomatology; plain radiographs were only 70-percent accurate. The isotope scan was also helpful in diagnosing other causes of pain, such as heterotopic bone formation. In general, the radionuclide exam provides a safe, noninvasive method of screening and confirming clinical or radiographic impressions of the patient with a symptomatic hip.

Gallium-67 scanning has been utilized as a method of differentiating the septic joint replacement from the loose prosthesis. In addition to being a marker of infection, ^{67}Ga is also a bone scan agent. Therefore, areas of increased blood flow or osteoblastic activity secondary to loosening may evoke increased uptake of gallium. However, as in technetium scanning, infection tends to evoke a broader, diffuse uptake than loosening; the differentiation is readily evident. Thus in the patient with a ^{99m}Tc scan suggestive of infection, the gallium scan is used as a follow-up study to confirm the suspicion of an infected joint (Fig. 2-15). Gallium-67 localization has been shown to occur in both septic and nonseptic areas of inflammation, i.e., bursitis or synovitis. 67-Gallium concentration in bone may reflect not inflammation but increased bone metabolism response to surgical trauma; comparison with a technetium MDP scan is therefore important, to assess the relative distribution patterns.[26] If the patterns of ^{99m}Tc MDP and ^{67}Ga uptake are incongruent, osteomyelitis is likely. If a congruent pattern is noted, infection is doubtful.[26] Intense focal uptake in a localized zone of osteomyelitis is an exception

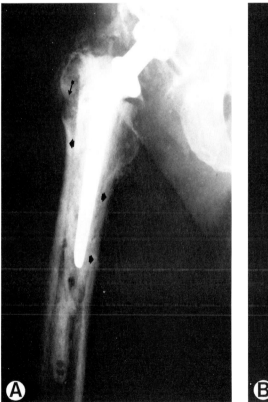 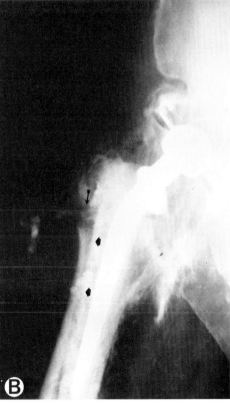

Fig. 2-15A. AP radiograph of a right total hip prosthesis demonstrates cortical destruction laterally (arrow); periosteal reaction (arrowheads); and overall modeling of the bone consistent with infection.

Fig. 2-15B. Sinogram demonstrates contrast tracking into the cortical break (arrow) and extending down the shaft (arrowheads).

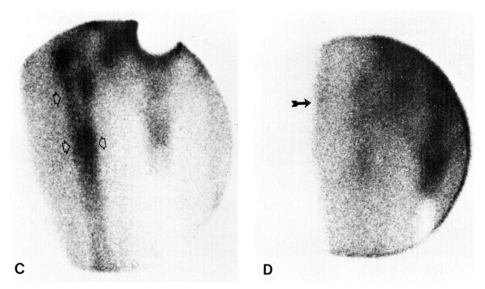

C   D

Fig. 2-15C. Technetium-99m bone scan demonstrates diffuse uptake in the trochanteric region, as well as around the shaft, suggestive of infection (arrowheads).

Fig. 2-15D. Gallium-67 scan demonstrates uptake in the adjacent soft tissues (arrow), as well as in the region of the sinus tract and distal shaft. This is consistent with infection.

to this pattern. Used in this complementary manner, the ^{67}Ga scan is important in the evaluation of possible infection related to the prosthetic hip. The efficacy of both scans provides a relatively accurate noninvasive method to determine the presence of loosening, infection, or other complications in the total hip replacement.

COMPUTED TOMOGRAPHY

The efficacy of computed tomography (CT) in the evaluation of total hip replacement has yet to be definitely established. However, if one extends the information obtained by CT when applied to other orthopedic areas, its potential contribution can be estimated.

In the evaluation of hip trauma, CT has been found to be especially helpful in evaluating the presence or absence of interarticular loose fragments, as well as the congruity of the joint space.[29] It also provides useful information concerning adjacent soft tissue and the quality of surrounding bone stock (Fig. 2-16). Applying this type of information to the patient with a total hip replacement, evaluation of heterotopic bone formation, soft-tissue plane displacement in areas of sepsis, evaluation of fibrous union and nonunion of trochanteric fragments, and evaluation of bone stock in the region of prosthetic components is currently feasible (Fig. 2-17). New algorithms are under development that will eliminate the artifacts caused by the dense metallic prosthesis; therefore, evaluation of the bone-cement interface may soon be possible. It is conceivable that CT may streamline the radiographic work-up of the prosthetic joint and may provide information that will eliminate the potential equivocal result.

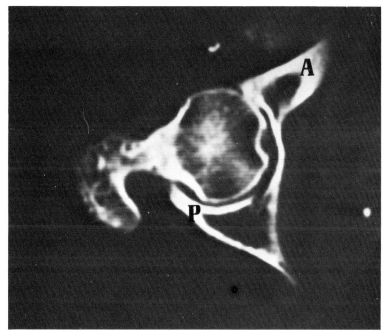

Fig. 2-16. CT of a normal hip demonstrating the anterior (**A**) and posterior (**P**) rims of the acetabulum. The fovea of the femoral head is well seen. CT is an accurate method for evaluating acetabular bone stock.

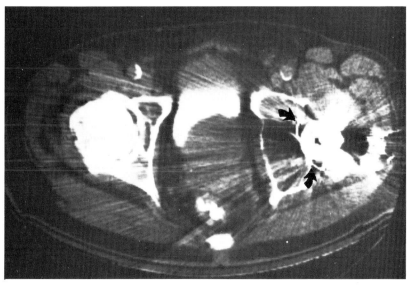

Fig. 2-17. CT of pelvis with left total hip replacement is limited by artifacts secondary to the high density metal femoral head. Nevertheless, bone stock as well as acetabular cup (curved arrows) can be evaluated.

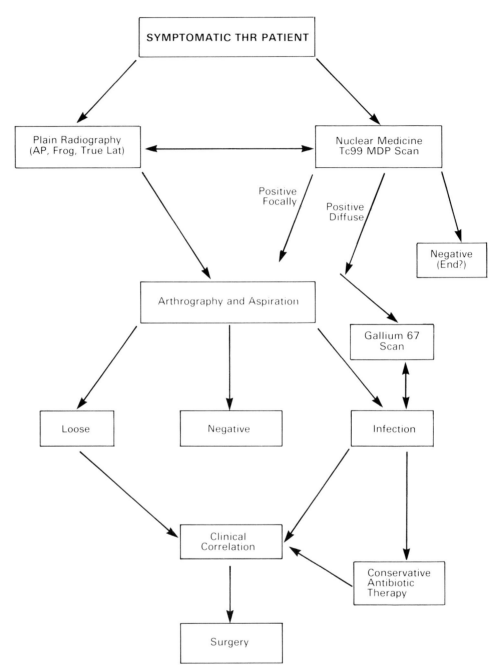

Fig. 2-18. Algorithmic evaluation of the total hip prosthesis.

SUMMARY

Efficacious radiographic examination of the total hip arthroplasty includes the complementary use of plain radiographs; arthrography and aspiration; radionuclide scanning; and clinical symptomatology. The latter component adds the proper bias level to the radiographic findings, allowing the clinician to elucidate a diagnosis and an appropriate therapeutic course. (An algorithm is provided (Fig. 2-18) to act as a rationale for radiographic evaluation of the total hip prosthesis.)

REFERENCES

1. Amstutz HC: Complications of total hip replacement. *Clin Orthop* 72:123–137, 1970.
2. Amstutz HC, Markolf KL, McNeice GM, et al: Loosening of total hip components: Cause and prevention. Proceedings of the Fourth Open Scientific Meeting of the Hip Society, 1976, pp 102–116.
3. Anderson GB, Freeman MA, Swanson SA: Loosening of the cemented acetabular cup in total hip replacement. *J Bone Joint Surg* 54B:590–599, 1972.
4. Anderson LS, Staple TW: Arthrography of total hip replacement using subtraction technique. *Radiol* 109:470–472, 1973.
5. Armbuster TG, Guerra J, Resnick D, et al: The adult hip: An anatomic study. Part 1: The bony landmarks. *Radiol* 128:1–10, 1978.
6. Beaubout JW: Radiology of total hip arthroplasty. *Radiol Clin North Am* 13:3–19, 1975.
7. Beckenbaugh RD, Ilstrup DM: Total hip arthroplasty. *Am J Bone Joint Surg* 60:306–313, 1978.
8. Campeau RJ, Hall MF, Miale A Jr: Detection of total hip arthroplasty complications with Tc-99m pyrophosphate. *J Nuc Med* 17:526, 1976.
9. Carlsson AS, Gentz C: Mechanical loosening of the femoral head prosthesis in the Charnley total hip arthroplasty. *Clin Orthop* 147:262–267, 1980.
10. Chao EY, Coventry MB: Fracture of the femoral component after total hip replacement. An analysis of fifty-eight cases. *J Bone Joint Surg* 63A:1078–1093. Sept. 1981
11. Coren GS, Curtis J, Dalinka M: Lymphatic visualization during hip arthrography. *Radiol* 115:621–625, 1975.
12. DeSmet AA, Kramer D, Martel W: The metal-cement interface in total hip prostheses. *Am J Roentgenol* 129:279–282, 1977.
13. Dolinskas C, Campbell RE, Rothman RH: The painful Charnley total hip replacement. *Am J Roentgenol* 121:61–68, 1974.
14. Drinker H, Turner RH, McKenzie JD, et al: Color subtraction arthrography in the diagnosis of component loosening in hip arthroplasty. *Orthopedics* 1(3):224–229, 1978.
15. Dussault RH, Goldman AB, Ghelman B: Radiologic diagnosis of loosening and infection in hip prostheses. *J Can Assoc Radiol* 28:119–127, 1977.
16. Freiberger RH, Kaye JJ: The adult hip, in Spiller J (ed): *Arthrography.* New York, Appleton-Century Crofts, 1979, 192–215.
17. Frey HS, Norman A: Radiographic subtraction by color addition. *Radiol* 84:123–124, 1965.
18. Gelman MI: Arthrography in total hip prosthesis complications. *Am J Roentgenol* 126:743–750, 1976.
19. Gelman MI, Coleman RE, Stevens PM, et al: Radiography, radionuclide imaging, and arthrography in the evaluation of total hip and knee replacement. *Radiol* 128:677–682, 1978.
20. Goergen TG, Resnick D: Evaluation of acetabular anteversion following total hip arthroplasty: Necessity of proper centering. *Br J Radiol* 48:259–263, 1975.
21. Guerra J. Armbuster TG, Resnick D, et al: The adult hip: An anatomic study, Part II: The soft-tissue landmarks. *Radiol* 128:11–20, 1978.
22. Harris, WH: Total joint replacement. *N Engl J Med* 297:650–651, 1977.
23. Hendrix RW, Anderson JM: Arthrographic and radiologic evaluation of prosthetic joints. *Radiol Clin of North Am* 19:349–364, 1981.

24. McInerney DP, Hyde ID: [99m]Tc pyrophosphate scanning in the assessment of the painful hip prosthesis. *Clin Radiol* 29:513–517, 1978.
25. Murray WR, Rodrigo JJ: Arthrography for the assessment of pain after total hip replacement. *J Bone Joint Surg* 57A(8):1060–1065, 1975.
26. Rosenthall L, Lisbona R, Hernandez M, et al: ^{99m}Tc-PP and [67]Ga Imaging following insertion of orthopedic devices. *Radiol* 133:717–721, 1979.
27. Salvati EA, Chuem IMV, Aglietti P, et al: Radiology of total hip replacements. *Clin Orthopaed and Rel Rsch* 121:74–82, 1976.
28. Salvati EA, Ghelman B, McLaren T, et al: Subtraction technique in arthrography for loosening of total hip replacement fixed with radiopaque cement. *Clin Orthop and Rel Rsch* 101:105–109, 1974.
29. Sauser DD, Billimoria PE, Rouse GA, et al: CT evaluation of hip trauma. *AJR* 135:269–274, 1980.
30. Weiss PA, Mall JC, Hoffer PB, et al: [99m]Tc methylene diphosphonate bone imaging in the evaluation of total hip prostheses. *Radiol* 133:727–729, 1979.
31. Weissman BN: Radiographic evaluation of total joint replacement, in Kelley WN, Harris ED, Ruddy S, et al (eds): *Textbook of rheumatology*. Philadelphia, WB Saunders Co, 1981, pp 2020–2054.
32. Willert HG, Ludwig J, Seinlitsch M: Reaction of bone to methacrylate after hip arthroplasty. *J Bone Joint Surg* 56A:1368–1372, 1974.
33. Williams ED, Tregonning RJ, Hurley PJ: [99m]Tc diphosphate scanning as an aid to diagnosis of infection in total hip joint replacements. *Br J Radiol* 50:562–566, 1977.
34. Williamson BR, McLaughlin RE, Wang GJ, et al: Radionuclide bone imaging as a means of differentiating loosening and infection in patients with a painful total hip prosthesis. *Radiol* 133:723–726, 1979.
35. Wilson JN, Scales JT: Loosening of total hip replacements with cement fixation. *Clin Orthop and Rel Rsch* 72:145–160, 1970.

Arnold D. Scheller, Jr. and
Joseph D'Errico

3

Hip Biomechanics and Prosthetic Design and Selection in Revision Total Hip Replacement

A rudimentary knowledge of hip kinematics and biomechanics is necessary for successful reconstructive hip surgery. A hip arthroplasty significantly affects the normal physiological stress patterns of the normal femur and acetabulum.

Each hip arthroplasty design induces a significant but variable change in stress when compared to others. An understanding of the particular changes for each hip design allows a deeper insight into artificial replacement of the hip. This deeper insight, along with proper patient selection and education, surgical technique, and meticulous rehabilitation, will substantially slow the increasing rate of revision total hip replacements.

When revision arthroplasty is indicated, utilization of a high-strength, super-alloy metal in an advanced design that has scientific and clinical documentation is crucial for a successful enduring result. In this chapter the traditional hip arthroplasty implants are discussed, and the philosophy for choosing a revision hip design is presented.

BIOMECHANICAL EVALUATION

The architecture of the human body is mechanically complex and subjects the hip joints to high forces. Many researchers have completed studies that determined the resultant loads on the femoral head during activity are several times higher than body weight.[45,46,50,51,61]

Hip joint load is a function of body weight, activity level, muscular force, and

49

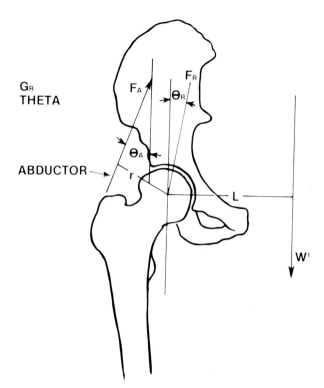

Fig. 3-1. Anatomical diagram at the hip joint used for static analysis in the one leg stance.

the distance from the body's center of gravity to the center of the femoral head. Therefore, to reduce the forces on the hip joint, it is necessary to revise one or all of these factors.

Greenwald has determined that a reduction of approximately 3 pounds of the joint load accompanies each pound of body weight lost.[26] Rydell demonstrated that the speed of walking affected the load on the hip joint.[51] Paul, using a dynamometer for ground-foot force measurements, has shown that the hip force increases from normal walking to fast walking.[46] He reasoned that the dynamic variation of ground-foot force increases with walking speed, and the longer stride length that accompanies faster walking gives greater offset from the joint axes of resultant ground-foot force line of action.

An anatomical model of the hip joint used for static analysis is shown in Figure 3-1. This diagram represents a simplified model, assuming no lateral shift of the pelvis or the shoulders. It is also assumed that the abductors are the only active muscles. The abductor distance, or moment arm (r); abductor muscle angle (θ_A); and the body weight moment arm (L) are measured from the x-ray of each individual case. The abductor moment arm (r) is defined as the distance from the center of the femoral head to the abductor muscle, measured along a line perpendicular to the angle of the abductors (θ_A). The body weight moment arm (L) is measured from the center of the femoral head to the center of gravity which corresponds with the center of the body. The force W^1 represents the body weight (W) less one leg. Therefore, the force W^1 will be five sixths of W ($\frac{5}{6}$ W).

The hip joint is analyzed in a static condition. A state of equilibrium must be created between the abductor muscle force (F_A) and the body weight force ($\frac{5}{6}$ W) and their respective moment arms. This principle is the same as employed with a laboratory balance: the forces multiplied by the distances from each side of the fulcrum (moment) must be equal. Should the moment on one side of the fulcrum be greater than the other, the system will not be at rest and is a dynamic situation. Equilibrium can be attained by changing the force or the distance the force acts from the fulcrum; however, the products of each side of the equation must be equal.

The equation for the anatomical model in Figure 3-1, using the femoral head as the fulcrum is:

$$F_{AV} \times r = \% \, W \times L$$

Since the distance from the center of the femoral head to the abductors (r) and the distance from the center of the body to the center of the femoral head (L) are measured from the roentgenogram, and W is the body weight, F_{AV} is the unknown in the equation; therefore:

$$F_{AV} = \frac{\% W \times L}{r}$$

F_{AV} is the vertical component of the abductor force F_A. It was necessary to find F_{AV} because F_A was exerting a force at an angle of θ_A degrees; therefore, the force vector is exerting a proportional load in the horizontal and vertical directions. Once F_{AV} is determined, F_A can be identified by the following equation:

$$F_A = \frac{F_{AV}}{\cos \theta_A}$$

θ_A can be measured directly from x-ray.

The horizontal force of the abductor muscle pull can also be calculated, using the following equation:

$$F_{AH} + F_A \sin \theta_A$$

Assuming that the body weight force only has a vertical component, the resultant force can be calculated with the Pythagorean theroem:

$$F_R - [(F_{AH})^2 + (F_{AV} + W)^2]^{\frac{1}{2}}$$

The direction of F_R can be calculated by:

$$\theta_R = \tan^{-1} \frac{(F_{AH})}{W + F_{AV}}$$

A rudimentary knowledge of normal hip biomechanics is necessary for a thorough understanding of arthroplasty composite failures. This understanding is valuable in analyzing the varying stem designs in their role as a factor of the arthroplasty composite.

EVALUATION OF FEMORAL STEM DESIGN

Total hip prostheses fixed with bone cement constitute a composite of metal, polymethylmethacrylate, and bone. The femoral component, the stiffest member of the composite, is the highest stressed member of the system.

The challenge in prosthesis design is to share the stresses between the implanted device and the bone. The viability of bone is affected by stress. In a primary hip replacement, the femur is stressed from the load acting on the femoral head in the hip joint. Subsequent to revision, the stress from the hip joint travels down the prosthetic shaft and is transferred to the bone. This pattern of stress transfer denies the proximal femur of physiologic stress. Mechanically, this is known as stress shielding.

Resorption of the medial calcar, as described by Charnley,[16] was found in 16.1 percent of 301 hips by Beckenbaugh.[6] The study was a follow-up of the Charnley total hip prosthesis.* The Charnley prosthesis has an insignificant collar that is not large enough either to reach cortical bone or to optimally load the proximal femur.

A number of theories have been postulated to explain proximal femoral calcar resorption associated with total hip replacement. According to Wolff's Law, an inadequate, physiologic stress to the femoral calcar could result in a disuse osteopenia from the stress shielding effect of the prosthesis. Others feel that excess stress in the femoral calcar causes microfracture and secondary reabsorption. There are also several other theories concerning resorption that are not stress-related, including: a compromised vascular supply to the calcar femoral; the cytotoxic effect of the cement; and granulation formation. The most widely accepted theory for resorption of the proximal femur is suboptimal stress in the calcar region secondary to the stress shielding from the femoral endoprosthesis.

When the proximal bone support fails, the remaining acrylic cement easily breaks away, leaving the stem of the prosthesis exposed and unsupported. Preservation of the cement mantle is extremely important to the success of total hip revisions. There certainly is enough evidence, clinically and theoretically, to relate total hip stem loosening with stem fracture (discussed more fully in Chapter 7).

An analytical study investigating the results of three common clinical modes of femoral failure is shown in Figure 3-2. Model I demonstrates good fixation and is an ideal for the other models. Model II shows an unsupported proximal stem with good distal stem fixation (cantilever). This is clinically analogous to a total hip prosthesis where the proximal femur has reabsorbed. A plot of the maximum stresses on the lateral side of the stem is shown in the adjacent graph. The heavy vertical line is the maximum fatigue value for a cast cobalt chrome (CoCr) material. It can be predicted that a fracture will occur in the area where the stress on the lateral stem approaches the fatigue value. Also shown is a roentgenogram revealing fracture in a clinical case where the proximal stem fixation was insufficient.

Model III shows a prosthesis that has fixation only at the distal tip. The midspan of the proximal stem is unsupported. Proximal-medial support is obtained from the bone and not from the cement. Again, the lateral stresses were plotted on a graph and the stem fracture was predicted from the analysis.

Model IV was done on a prosthesis that was totally loose within the femur.

*Chas. F. Thackray Ltd.

The only support was from impingement on the proximal medial cortex and the distal lateral cortex of the intramedullary canal.

The theoretical data was again plotted on a graph and the susceptible failure zone was identified. Roentgenograms verified the clinical relevance of the model (Fig. 3-2)

This exercise demonstrates the necessity of good cement fixation for successful total hip revisions. A requirement in designing a successful total hip prosthesis is a provision for protection of the cement. The cement is the most fragile component of the bone-metal-acrylic composite.

In order to map the future for a new total hip design, it is important to review the history of the total hip prosthesis. The first total hips introduced in the United States were the Charnley Total Hip,* the Müller device, and the Aufranc-Turner† and Harris Hip.†

The Charnley device is a varus design prosthesis with a neck-stem angle of 130°. The stem is generously curved in the proximal region and has a 22.0 mm head diameter. The first prostheses were stainless steel and later introduced in cast CoCr. The stem geometry cross-section, shown in Figure 3-3, is rounded on the medial side and flat on the lateral side of the prosthesis. Originally, the prosthesis was available in only one size. Later designs, like the Round-Back and Cobra, were revised to have a rounded lateral geometry. The Charnley designs have a small collar of insignificant size.

Resorption of the proximal femur was reported to be 16.1 percent with the Charnley prosthesis by Beckenbaugh.[6] Marmor recognized that the loss of proximal fixation contributed to the bending of the stainless Charnley prosthesis.[39]

Failures of the Charnley prosthesis are mostly attributable to the material. The Charnley was first manufactured of cast stainless steel, the yield strength of cast stainless steel is reported to be 30,000 psi. Loads of this magnitude in the hip joint are not uncommon.

When stressed past the ultimate stress, Charnley stems have fractured. The fracture site is many times located at the lateral tangent point on the stem where the curvature of the proximal stem blends with the straight distal stem section. Peak stresses have been recognized to occur at this area by both theoretical and experimental test studies.[55,60]

The extreme varus stem-neck angle of the Charnley design contributes to the high stress on the lateral stem. The varus angle increases the moment arm, multiplying the effect of the hip joint load.

The Müller prosthesis featured a diamond-shaped cross-sectional stem geometry as shown in Figure 3-3. Curvature of the stem in the medial-lateral direction was banana-shaped, but not as severely curved as the Charnley design. Again, the small collar of the Müller was not large enough to rest on cortical bone. Three neck lengths were available to aid in accurately reconstructing length. A 32.0 mm head diameter was incorporated to provide greater range of motion. Cast CoCr was the original material for this design.

The cross-sectional area of the Müller design is rather small. The design contradicts the laws of mechanics for a device that is intended to resist bending.

*Chas. F. Thackray, Ltd.
†Howmedica Inc.

Schematic—Support Condition

Good Fixation—Safe Condition

A. Stem Firmly Affixed

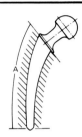

Proximal Loosening

A. Proximal Stem Unsupported
B. Distal Stem Affixed

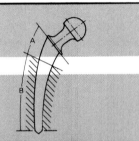

Partial Fixation
with Varus Positioning

A. Proximal Medical Support
B. Unsupported Midspan
C. Distal Stem Affixed

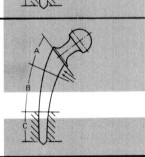

Complete Loss of Fixation

A. Proximal Medical Support
B. Unsupported Midspan
C. Distal Lateral Edge Support

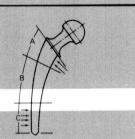

Howmedica Inc. 1981

Fig. 3-2. Three forms of incomplete femoral component support which could contribute to possible fatigue fracture (Courtesy Howmedica Inc.).

Computer Stress Prediction   Clinical Indication

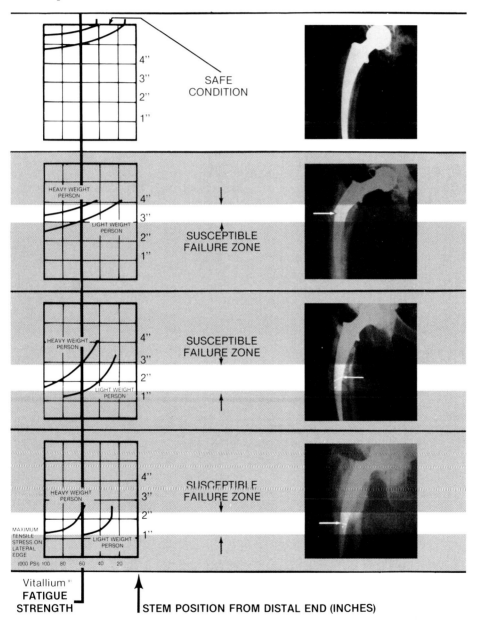

SAFE
CONDITION

SUSCEPTIBLE
FAILURE ZONE

SUSCEPTIBLE
FAILURE ZONE

SUSCEPTIBLE
FAILURE ZONE

HEAVY WEIGHT PERSON
LIGHT WEIGHT PERSON

MAXIMUM
TENSILE
STRESS ON
LATERAL
EDGE

(000 PSI) 100   80   60   40   20

Vitallium ®
**FATIGUE
STRENGTH**

STEM POSITION FROM DISTAL END (INCHES)

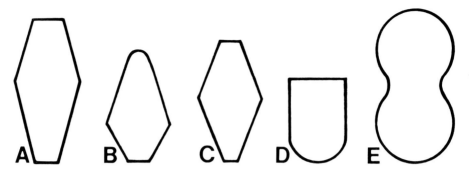

Fig. 3-3. Cross-sectional geometry and section modul: (A) Autrane-Turner, (B) Müller, (C) Harris, (D) Charnley, (E) CAD® Total Hip.

The greatest mass of material is located in an area where the stresses are least. Likewise, on the lateral edge, where the stresses are the greatest, there is little material to resist overload. The ability of a beam to resist bending is determined in part by the *section modulus*, which is calculated by multiplying the cross-sectional area by the distance from the neutral axis to the center of mass. Figure 3-3 illustrates the cross-sectional geometries and the section moduli for each design. The diamond-shaped design allows for the greatest mass of the material to be in a functionally poor area. The largest sectional area in the diamond design lies almost directly on the neutral axis. Reviewing the location of the material as it relates to section moduli, the largest mass of material should be as far away from the neutral axis as possible to best resist bending.

The sharp edges on the medial and lateral side of the stem create stress risers in the cement. These concentrations of stress result in the breakdown and deterioration of the cement bed. The loss of cement fixation contributes to the acceleration of stem loosening and fatigue failure of the prosthesis. As previously shown, the stem stress is greatly increased when fixation of the stem is lost.

Aufranc and Turner introduced their total hip prosthesis with a similar diamond-shaped cross-sectional design as Müller (Fig. 3-3). They also chose the 32.0 mm head diameter, and added an elliptically shaped, cross-sectional neck design for even greater range of motion. A platform was added to the lateral collar to allow for driving the component into the intramedullary canal. An undercut beneath the collar was provided to create an interlock between the cement and the prosthesis, to obviate proximal motion. Curvature in the stem was very slight, creating a relatively straight prosthesis. Three neck lengths were available for leg length adjustment. The short neck design was available in a shorter stem length, for the smaller patient. Again, cast CoCr was the original metal of choice for manufacture of the design.

The Harris design incorporates a modified diamond-shaped stem (Fig. 3-3) with slight curvature in the medial lateral plane. Harris chose a 26.0 mm head diameter to gain greater range of motion than the 22.0 mm design. An advantage to the smaller femoral head size was a correspondingly small requirement for acetabular component size, for increased ease of reconstruction in those patients who did not have adequate bone stock for a larger acetabular cup.

Breakage of the Aufranc-Turner (A-T) and Harris total hip stems has been significantly lower than those of the Müller and Charnley designs for a comparable implant time.[5,22,24,34,54] The only mechanical reason that could be offered is that the section modulus is greater in those two designs than the Müller and Charnley. The A-T and Harris stems also have a more valgus stem-neck angle of 135°, thereby reducing the stress on the stem.

The recognition of failed and fractured total hip stems led to the development of newer total hip designs. Müller maintained the shape of his prosthesis, but introduced a new super-alloy material. This design change resulted in the treatment of the symptoms, but did not treat the cause. The early Müller prosthesis fractured because it became loose; the sharp edges and diamond design created high stresses in the cement and caused it to fail. Charnley responded by offering his Cobra* prosthesis. He basically maintained the original design concepts but increased the prosthesis size.

The introduction of the CAD† total hip prosthesis in 1974 provided a revolutionary new concept that fostered a new generation in total hip design. The CAD total hip was the first femoral stem to have a totally rounded cross-section without sharp corners. The cross-sectional area was much larger than the original total hip stems (Fig. 3-3). The intended purpose of the large stem was to fill the intramedullary canal with metal, minimizing the amount of cement to be used.

Crowninshield later reported that increasing the cross-sectional size of the femoral stem not only decreased the compressive stress in the cement but also the tensile stress in the stem.[20] A 20-percent increase in the stem's cross-section resulted in a 5-percent decrease in stress in the cement, and 12-percent decrease in the tensile stress of the stem. Rounding the medial and lateral borders of the stem further decreased the stress in the cement by enlarging the cross-sectional area of the stem.

The diamond-shaped design had a knife-like edge pressing against the cement. Stress is a function of load and the area that the load acts upon. When the area is small, the stresses will be high, when compared to a broader surface under the same load. Rounding the medial border added even more surface area than would have been realized if a flat, rectangular cross-section was used. It also allowed for a smoother transition at the corners, minimizing stress concentrations. The tear-drop in the CAD stem was designed to provide an interlock with the cement and to minimize the shear stresses (Fig. 3-3). The CAD total hip was the first prosthesis to have several different sizes available to the surgeon. This system approach made it possible for the orthopaedist to better fit the prosthesis to the patient.

It became obvious from the earlier experiences that it was necessary to reduce the stress in the total hip stem and protect the cement, in order to ensure a successful prosthesis. Reduction of the stresses in the stem can be handled by two methods: (1) Increasing the *cross-sectional geometry* of the stem allows the prosthesis to endure higher loads without jeopardizing the integrity of the implant. (2) Employing a material with *improved mechanical properties* will allow the prosthesis to carry higher stresses with less incidence of failure.

Although increasing the cross-sectional geometry and using a stronger material does not lessen the stress on the prosthesis, it does satisfy the basic intention of increasing the expected prosthesis life by allowing it to endure the activities of the body without failure.

A physiologic method of reducing the stresses in the stem is by lessening the

*Codman & Shurtleff, Inc.
†Howmedica, Inc.

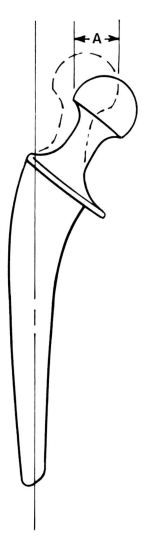

Fig. 3-4. Moving the neck-stem angle in the valgus direction reduces the moment arm, thereby minimizing bending stress on the prosthesis stem.

resultant load on the prosthesis (weight reduction), or by sharing the load with a surrounding structure (crutches). Certainly, the easiest thing to do is to have the patient lose weight and/or use crutches or a cane.

Moving the neck-stem angle of the prosthesis into a valgus position will reduce the stresses on the stem (Fig. 3-4). When the prosthesis neck-stem angle is moved valgus, the moment arm is reduced, the resultant stresses in the stem are decreased, and the actual head force increases, as shown by earlier equations (Fig. 3-5). The reduction of stress in the stem, however, does not occur without decreasing the stability of the total hip arthroplasty. This revision in the anatomical structure results in an imbalance of the mechanical model, increasing the stress in the abductors and hip instability (Fig. 3-5). For a young patient with good muscle tone, this is a small price to pay for longer stem life. However, the older patient who has been inactive for several years because of hip pain will have more difficulty maintaining a normal gait when the hip is reconstructed with a valgus neck-stem prosthesis.

Reduction of total hip stem load can also be accomplished by transferring a portion of the load to the cortical wall of the femur. A collar large enough to attain collar-calcar contact is necessary for maximizing load transfer to the bone. Proponents of the large collar design prosthesis believe that the load shared by the proximal femur is important to bone life. A common theory for the cause of proximal bone resorption subsequent to prosthetic revision is stress-shielded bone causing localized disuse osteoporosis. If disuse osteoporosis is indeed a factor in the proximal femoral resorption, it would be beneficial to provide additional stress to the proximal femur.

Large collars are not the only approach to stressing the proximal femur. Several designs have been introduced that are totally collarless, yet they are claimed to stress the proximal femur. The concept behind these designs is to load the bone from within the intramedullary canal through hoop stresses. *Hoop stress* is analogous to the reaction of a metal ring around an old rain barrel (Fig. 3-6). When the barrel is empty, there is relatively little stress on the ring. When the barrel is filled with water, the ring is highly stressed in an effort to hold the staves together. Hoop stresses are circumferential tensile stresses different from the physiologic compressive stresses that the calcar femorali is normally subjected to.

This principle relates to the collarless hips that have tapered stems, becoming increasingly smaller toward the distal end. The intramedullary canal is reamed with the same taper as the femoral component. When the stem is implanted, the sides of the prosthesis will be *congruous* to the walls of the intramedullary canal. When the

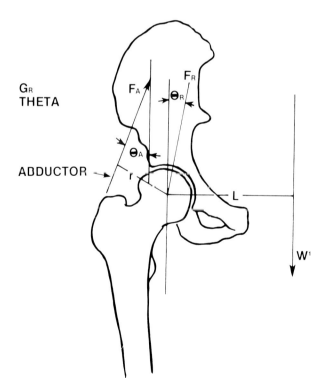

Fig. 3-5. When the femoral head is moved toward valgus, the abductor distance "**r**" decreases while the body weight distance "**L**" increases. This change in moment arm forces the abductor muscles to work harder because of the greater leverage attained by the body weight force.

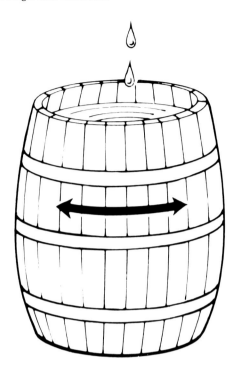

Fig. 3-6. The metal rings around a barrel endure circumferential tensile stress, or hoop stress, when the barrel is filled.

hip is loaded, the effect will be similar to the rain barrel that is filled with water. As the load increases on the hip stem, more stress will be transferred to the bone (Fig. 3-7), by wedging of the prosthesis in the canal. The controversy of the collar-calcar contact in total hip design will continue until significant clinical data is accumulated showing favor to one side. In vitro bench studies[43] and theoretical analyses[20] have been generated to favor the large collar designs.

Crowinshield, utilizing finite element analysis, demonstrated that any and all femoral endoprostheses will cause a reduction in the physiologic stress in the calcar femorali.[20] His work emphasizes that the collarless prosthesis decreases this physiological stress more than the collar prosthesis. Oh and Harris, utilizing strain gauge analysis, duplicated the finite element analysis study and demonstrated a significant difference in stress distribution in those prostheses with collars and those without collars.[43] The data from the strain gauge analysis demonstrated:

1. That the prostheses with large collars transferred approximately 33 percent of the anatomic stress into the bone at the osteotomy site. Prostheses with insignificant collars (not extensive enough to reach the cortex) imparted no stress to the proximal femur.
2. In the anatomic model, the data showed that the stress was highest in the proximal femur and decreased distally to the anterior bow. When a prosthesis was implanted, the stresses in the proximal femur were lower than the stresses in the bone at the distal tip of the prosthesis.
3. The study determined that there was little difference in the bone stress when a large, stiff femoral stem was implanted as compared to a smaller, more flexible prosthesis.[43]

Markolf analyzed micro motion in the collar-calcar area and flexural bending as a function of collar size and noted that with adequate collar-calcar contact, micro motion and flexural bending were decreased by one half.[38] Although these in vitro studies do not reproduce the anatomy and physiology of the reconstructed hip joint, the comparative data received from each model demonstrated the important differences in design concepts as they related to bone stress.

Material choice is another area of controversy in total hip design. Cast CoCr alloy has been the material of choice in total hip stems since the introduction of total hip prostheses in the United States. True, some prostheses were manufactured of stainless steel alloy; however, few designs remain in this metal. The few that are manufactured in stainless steel represent a small percentage of total hips being implanted in the United States.

Just as the design of total hip stems changed with the recognition of fractured stems, manufacturers also developed stronger metals to fabricate total hip stems. High-strength alloys with fatigue endurance limits exceeding 100,000 psi are now available from several manufacturers. The higher fatigue strength of the new materials permits more liberty in the design of total hips, in order to decrease cement stress and increase bone stress (to prevent loosening).

Cast CoCr alloy is reported to have a fatigue endurance limit of approximately 45,000 psi.[58] Therefore, the high-strength alloy offers more than twice the fatigue endurance protection than the cast CoCr material. To the designer of total hips, this means that the fatigue endurance limit of any given design could be doubled by manufacturing the same design in a high-strength alloy material.

Fatigue strength, fatigue endurance, and endurance limit all refer to the same material property: the maximum stress that can be endured for an indefinitely large number of times without producing fracture of the material. In most cases, the

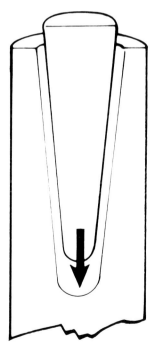

Fig. 3-7. The prosthesis has a constant taper that is congruous to the cement bed. As the prosthesis is loaded, stresses are transferred from the prosthetic hip stem by wedging it into the cement mantle.

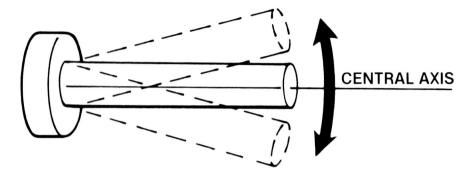

Fig. 3-8.   Reverse bending. The material is deflected equidistantly to opposite sides of the central axis. Unidirectional bending deflects the material to only one side of the central axis.

stress is applied by moving the material in reverse bending (Fig. 3-8). In reverse bending, the material is forced to cross a central axis on both sides. Unidirectional bending forces the material to yield to only one side of the axis.

When the test is conducted, the load is introduced to the test specimen at rest while it lies on an axis. The force of the load causes the material to bend away from the axis. When the force is removed, the material will return back to a rest position on the axis. This is unidirectional bending.

Reverse bending follows the same pattern as unidirectional bending, but the material is not allowed to return to the rest position on the axis. Instead, a force is applied on the other side of the specimen 180° away from the first load. This second force is opposite in location and equal in magnitude to the first force. This causes the metal to bend in a direction opposite to the first bend and at an equal distance away from the axis.

The *endurance limit* is a function of time (number of cycles) and stress. It is apparent, then, that the number of cycles, or the implant life, could be increased if stress is lowered. However, the figure most useful when designing total hips is the *endurance strength.* The endurance strength is the maximum stress a material will endure for a given number of cycles. Reverse bending is usually implied unless otherwise stated. When defining the endurance strength, 10^7 cycles is the accepted number of cycles usually employed. Endurance strength relates to the material alone; the values for endurance strength, therefore, do not take into consideration the geometry of the prosthesis.

The *modulus of elasticity* is another mechanical property of metals that is important to the design of total hips. The modulus of elasticity, or Young's Modulus, is a ratio between stress and strain.[48] Simply, it is the ratio of load (stress) and the amount of deformation (strain) caused by that load. Large values for Young's Modulus indicate that the material is stiff; lower values mean that it is flexible and yields more easily to a load. The modulus of elasticity is particularly of interest in designing total hips because of the composite structure of bone, methylmethacrylate, and prosthesis that is created with revision arthroplasty. In a composite, the stiffest member will endure the greatest amount of stress. The stiffest member of the composite in a total hip replacement is the prosthesis.

The bar graph in Figure 3-9 shows the modulus of elasticity for CoCr alloys, cortical bone, Simplex P Bone Cement* and titanium alloy. The varied difference between the bone, acrylic bone cement, and the implant metals is most noticeable. Cortical bone has a value ten times greater than acrylic bone cement. Likewise, the modulus of elasticity of CoCr is approximately ten times greater than that of cortical bone. Titanium alloy offers a reduction of approximately 50 percent in the modulus of elasticity of CoCr. Proponents of the use of titanium alloys believe the lower modulus material decreases the stress in the prosthesis and increases the stress in the proximal femur. However, a comparative analysis of the proportional difference of titanium alloy and CoCr alloy to cortical bone reveals that the relative elastic moduli are changed by 10 percent with titanium alloy. Titanium alloy $(E = 16 \times 10^6)$ is 20 percent of the elastic modulus of cortical bone $(E = 3 \times 10^6)$. Likewise, CoCr alloy $(E = 32 \times 10^6)$ is 10 percent of the elastic modulus of cortical bone $(E = 3 \times 10^6)$. Although the difference of moduli between the two metals is 50 percent, the magnitude of the change relative to cortical bone is only 10 percent.

Crowninshield conducted a three-dimensional finite element analysis comparing the design of femoral components with respect to length, cross-sectional size, material properties and collar/collarless prostheses.[20] He found that stress in the prosthesis stem decreased by 26 percent when the modulus of elasticity was lowered 50 percent, while the maximum compressive stress in the cement increased by 46 percent.

The more flexible titanium alloy stems changed the proportional share of stress to the individual members of the bone-cement-prosthesis composite. In so doing, stress was transferred from the femoral component to the cement. Bone cement is

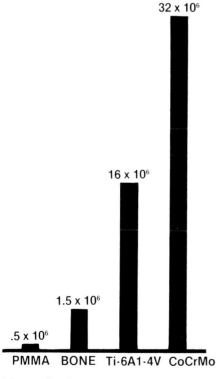

32×10^6

16×10^6

1.5×10^6

$.5 \times 10^6$

PMMA   BONE   Ti-6A1-4V   CoCrMo

Fig. 3-9. Modulus of elasticity (Young's Modulus).

*Howmedica, Inc.

commonly recognized as the weak link in the bone-cement-prosthesis composite. It has been the ambition of total hip designers to include geometries in total hip stem designs that would be compatible with cement and extend the useful life of the cement, as increasing the stress in the cement is too high a price to pay in total hip design. Crowninshield further recommends that increasing the stem length from 100 mm to 130 mm lessens the stress in the cement. He also recognized a reduction in cement stress when a prosthesis with a large collar was employed.[20]

The only argument against large collars on total hip prostheses is that some believe that good collar-calcar contact is impossible to attain in surgery.[38] No arguments exist that state collar-calcar contact is absolutely impossible to attain in surgery. No arguments exist that state collar-calcar contact is detrimental to proximal femoral bone life or the integrity of the prosthesis. This being the case, it would seem logical that a large-collared total hip should be used to achieve collar-calcar contact. Prostheses without a significant collar suffer from proximal bone resorption. Therefore, no real risk is present when using the large-collar prosthesis.

In summation, the prudent choice for a successful total hip stem is a prosthesis with: (1) A cross-sectional stem design that minimizes all stress concentrations in both the prosthesis and the cement. (2) A large collar on the prosthesis to transfer stress from the stem and cement to the bone; reduction of stem stress can extend the useful life of a prosthesis. Relief of stress in the cement will retard fracture of the cement and delay stem loosening. If, in fact, resorption of the proximal femur is a result of too little stress, a large collar can give additional stress to the bone. (3) The use of a new high-strength alloy is a necessity. Combination of good stem design with high-strength material will increase the life of the total hip prosthesis. The high-strength alloys are more than twice as strong as the cast alloys and almost 33 percent stronger than the titanium alloys. (4) Longer stem lengths have been shown to reduce the stress in the cement mantle because they have a larger surface area to distribute the stresses.

Prophylactic measures in preventing femoral stem loosening and eventual stem fracture are crucial. These include proper patient selection and education, strict surgical technique, meticulous cementing technique, and the choice of an advanced design prosthesis fabricated in one of the high-strength metals. Utilizing these measures will decrease the incidence of failure of the total hip arthroplasty.

FEMORAL COMPONENT SELECTION IN REVISION TOTAL HIP REPLACEMENT

The choice of a femoral component for revision surgery is crucial; secure, enduring fixation is fundamental to the concept of joint arthroplasty. The setting is less than ideal and a "realistic" insight into the pathologic osseous "real estate" aids one in reconstruction. The surgeon does not have the advantage of the same virgin medullary canal constrained within a strong cortical tube encountered during the initial reconstructive procedure.

The changes in the normal anatomy and physiology of the proximal femur which present to a surgeon at revision are numerous, and have a bearing on the success of the procedure. There is usually a serious depletion of bone stock in the proximal femur as a result of resorption due to stress shielding, movement, sepsis, osteolysis, perforation, or actual fracture.

Calcar resorption is a frequent observation in failed femoral stems. Cupic, in an analysis of Charnley's original series with a follow-up of 11.5 years, noted 1 to 5 mm of calcar resorption in 74.7 percent of the cases.[21] Theoretically, most feel this phenomena is due to stress shielding.[43] The revision component will almost invariably be seated more distal on the femoral neck, towards the lesser trochanter. Accordingly, a longer neck prosthesis, calcar replacement, or proximal femoral replacement may be needed to approximate physiologic reconstruction of the mechanics of the hip.

After removal of the initial implant and surrounding cement mantle, the surgeon is confronted with a pathologic cortical tube of bone encompassing the proximal third of the femur, as described by Amstutz.[1] Trabecular bone has disappeared as a result of previous reaming, implant movement, resorption, granuloma formation, and/or sepsis. The canal has enlarged; the cortex is thinned and sometimes even perforated. This sclerotic cortical tube extends distally in the femur to the most distal extent of the original implant and surrounding cement mantle (Fig. 3-10). The choice of a proper revision implant to deal with calcar resorption, increased intermedullary canal size and a pathologic cortical tube extending through the proximal third of the femur is crucial for a successful enduring result.

Just as there is significant change in the anatomy and physiology, there is a significant change in the biomechanics of the proximal femur. There is a significant change in the geometry of the femur at the junction between the pathological cortical tube and the distal, normal long-bone architecture. This is of mechanical significance because an inherent stress-raiser exists at the juncture of abnormal and normal osseous geometry. In any structure, internal stresses are increased in areas where there is a change in geometrical shape. Examples of this stress-raiser effect

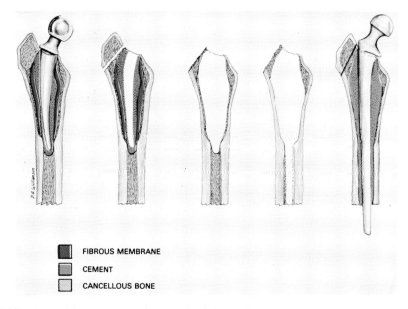

■ FIBROUS MEMBRANE

▨ CEMENT

▨ CANCELLOUS BONE

Fig. 3-10. In revision surgery, the proximal femoral canal is enlarged and the cortex is thinned. This sclerotic cortical tube extends distally in the femur to the most distal extent of the original implant and surrounding cement mantle.

are a drill hole in bone or the juncture of the straight and curved portions of a femoral component stem.[48] Therefore, in reconstruction of the femur at revision surgery, it is necessary to realize that the stresses in the bone are increased at the junction between abnormal and normal bone and that the stem should bypass this inherent stress-raiser.

Using the analogy between the diaphysis of the femur and a cylinder, one can analyze this inherent stress-raiser in engineering principles. In a structure with a stress-raiser, the internal stress becomes "normal" a certain distance from the raiser. In a cylinder, this distance from the stress raiser is two times the width of a cylinder.[48] Therefore, in a femur, normal internal stresses would be expected to occur distal to the pathologic proximal femur by a distance of two times the width of the bone.[4,32,48] A stem that reaches this distal point in the intra-medullary canal then becomes part of a total hip composite that is stressed by more normal internal stresses than a stem that ends proximally at the inherent stress-raiser area. The revision arthroplasty would then better endure, since the composite is more physiologically stressed.

Miller, in Chapter 8, describes the difficulty in obtaining fixation of components during revision surgery. He notes, "The most serious deficiency in the proximal femur is the almost complete absence of interstices or cancellous bone and, thus, little or no opportunity for micro-interlock." Pressurization and micro-interlock fixation can only be attained by going distally into the virgin intramedullary bed. Proximally, in the pathologic cortical tube, fixation is only obtained by bulk filling. In order to assure the most rigid fixation possible, the femoral stem should traverse the proximal cortical tube and any cortical defects, and penetrate the virgin cancellous bed distally, for micro-interlock fixation.

Empirically, surgeons have utilized femoral stems of approximately 110 mm to obtain adequate fixation in virgin bone during primary arthroplasty. At revision, the pathologic cortical tube, created by removal of the 110 mm stem and distal 10 to 20 mm cement plug, extends about 120 to 130 mm. We feel that adequate micro-interlock fixation can be obtained by extending distal to the cortical tube by a distance of at least 100 mm. Stem lengths of 220 to 300 mm may be required for adequate fixation, depending on femoral anatomy.

There are advantages and disadvantages to the use of a longer stem total hip replacement at revision. One disadvantage is that increased stem length potentially stress-shields the proximal femur and theoretically increases proximal resorption. Another disadvantage is more bony real estate is sacrificed and stressed in an unphysiologic mode. There is an increased technical difficulty in revising a long stem prosthesis, as opposed to a more conventional length. The clear advantages to increased stem length are protection of the cement and stem.[20] Fixation is improved because of the increased length and micro-interlock fixation, which can be obtained in the distal virgin bed. Finally, the longer stem bypasses the inherent stress-raiser and reaches bone that has a more normal internal stress. We feel that the advantages far outweigh the disadvantages in utilizing a longer stem for reconstruction of the proximal femur at revision surgery.

Experience has shown us that the variety of pathology encountered in the proximal femur at revision dictates a wide selection of implants. Femoral implants should be available with variable head diameters, neck sizes, calcar build-ups, and stem lengths. Variable head sizes are crucial in cases where an acetabular component

Jr. and Joseph D'Errico

need not be exchanged. Various neck lengths allow more freedom in reconstructing the normal biomechanical properties of the hip. Calcar build-ups, whether calcar replacements or proximal femoral replacements, avoid the problems of extreme limb shortening or of an exceedingly long neck prosthesis. These build-ups also more anatomically reconstruct the proximal femur. Variable stem sizes permit the surgeon to fit the smaller femur or deal with excessive anterolateral femoral bow.

A revision prosthesis should be chosen by evaluation of the preoperative x-rays and intraoperative anatomy. Preoperative x-rays should be analyzed for the degree of calcar resorption, evidence of cortical perforation of fracture, and the distal extent of the primary stem and surrounding cement mantle. Prosthetic templates can be especially helpful in predicting the revision implant needed. Intraoperatively, the femoral environment becomes clearer and the necessary implant for reconstruction can be chosen. A number of points to aid the surgeon in this decision are outlined in Chapter 4.

We have chosen a system of implants in a high-strength forged metal to meet the demands of revision surgery. This system includes the Aufranc-Turner long stem, ATS long stem THR,* Harris calcar replacement, and the Müller proximal femoral replacement (Fig. 3-11). In difficult revisions, custom-made modifications

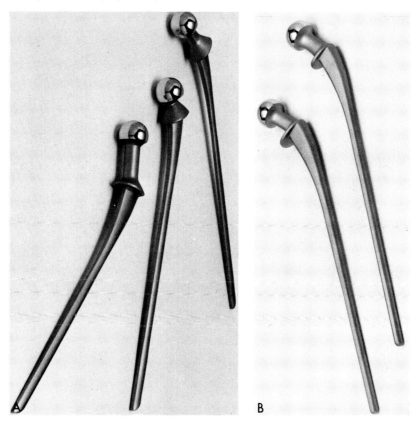

Fig. 3-11A. The Aufranc-Turner long stem implant.

Fig. 3-11B. The ATS long stem implant.

*Howmedica Inc.

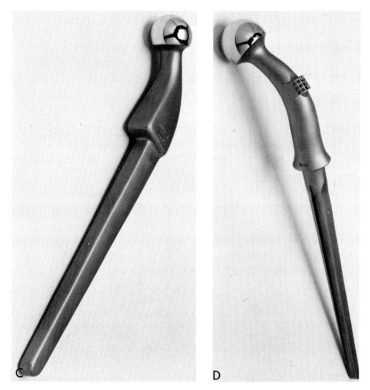

Fig. 3-11C. The Harris calcar replacement.

Fig. 3-11D. The Müller proximal femoral replacement.

of the above implants may be necessary. In these cases, consultation with an experienced engineer will aid in choosing the most acceptable design, metal, and method of manufacturing.

In summary, a femoral revision component should be chosen that will adequately replace any resorbed femoral calcar without utilizing an excessively long neck. The component should be fabricated from a high-strength metal alloy, preferably a forged CoCr alloy. The revision stem should traverse the distal extent of the proximal cortical tube by a distance of at least twice the width of bone to avoid the proximal stress raiser, and be at least 100 mm longer than the primary stem to obtain sound fixation.

ACETABULAR COMPONENT SELECTION IN REVISION TOTAL HIP REPLACEMENT

The objective of acetabular reconstruction is to restore the hip biomechanics as closely to normal as possible. The acetabular reconstruction depends on the mechanism of failure, surgical anatomy, and the integrity of osseous architecture after removal of the initial component and cement. (The reader is referred to Chapter 5 for a detailed guide to acetabular reconstruction.)

The acetabulum may have to be medialized or lateralized, for proper reconstruction. Bone grafting may be needed to form an adequate osseous support for the composite. At revision, the bony acetabulum is larger and deeper. Occasionally perforation or protrusio may exist. We advocate filling the large acetabular cavity with a correspondingly large-sized polyethylene component, allowing for at least a 2 mm mantle of cement. Cement is the weak link in the reconstructed composite; the use of excess amounts to fill large voids will weaken the composite. An array of the variable-sized acetabular components should be available, and are seen in Figure 3-12. Cement pressurization may also be decreased with the use of a small cup and excess cement.

Acetabular defects and perforations should be obturated and bone grafted to prevent intrapelvic protrusion of cement. Small defects can be treated with a Charnley cement restrictor and bone graft; larger defects may need mesh and bone graft (Fig. 3-13). An Oh-Harris protrusio ring (Fig. 3-14) is useful for lateralizing an acetabulum with a large medial wall defect.

Meticulous technique, creativity, and ingenuity are necessary to successfully reconstruct an enduring acetabulum. The key steps before choosing an acetabular implant for revision are: (1) fill the bony cavity with as large a polyethelene component as possible, allowing for a minimum 2 mm mantle of cement; (2) obturate and graft acetabular perforation; and (3) bone graft gross osseous defects.

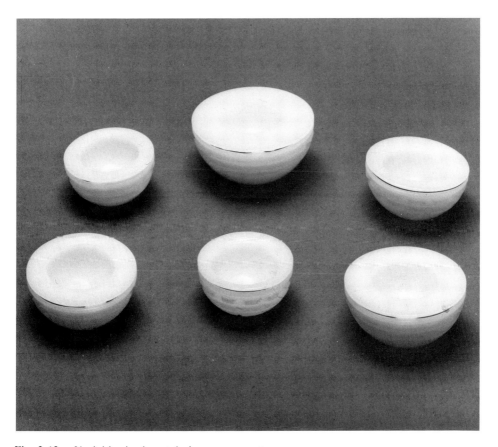

Fig. 3-12. Variable-sized acetabular components.

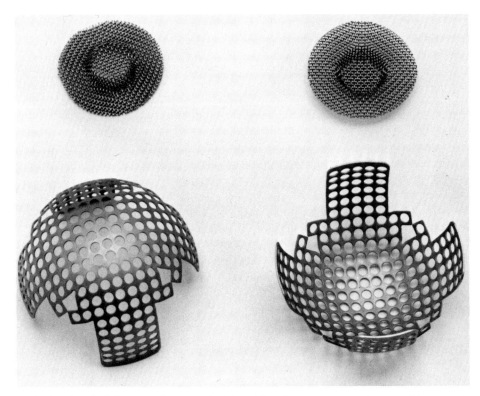

Fig. 3-13. Small defects can be treated with a Charnley cement restrictor and bone graft; larger defects may need mesh and bone graft.

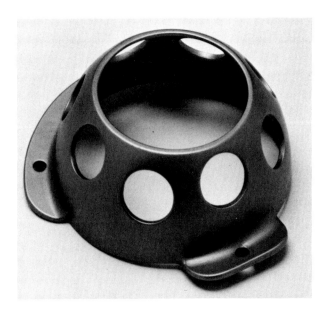

Fig. 3-14. The Oh-Harris protrusio ring.

REFERENCES

1. Amstutz HC: Personal communication.
2. Amstutz HC: Loosening of total hip femoral components: Cause and prevention, in *The Hip: Proceedings of the Fourth Open Scientific Meeting of the Hip Society.* St Louis, CV Mosby, 1976, pp 102–116.
3. Andriacchi TP, Galante JO, Belytschko TB, et al: A stress analysis of the femoral stem in total hip prosthesis. *J Bone and Joint Surg* 58A:618–624, 1976.
4. Bartel DL: Theoretical modeling: Stress analysis effect of geometry. Proceedings of the Workshop Mechanical Failure of Total Joint Replacement. American Academy of Orthopaedic Surgery, Document 916-78, p 141, June 1978.
5. Bechtol CO: Failure of femoral implant components in total hip replacement operations. *Orthop Rev* 4:23–29, 1975.
6. Bechenbaugh RD, Ilstrup DM: Looking back at total hip arthroplasty. A review of thirty-three hips four to seven years after surgery with special emphasis on loosening and wear. Paper presented at the 45th annual meeting of the American Academy of Orthopaedic Surgery, Dallas, 1978.
7. Blacker GJ, Charnley J: Long-term study of changes in the upper femur after low-friction arthroplasty. Paper presented at the 44th annual meeting of the American Academy of Orthopaedic Surgery, Las Vegas, 1977.
8. Blackwell RS, Pillar RM: Fatigue in a hostile environment. *Ind Rsch* pp 89–93, March, 1977.
9. Bocco F, Langan P, Charnley J: Changes in the calcar femoria in relation to cement technology in total hip replacement. *Clin Orthopa* and 128:287–295, 1977.
10. Brockhurts PJ, Svensson NL: Design of total hip prosthesis—the femoral stem. *Med Prog Technol* 5:83–102, 1977.
11. Carlsson AS, Gentz CF, Stenport J: Fracture of the femoral prosthesis in total hip replacement according to Charnley. *Acta Orthop Scand* 48:650–655, 1977.
12. Chao EYS, Coventry MD, Rostoker W, et al: Biomechanical analysis of fractured femoral components. Paper presented at the First International Hip Society Meeting, Kyoto, Japan, October, 1978.
13. Chao EYS, Coventry MD: Fracture of the femoral component after total hip replacement: An analysis of fifty-eight cases. *J Bone and Joint Surg* 63A: 1078–1093, 1981.
14. Charnley J: Low-friction arthroplasty of the hip, in *Low-Friction Priciple* (ed 1). Berlin Heidelberg New York, Springer-Verlag, 1979, pp 3–19.
15. Charnley J: A biomechanical analysis of the use of cement to anchor the femoral head prosthesis. *J Bone and Joint Surg* 47B:354–363, 1965.
16. Charnley J: Fracture of femoral prostheses in total hip replacement: A clinical study. *Clin Orthop* 111:105–120, 1975.
17. Charnley J, Follacci FM, Hammond BT: The long-term reaction of bone to self-curing acrylic cement. *J Bone and Joint Surg* 50B:822–829, 1968.
18. Clarke IC, Gruen T, Matos M, et al: Improved methods for quantitative radiographic evaluation with particular reference to total hip arthroplasty. *Clin Orthop* 121:83–91, 1976.
19. Collis DK: Femoral stem fracture in total hip replacement. *J Bone and Joint Surg* 59A:1033–1041, 1977.
20. Crowninshield RD, Brand RA, Johnston RC, et al: An analysis of femoral component stem design in total hip arthroplasty. *J Bone and Joint Surg* 62A:68–78, 1980.
21. Cupic Z, Charnley J: Etiology and incidence of dislocation in Charnley low-friction arthroplasty. Internal publication No. 46, Center for Hip Surgery, Wrightington, Wigan, England, 1974.
22. Ducheyne P, Aernoudt E, Martens M, et al: Fatigue fractures of the femoral component

of Charnley and Charnley-Müller type total hip prostheses. *J Biomed Mat Res* 9:199–219, 1975.

23. Fornasier VL, Cameron HU: The femoral stem/cement interface in total hip replacement. *Clin Orthop and Rel Rsch* 116:248–252, 1976.

24. Galante JO, Rostoker W, Doyle JM: Failed femoral stems in total hip prostheses. A report of six cases. *J Bone and Joint Surg* 57A:230–236, 1975.

25. Goel VK, Svensson NL: The finite element stress analysis of a human femur fitted with Charnley prosthesis. Paper presented at the Sixth Australian Conference on the Mechanics of Materials, Christ Church, New Zealand, August, 1977.

26. Greenwald SA, Nelson CA: Biomechanics of the reconstructed hip. *Orthop Clin N Amer* 4:435–447, 1973.

27. Gruen TA, McNeice GM, Amstutz, HC: Modes of failure of cemented stem type femoral components—A radiographic analysis of loosening. *Clin Orthop and Rel Rsch* 141:17–27, 1979.

28. Hamati YI, Scott R, Stillwell WR, et al: Long-term follow-up on long stem total hip replacement. (Submitted for publication to the *J Bone and Joint Surg* 1980.)

29. Harris WH, Schiller AL, Scholler JM, et al: Extensive localized bone resorption in the femur following total hip replacement. *J Bone and Joint Surg* 58A:612–617, 1976.

30. Harris WH, White RE, Mitchell S, Barber F: A new technique for removal of broken femoral stems in total hip replacement: A technical note. *J Bone and Joint Surg* 63A:843–845, 1981.

31. CAD total hip presentation, Howmedica, Inc., 1976.

32. Huiskes R: Some fundamental aspects of human joint replacement: analysis of stresses and heat conduction in bone-prosthesis structures. *Acta Orthop Scand,* Suppl No 185: 1980.

33. Huiskes R, Elangovan PT, Banens JPA, et al: Finite element computer methods of design and fixation problems of orthopaedic implants. The Netherlands, Lab of Exp Orthop, Dept. of Orthopaedics, University of Nijmegan, 1978.

34. Jaeger JH, Gaesener R, Briot B, et al: Fracture of total hip arthroplasties at the level of the femoral component. *Acta Orthop Belg* 40:861–876, 1974.

35. Kwak BM, Lim OK, Kim YY, et al: Study on the effect of cement thickness in an implant by finite element stress analysis. *Internat Orthop* June, 1978, pp 315–319.

36. Markolf KL, Amstutz HC: A comparative experimental study of stresses in femoral total hip replacement components: the effects of prostheses orientation and acrylic fixation. *J Biomech* 9:73, 1976.

37. Markolf KL, Amstutz HC: Stem fracture in total hip replacement. AAOS Committee of Biomechanical Engineering Exhibit, Academy Meeting, Las Vegas, February 1–3, 1977.

38. Markolf KL, Amstutz HC Hirchowitz DL: The effect of calcar contact on femoral component micromovement: a mechanical study. *J Bone and Joint Surg* 62A:1315–1323, 1980.

39. Marmor L: Femoral loosening in total hip replacement. *Clin Orthop* 121:116–119, 1976.

40. Martens M, Aernoudt E, DeMeester P, et al: Factors in the mechanical failure of the femoral component in total hip prosthesis. *Acta Orthop Scand* 45:693–710, 1974.

41. McNeice GM, Amstutz HC: Finite element studies in hip reconstruction, in Komi PV (ed): *Biomechanics V-A Proceedings of the Fifth International Congress of Biomechanics, Jyvaskyla, Finland, 1975.* Baltimore, Maryland, Baltimore University Park Press, p 394, 1976.

42. Nicholson, OR: Failed femoral stems in total hip prostheses. Proceedings of the New Zealand Orthopaedic Association. *J Bone and Joint Surg* 58B:262, 1976.

43. Oh I, Harris WH: Proximal strain distribution in the loaded femur. An in vitro comparison of the distributions in the intact femur and after insertion of different hip replacement femoral components. *J Bone and Joint Surg* 60A:75–85, 1978.

44. Park HW, Scheller AD, Harris JM: Mechanical analysis of femoral hip arthroplasty composites as a function of stem length. (Submitted for publication to *Clin Orthop*, 1980.)

45. Paul JP: Load actions on the human femur during walking and some stress resultants. Exper Mech 121–125, 1971.

46. Paul JP: Force actions transmitted by joints in the human body. *Prox R Soc Lond* 192B:163–172, 1976.

47. Rhinelander FW: Tibial blood supply in relation to fracture healing. *Clin Orthop* 105:34–81, 1974.

48. Roark RJ, Young WC: *Formulas for Stress and Strain*, (ed 5. New York, McGraw-Hill Book Co, 1975.

49. Rostoker W, Chao EY, Galante JO: Defects in failed stems of hip prostheses. *J Biomed Mat Res* 12:635–651, 1978.

50. Rybick EF, Simoner FA, Weis EB Jr: On the mathematical analysis of stress in the human femur. *J Biomech* 5:203–215, 1972.

51. Rydell N: Intravital measurements of forces acting on the hip joint, in Evans FG (ed): *Studies on the Anatomy and Function of Bone and Joints*. New York, Springer-Verlag, 1966, pp 52–68.

52. Salvati EA, Im VC, Aglieti P: Radiology of total hip replacements. *Clin Orthop* 121:74–80, 1976.

53. Scales JT: Fractures of the femoral component—the need for fatigue studies. Paper presented at the 42nd Annual Meeting of the American Academy of Orthopaedic Surgery, San Francisco, January 1975.

54. Scheller AD, Hamati YI, Stillwell WT et al: Femoral component fracture in total hip replacement. (Submitted for publication to the *J Bone and Joint Surg* September, 1979.)

55. Svensson NL, Valliappan S, Wood RD: Stress analysis of human femur with implanted Charnley prosthesis. *J Biomech* 10:581–588, 1977.

56. Teuber E, Kottmann B: Vergleichende Analyse der Shaftgeometrie Haufig Verwendeter Endoprosthesen fur das Huftgelenk. *Chirurg*, 47:674–681, 1976.

57. Walker PS: *Human Joints and Their Artificial Replacements*. Springfield, Ill: Charles C Thomas, 1977.

58. Walker PS: The Optimum Use of Materials in Total Hip Design, in *The Hip*: Proceedings of the Fifth Open Scientific Meeting of the Hip Society. CV Mosby Co, 1973, pp 46–66.

59. Weber FA, Charnley J: A radiological study of fractures of acrylic cement in relation to the stem of a femoral head prosthesis. *J Bone and Joint Surg* 297–301, 1975.

60. Weightman B: The stress in total hip prosthesis femoral stems: a comparative experimental study, in Schaldach M, Hohmann D (eds): *Advances in Artificial Hip and Knee Joint Technology*. New York, Springer-Verlag, 1976.

61. Williams JF, Svensson NL. A force analysis of the hip joint, *Biomed Eng* 3:365–370, 1968.

62. Wroblewski BM: The mechanisms of fracture of the femoral prosthesis in total hip replacement. *Internat Orthop* 3:137–139, 1979.

63. Zeide MS, Pugh J, Jaffee WL: Failure of femoral component in total hip replacement arthroplasty: a case study failure analysis. *Orthop* 1:291–293, 1978.

64. Zickel RE, Amstutz HC: Metal and orthopaedic surgery. Committee on Biomedical Engineering Exhibit, AAOS Annual Meeting, San Francisco, February 1978.

Roderick H. Turner and
Roger H. Emerson, Jr.

4

Femoral Revision Total Hip Arthroplasty

As stated in the preface to this volume, more than 760 revision hip arthroplasties have been performed at our hospital during the past 10 years.

Approximately 300 of these 760 revisions have involved the removal of a cemented femoral implant with an intramedullary stem. This chapter will present the basic techniques evolved by the senior author (R.H. Turner) for femoral cement removal and component replacement in operations performed mainly on patients in group 1, as noted in the Preface.

The reasons for femoral revision arthroplasty include: femoral component loosening,[2,7,8,10,33,35,39,47] recurrent dislocations,[2,9,19,39] femoral shaft fractures,[16] infections,[2,7,39] and femoral stem failure.[3,5,14,62] The special issues of infection, femoral shaft fracture, and femoral implant failure are the subjects of individual chapters later in this text.

Beckenbaugh and Ilstrup,[2] in a series from the Mayo Clinic, noted that the "unsatisfactory results [in total hip replacement] were associated mostly with pain from femoral loosening in hips not yet treated by re-operation." After 5 years of follow-up, they reported that 24 percent of their patients had roentgenographic evidence of femoral loosening. However, only 8 percent (5 of 61) of those showing femoral loosening had come to revision. The Mayo Clinic series further documented that roentgenographic evidence of femoral loosening was as high as 50 percent in patients in whom the diameter of the prosthesis was less than half the width of the femoral canal. As will be discussed in later chapters, this greater incidence of loosening is probably related to poor cement pressurization. McBeath et al,[35] after 3 years of follow-up, reported 15.9 percent femoral loosening. Roentgenographic loosening preceded clinical symptoms by 8 months in their series. Marmor studied a series of 160 Charnley total hip replacements; 10 patients developed femoral loosening between 6 months and 5 years following surgery.[33] Marmor pointed out

75

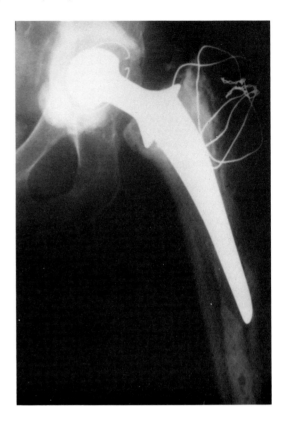

Fig. 4-1. The femoral stem here is translated into varus with a medial radiolucent "windshield-wiper" effect distally and a corresponding radiolucency proximally and medially. Note subsidence into the medial calcar of the femoral neck.

that femoral loosening usually begins with a radiolucent shadow on the lateral side of the bone-cement interface, followed by a sinking of the prosthesis into the concave side (Fig. 4-1). Lazansky has reported six cases of femoral loosening due to subsidence, and three cases associated with fracture of the acrylic cement.[26] The incidence of cement fracture has been reported from 1.5 to 8 percent.[2,15,56] Cement fractures are fatigue fractures and they usually occur within 2 cm of the tip of the prosthesis.[15,56] Salvati has reported radiolucent lines around 60 percent of femoral stems, two-thirds of which were less than 1 mm.[47] Most of the radiolucent lines were in the proximal aspect of the shaft in this series. Amstutz et al followed 339 total hip arthroplasties from 2 to 5 years (average, 3 years), and found a 19.5 percent incidence of mechanical loosening by radiographic criteria, via detailed zonal analysis.[1] From their study, they were able to define four modes of failure of cemented stems, discussed in detail in Chapter 7.

A less common cause for failure on the femoral side is recurrent dislocation. The dislocation rate following total hip replacement (THR) has been reported to be between 1 and 3 percent.[2,39,44,56] Recurrent dislocations are less common, reported at 0.5 percent.[39] Femoral component malposition requiring revision surgery is less common than acetabular malposition.[2,39] When the femoral component is responsible for the recurrent dislocations, Lowell feels that retroversion is the abnormality most often identified.[29]

This chapter will attempt to outline a systematic approach to femoral component revision. The surgeon has a great responsibility, because he or she must produce a durable joint arthroplasty when previous attempts to achieve rigid fixation in healthier proximal femoral bone than will be encountered at the time of attempted revision surgery have failed. Conversion of a previous hip operation to a primary total hip replacement has a higher incidence of complications.[7,10] Similarly, revision of a failed femoral component is fraught with technical challenges and presents several unique surgical tasks. Planning and execution of femoral component revision will be discussed in seven sequential steps:

1. Pre-operative analysis and planning;
2. Surgical approach, trans-trochanteric;
3. Surgical exposure and techniques;
4. Femoral component and cement removal;
5. Femoral component selection and implantation;
6. Cementing techniques; and
7. Wound closure and trochanteric fixation.

PRE-OPERATIVE ANALYSIS AND PLANNING

The diagnosis of a failed femoral component requires a careful physical examination. Although most patients present with hip pain, some patients with impending mechanical loosening or failure of a femoral stem can be clinically asymptomatic.[2,15,47] The presence of a radiolucent line adjacent to a total hip prosthesis does not in itself indicate that loosening is the source of the patient's complaint. In general, the pain of a loose femoral stem is specifically associated with weightbearing, and is accentuated by rotational stresses. Pain from a loose femoral component is frequently appreciated in the mid-thigh area, and is worse after the initiation of weightbearing, often subsiding after the first few steps. Wilson and Scales have reported that a palpable "klunk" is more likely to be associated with a loose acetabular component.[61] The patient with a failing femoral stem will frequently have a good range of motion, but will develop an antalgic decrease in straight leg-raising on the affected side, as well as atrophy of the quadriceps and a positive Trendelenburg gait. If pain is completely unrelieved by rest, one must suspect that sepsis may accompany losening.

Plane x-rays of the hip will frequently be all that is necessary to make a presumptive diagnosis of a failed femoral component. The width and location of any radiolucencies, whether they are between the cement and the prosthesis or the bone and the cement, should be noted (see fig. 4-1). When fatigue fractures of cement occur, they are usually located within 2 cm of the distal tip of the stem. In a study by Weber and Charnley,[56] the incidence of cement fracture was 1.5 percent, and usually occured within the first 6 months after surgery. These authors felt that the cause was proximal loosening, causing the stem to become end-weight-bearing and the cement therefore to fail in tension (see Fig. 4-2). These authors believe that the prosthesis can frequently "subside" to a more stable position, and thus would not necessarily be doomed to failure. Ling has reported a 32 percent incidence of "radiological subsidence" in patients with Exeter-type double-tapered collarless femoral components.[28] We regard subsidence as a potential early sign of femoral bone-cement interface failure. Ling joins the other British authors cited earlier in regarding subsidence as a fairly innocent phenomenon of micromotion and settling

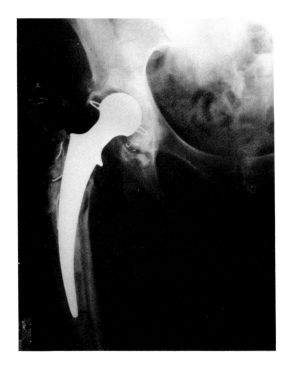

Fig. 4-2. Cement fracture at tip of prosthesis.

which only infrequently proceeds to clinical failure of the femoral bone-cement composite.[56] Gruen et al have studied the plane radiographs of 301 patients who underwent 389 total hip arthroplasties followed for 3 years.[15] They divided the proximal femur into seven zones, and followed: the change in width of radiolucent lines; sclerotic bone reaction; widening of the acrylic cement fracture gap; fragmentation of the cement; gross movement of the femoral component; and stem fracture. They isolated four modes of failure (Fig. 4-3):

1. Pistoning failure
   • in which the stem pistons within the cement
   • in which the prosthesis and the cement mantle piston within the proximal femoral shaft
2. Medial mid-stem pivot
   • in which the distal stem goes laterally and the proximal stem collapses medially
3. Calcar pivot
   • in which there was good fixation on the calcar with a windshield-wiper pattern of loosening at the tip of the prosthesis
4. The bending cantilever
   • in which there is firm fixation of the tip of the prosthesis with loss of support proximally

They specifically noted that the fourth mode of failure was highly predictive of eventual mechanical failure of the stem. The most common mode of failure in femoral-cement interface failure was pistoning of the prosthesis and cement within the shaft. Radionuclide technetium bone scans will usually be positive when there is failure of the bone-cement interface; positive scans, however, are significant only after 1 year following the last hip operation. Hip aspiration and arthrography are performed on a routine basis as part of the pre-operative evaluation of the painful total hip arthroplasty. In studies by Salvati et al, a positive arthrogram was felt to be of diagnostic value, but a negative arthrogram did not rule out an abnormality of the fixation of the components.[45,46] Murray and Rodrigo compared 25 painful hips to 53 asymptomatic hips.[38] Their study showed that a positive arthrogram, that is, radiographic contrast material between the bone-cement or the bone-prosthesis interface, did not correlate completely with the patient's presenting symptoms. Findings at surgery in their study differed from the arthrographic findings in 42 percent of the cases. These authors have clearly documented that there can be both false-positive and false-negative arthrograms. Aspiration of the painful total hip under fluoroscopic control to document the absence or presence of sepsis is an important part of pre-operative planning. The addition of contrast material following aspiration of the hip for culture adds little risk and yet yields an arthrogram as one more piece of information on which to base a treatment plan. Drinker et al have described color-subtraction arthrography, further refining the accuracy of the arthrogram as compared to black-and-white subtraction techniques.[9] Weissman has likewise cited color-subtraction arthrography as providing the advantages of "immediate viewing of the subtracted image and decreased cost."[58] For further details on radionuclide scanning and on arthrography, see Chapter 2.

There exists a group of patients who have radiographic evidence of impending femoral component failure but are nevertheless asymptomatic. This patient group presents a dilemma, in that revision surgery is ordinarily reserved for those with significant pain. There is a sub-group of patients who have massive bone osteolysis around their femoral stems, as reported by Harris (see Fig. 4-4).[19] In his evaluation of four such cases, he was unable to find evidence of infection or tumor. At revision, the pathology revealed massive accumulations of histiocytic macrophages and rare foreign body giant cells, without any acute or chronic inflammation. Also present were refractile bodies measuring from 15 to 30μm, surrounded by these

I	Ia	Pistoning: Stem within Cement	
	Ib	Pistoning: Stem within Bone	
II		Medial Midstem Pivot	
III		Calcar Pivot	
IV		Bending Cantilever (Fatigue)	

Fig. 4-3. Modes of femoral stem fracture. (From Gruen TA, McNeice GM, Amstutz HC: Modes of failure of cemented stem-type femoral components. *Clin Orthop* 141:17–27, 1979. Reprinted with permission from JB Lippincott Co., East Washington Square, Philadelphia, Pennsylvania.)

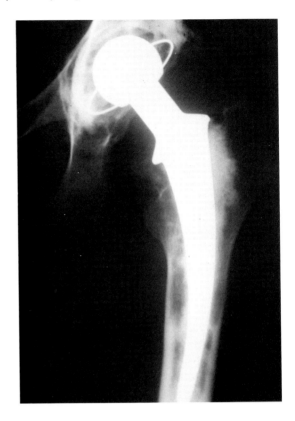

Fig. 4-4.   Massive osteolysis around the femoral stem.

macrophages. Similar bodies seen in experimental animals have been shown to be particles of polymethylmethacrylate.[50] Harris writes that gross motion coupled with fragmentation of the cement is the cause of this massive bone resorption. He believes these patients should be treated by removal of all of the soft granulomatous material followed by revision with a long-stem prosthetic component. Follow-up of 13 to 18 months in his four cases revealed no further evidence of similar resorption of bone.

The other situation when revision surgery may be warranted before pain develops is in the patient with bony resorption around the calcar and medial neck of the prosthesis, placing the femoral stem in jeopardy because of complete loss of proximal and medial support. This is the mode IV failure patter of Gruen et al,[15] which preceded stem fracture in a significant percentage of cases studied. The patient should, at the very least, be protected with a cane or crutches and carefully followed. In general, progressive loss of bone stock which would compromise revision surgery is an indication for earlier surgical intervention. The judgement decision to revise such a hip is difficult and must be made on a case-by-case basis.

Recurrent dislocation attributable to malpositioning of the femoral component is not common, but retroversion of the femoral neck can lead to this complication.[29] Anterior/posterior (AP) and true lateral x-rays of the hip and pelvis, as well as internal and external rotation views of the femur, will help to determine the orientation of the femoral component in the shaft. Fluoroscopy of the hip can further aid this determination. If dislocations continue to occur without obvious etiology, exploration of the hip may be necessary in order to observe the components directly. Revision of a malpositioned femoral component is usually a major challenge because the components tend to be rigidly fixed in the femoral shaft, and the cement-bone interface is usually healthy.

Deciding the mechanism of femoral component failure directs the surgeon during the reconstruction. In addition, the surgeon must have an appreciation of the state of the soft tissues about the hip, the adequacy of bone stock, and the degree of difficulty required to extract the failed femoral component. X-rays (AP and lateral) of the upper femoral shaft should be scanned for femoral component position, cortical thickness, areas of osteolysis, fractures, cortical perforations, and width of the femoral canal. If there are deficiencies in the femoral shaft, the surgeon should prepare to have either autologous or homologous bone graft available at the time of surgery (Figs. 4-5A through 4-5E). The state of the greater trochanter should be established; please refer to Chapter 11 for a thorough discussion of trochanteric problems.

The patient requires a complete medical evaluation permitting him or her to safely undergo long surgery with the potential for large turnover in blood volume. The patient's leg lengths and neurovascular status should be established pre-operatively for later comparison.

The type of total hip components in place must be ascertained. If the acetabular component is not to be revised, appropriate revision femoral components that fit the acetabular component must be available in a full selection of neck lengths. If not revised, the acetabular side must be carefully protected from damage during femoral revision.

The state of the overlying skin should be assessed; on occasion a plastic surgery consulation will be necessary to improve the skin which may have become densely adherent to bone, such as the greater trochanter of ilium. Because primary skin closure is absolutely essential after revision total hip surgery, it is sometimes necessary to have a preliminary plastic surgical procedure, such as a rotational flap, performed to provide a healthy soft-tissue bed. Definitive revision surgery should be delayed by at least 3 months following any preliminary plastic surgical procedures.

SURGICAL APPROACH—TRANS-TROCHANTERIC

Our experience is that osteotomy of the greater trochanter is necessary in virtually all cases of femoral component revision. The consensus from the ortho-paedic literature is the same.[3,10,20,26,37,49,53] The advantages of trochanteric removal include better overall exposure and ease of insertion of the new components. Eftekhar et al,[10] in reviewing 70 total hip arthroplasties in cases of previous surgeries, felt that trochanteric removal was absolutely necessary. Thompson and Culver reviewed a comparable series of 126 cases in which the trochanter was removed, and 99 cases where the trochanter was not transplanted.[53] They felt that removal of the trochanter was especially valuable in approaching previously operated hips because of a decreased incidence of complications. These complications included: penetration of the femoral shaft; fracture of the greater trochanter; greater than 2½ hours of operating time; and greater than 6 units of blood loss.

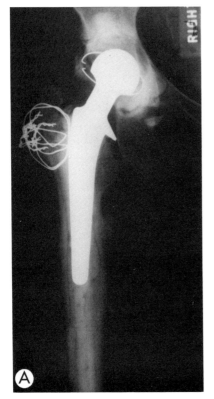

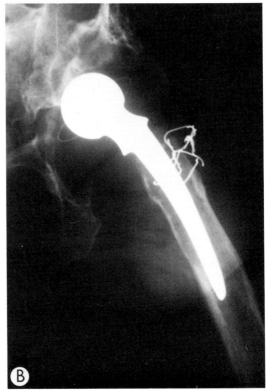

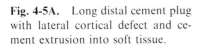

Fig. 4-5A. Long distal cement plug with lateral cortical defect and cement extrusion into soft tissue.

Fig. 4-5B. Marked thinning of proximal femur. Radiolucent cement was used in this case.

Fig. 4-5C. Perforation of femoral shaft by prosthesis.

Fig. 4-5D. Failed femoral stem with proximal shaft fracture.

Fig. 4-5E. Small femoral canal that will not accommodate standard component stem.

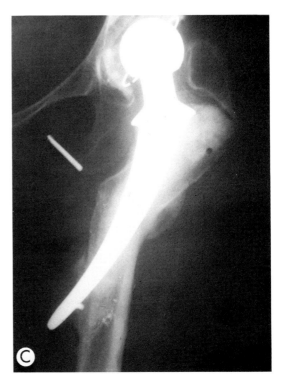

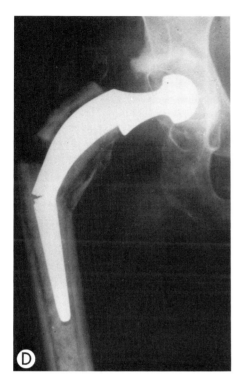

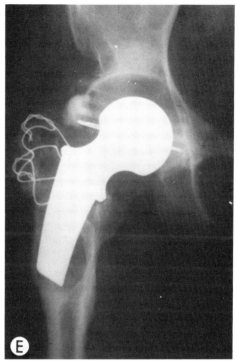

There were 19 complications related to exposure in the 99 cases where the trochanter was not osteotomized. In reviewing the patients with complications, Thompson and Culver were able to identify a group that had a fixed 30° or greater flexion contracture, and a fixed 10° or greater external rotation contracture that were at particularly high-risk for problems related to exposure. Charnley feels that it is easier to get a valgus position of the femoral component with the trochanter removed.[3] Hips that require revision surgery have a poorer average range of motion than hips undergoing primary hip surgery; removal of the greater trochanter permits greater ease in accomplishing complete capsulectomy and debridement of scar about the hip, which in turn permits a better post-operative range of motion, as well as greater ease in regaining any lost leg length.[51] The incidence of trochanteric nonunion is 1.8 percent, and delayed union 2.7 percent, in the series by Lazansky.[26] In comparing a group of patients with bilateral primary total hip replacements in which the trochanter was removed on one side, Weisman et al report that patients subjectively prefer the side in which the trochanter was not transplanted.[59] Nevertheless, there was no difference in the Harris hip scores comparing side to side. Despite this preference, for the special situation of revision surgery the advantages of trochanteric osteotomy far outweigh its disadvantages. Chapter 11 provides a detailed discussion of the indications for trochanteric transplantation in both primary and revision hip surgery.

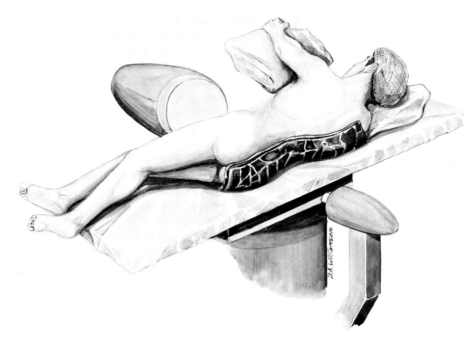

Fig. 4-6.   Patient positioned with vacuum-pack support and C-arm fluoroscopic X-ray unit.

SURGICAL EXPOSURE AND TECHNIQUES

The patient is anesthetized. Special monitoring lines should be established according to the patient's medical history and the need for specific blood transfusion techniques, as discussed in Chapter 15. If pre-operative planning suggests a lengthy revision procedure, it is our practice to request a central venous pressure line.

The patient is placed in the lateral position and the nonsurgical leg is flexed about 20°. We recommend using a C-arm portable fluoroscopic x-ray unit in conjunction with either a pedestal-type table or a table equipped with an extension on the foot-end. These tables permit biplane fluoroscopic monitoring of the femur during any phase of the revision surgery. Accordingly, the patient is secured on a radiolucent vacuum-pack body support rather than the usual kidney-rest type supports (see Fig. 4-6). Cement removal, cement plugging, cement pressurization, and femoral component positioning are all safer and more precise when done under precision biplane fluoroscopic control.

The hip and leg are then prepped and draped; the leg is positioned free, to permit easy manipulation. The operative field should include the iliac crest in case autogenous bone graft needs to be harvested during the operation. The sterile, prepped operative field should extend distally down the entire lateral shaft of the femur to 4 inches below the knee to cope with potential distal femoral cement problems. The normal tissue planes surrounding the hip are distorted in most cases of revision surgery. As Dr. Aufranc has stressed in his introductory remarks, it is necessary to start the dissection about the hip in an area of normal tissue both distally and proximally, and then trace the normal anatomic planes into the area of maximum scarring.

The skin incision is lateral and comes straight up the shaft of the femur, curving gently over the greater trochanter to arch towards the posterior superior iliac spine (Fig. 4-7). The incision can be extended distally to expose the entire shaft of the femur if necessary. Previous incisions that are less than 1 year old should be included as part of the revision incision if at all possible. The older the scar, the more safety there is in creating parallel incisions. Complications have been very rare with parallel incisions about the hip, given ample subcutaneous tissue between the incisions and at least 12 months since prior surgery.

The subcutaneous tissues are divided down to the fascial layers and the tensor fascia is opened along the line of the skin incision (Fig. 4-7). The dissection is then brought proximally over the greater trochanter and the fibers of the gluteus maximus are bluntly separated parallel to their long axis. If a previous trochanteric osteotomy has been performed, the fixation wires will be uncovered and removed in the bursal sac beneath the tensor fascia. Careful study of the pre-operative x-rays will help to reveal the location of the wires. If the wires have fragmented, it is not necessary to remove them in their entirety. An important and constant landmark in dissecting about the hip in densely scarred situations is the insertion of the gluteus maximus tendon into the linea aspera of the femur.

After wire removal, the anterior and posterior borders of the gluteus medius are identified. The vastus lateralis is cut with cutting electrocautery from the vastus tubercle, leaving a 1 cm fascial cuff for later reinsertion (Fig. 4-8). The trochanter is further defined anteriorly along the base of the hip capsule between the gluteus minimus and the origin of the vastus intermedius. Posteriorly, any remnants of the short external rotators (which are usually ill-defined, due to prior surgery) are sectioned from the back of the trochanter and reflected posteriorly to protect the sciatic nerve. A blunt curved instrument is passed underneath the greater trochanter between hip capsule and abductor muscle mass to define the plane for trochanter osteotomy. Where possible, the osteotomy should be planned so that an adequate cancellous bone bed is preserved for later reattachment. Trochanteric osteotomy

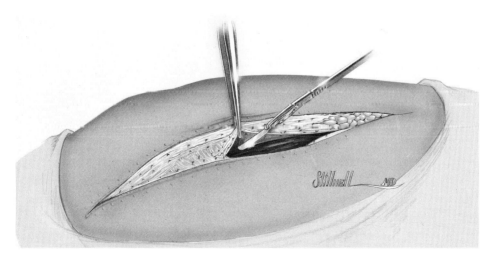

Fig. 4-7. In revision hip surgery the dissection should be started distally in an area of normal tissue and then the anatomic plains traced proximally.

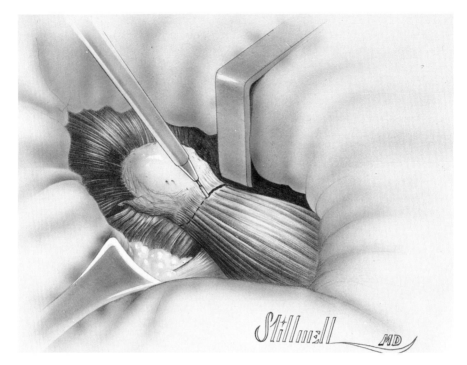

Fig. 4-8.   The vastus lateralis is divided at its origin leaving a small cuff for later repair.

can be performed with a broad osteotome, curved gouge, or gigli saw, depending upon the preference of the operator (Fig. 4-9). Care must be taken to leave the entire insertion of the gluteus minimus tendon on the greater trochanteric fragment. The greater trochanter is then retracted cephalad and the hip capsule is delineated. The abductors can be held in a retracted position above the level of the acetabulum

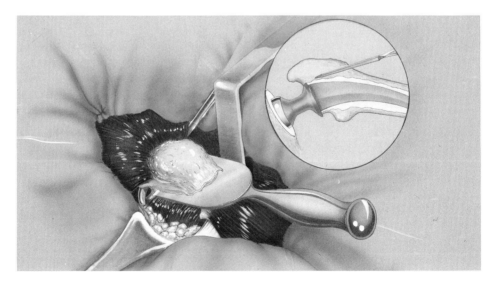

Fig. 4-9.   The trochanteric osteotomy must be planned to permit secure reattachment later.

with a broad abdominal retractor with two Steinman pins driven through the ilium superior to the acetabulum. These fixation pins should penetrate both tables of the ilium for secure fixation. Care should be taken not to disturb the cement fixation of the existing acetabular component in performing pin insertion, in case it is decided not to revise the acetabulum. At this point, a specimen of the hip joint capsule should be sent for a culture (Fig. 4-10). If joint fluid is encountered, it is sent both for immediate Gram stain and for culture. Intravenous antibiotic treatment is then begun by the anesthesiologist with 2 g of cefamandole. After cultures are obtained, wound towels are sewn to the tensor fascia and moistened with irrigation solution containing topical antibiotics.

A complete capsulectomy is recommended in revision hip arthroplasties to complete a wide exposure of both the acetabulum and the femur. Removal of the capsule may be difficult because of heterotopic ossification within its substance. A frequent area of difficulty is the posterior capsular dissection: the sciatic nerve may adhere to the capsule, and there often is found a deficiency of posterior soft-tissue due to prior surgery. If there is distortion of the posterior anatomy, the sciatic nerve should palpated, exposed, and carefully protected. Prior to dislocating the hip, the leg-length should be measured to establish a baseline for comparison later in the operation when the new components are inserted. The simplest way to measure intra-operatively is from the Steinman pins retracting the greater trochanter to a fixed mark on the lateral cortical bone of the femur. This measurement should be written down so that it can be referred to at the end of the procedure. When there has been chronic and severe shortening of the extremity, as with congenital dysplasia, lengthening the leg to achieve equality with the other side is not valuable if it means tenuous trochanteric fixation. It is usually possible to gain from 2 to 3 cm of length without special techniques. Attempts to gain more than 3 cm of leg length are rarely indicated unless the patient pre-operatively has either piston mobility or significant subsidence of a femoral component in the medullary canal.

The hip is dislocated by flexing, externally rotating, and adducting the leg over

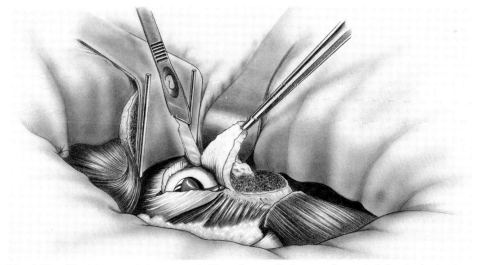

Fig. 4-10. The hip capsule is removed. Note the two Steinman pins and abdominal retractor holding the greater trochanter.

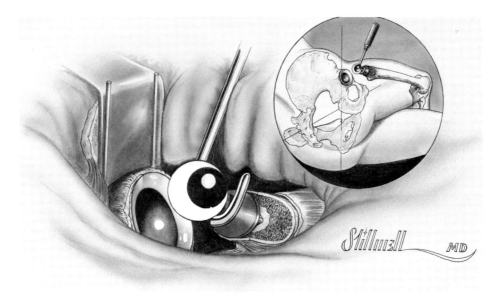

Fig. 4-11.   The hip is dislocated by flexion, adduction, and external rotation. A bone hook placed under the prosthetic femoral neck helps to lift the femoral component out of acetabulum eliminating torque forces on the proximal femur.

the side of the operating table into a sterile pouch or into a large sheet folded in a pouch-like configuration. A bone hook is placed around the femoral neck to assist in dislocation (Fig. 4-11). It is important to avoid dislocation by simple manual manipulation of the leg; this can lead to femoral shaft fracture. A broad Bennett retractor can be placed underneath the proximal femur to help deliver the femoral neck into the field. Prior to any attempts at removing the component, the soft tissues about the proximal femur and the collar of the prosthesis must be dissected away, exposing the cement-bone and the cement-prosthesis interface. These should be carefully inspected for evidence of fragmentation as well as for gross motion. Blood can frequently be expressed from any loose interfaces between the prosthesis and cement or between cement and bone.

FEMORAL COMPONENT AND CEMENT REMOVAL

In most instances the prosthesis can easily be disimpacted by repeated blows with an impactor or a bone tamp from below the femoral head (see Fig. 4-12). Removal of the femoral component provides additional exposure for a final circumferential capsulectomy of the hip.

Femoral cement removal is the most difficult part of revision surgery.[11] In the case of a septic femoral component, the cement should be removed in its entirety as part of the debridement. However, in septic situations the cement is usually loose and comes out easily. In the nonseptic situation, the cement can either be grossly fragmented and therefore quite loose, with a granulomatous membrane at the bone-cement interface; or, it can be partially adherent to bone. As much cement as possible should be removed, both to permit insertion of the new component and to provide an optimal surface for maximum interdigitation between new cement and bone. It is especially important to remove the mentioned interface membrane, which is usually densely adherent to the endosteal surface of the femur.

The acrylic cement can be removed with hand and/or power instruments. Both capabilities should be available for any given revision procedure. In general, the authors have found that hand instruments are adequate for removing the proximal cement, but power instruments are necessary for the distal cement (Figs. 4-13A, 4-13B). A head-mounted fiberoptic light source should also be available to permit direct visualization down the medullary canal of the femur. Extra-long currettes, long thin osteotomes, and extended suction equipment are also helpful (Fig. 4-14). The leg is positioned over the side of the operating room table in a sterile bag with the hip flexed, adducted, and externally rotated. The surgeon is seated in a comfortable position to allow direct visualization down the femoral shaft. It is important in the positioning and draping of the patient to allow for free adduction of the hip: this is necessary for easy visualization during the removal of cement and the interface membrane.

The task of cement removal is divided, conceptually at least, into two parts: first, the proximal cement which is accessible; and second, the distal cement, which usually is inaccessible. The proximal cement can be fragmented, using thin, hand-held osteotomes; fragments are then removed under direct vision (see Fig. 4-15). The headlight adequately illuminates 4 to 6 inches of the proximal shaft. The interface membrane discussed above can actually guide the dissection of the cement away from bone. Occasionally the entire cement mantle can be removed in total, especially in infected cases. More often, the deeper and more distal cement remains behind and must be removed as a separate maneuver.

The technique originally advocated by Müller[37] and others for removing deep cement was to create a window or gutter in the anterior or lateral shaft of the femur. Such violation of the femoral bone stock should be necessary only in extreme and unusual cases. Creating windows and gutters seriously compromises the mechanical strength of the femoral shaft and should be avoided whenever possible.

Several types of guides and instrumentation systems have been designed for using power to remove the deeper cement. Eftakhar has reported a drill guide which

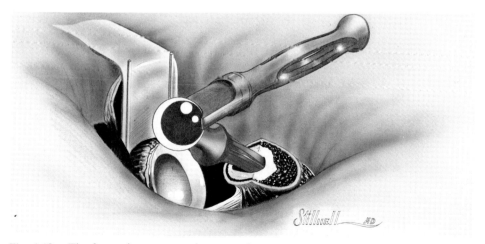

Fig. 4-12.   The femoral component is removed.

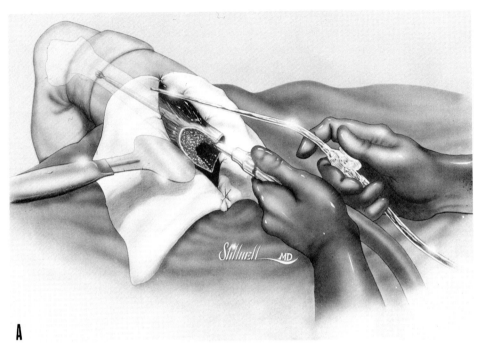

A

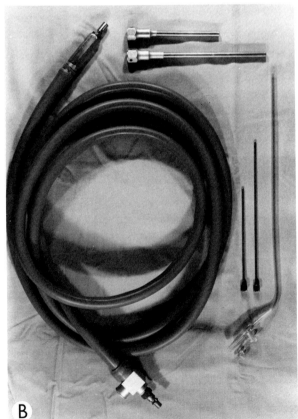

Fig. 4-13A. High-speed cutting tool in the femoral canal. Long-tipped suction equipment is required.

Fig. 4-13B. Midas Rex motor with 12.5 cm and 19 cm sleeves, cutting tools, and long, disposable suction tip.

B

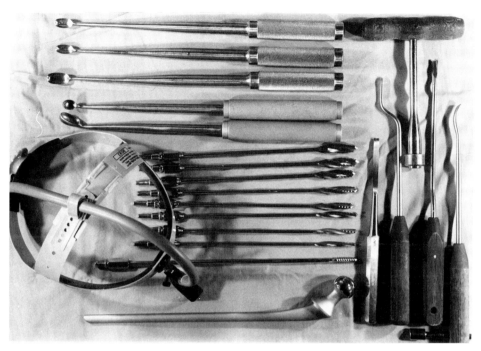

Fig. 4-14. Extra long currettes, osteotomes, hand reamers, and fiberoptic headlight. If power-reaming is performed, flexible reamers are used.

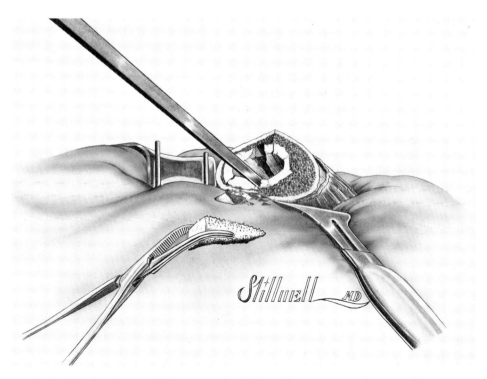

Fig. 4-15. Proximal cement is fragmented with hand instruments and removed.

clamps onto the femur and permits the use of a conventional drill to break up cement.[11] He recommends using AP and lateral x-ray control as a guide to the reaming process. Razzano found that carbide drill bits are superior for cement removal, as these bits cut into the cement as opposed to fracturing it.[42] He believes that fracturing the cement potentially exposes the femoral shaft to a spiral fracture. Harris[20] and Turner[54] have advocated cement removal with the Midas Rex pneumatic cutting tool, a high-speed drill that revolves at 75,000 rpms. We have found it to be the most effective cement removal drill available; it is especially useful in removing the cement from the isthmus of the femoral canal. Frequent and copious irrigation is necessary to maintain the cutting tips as cool as possible, as well as to remove cement debris (Figs. 4-13A, 4-13B). Disposable sterile plastic sigmoidoscopic suction-tips permit repetitive suction deep in the shaft. Harris recommends elevation of the proximal third of the quadriceps from the femoral shaft to permit better directional control of the high-speed cutting tool.[20] Our practice has been to drill away cement with the Midas Rex drill under precise biplane fluoroscopic control by means of the portable C-arm unit.[54,55] This combination of high-efficiency tools permits direct visualization during the reaming process and therefore eliminates the need for gutters and windows, as well as for any routine extensive stripping of the quadriceps. Scott et al, in an evaluation of post-operative fractures, noted that three of five fractures that occured at or just below the distal tip of the total hip prothesis occurred through cortical windows, which had been made to remove cement.[48] Refer to Chapter 6 for more details and for other negative consequences of violating the integrity of femoral cortical bone.

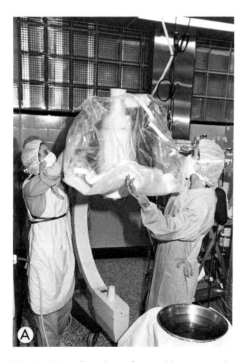

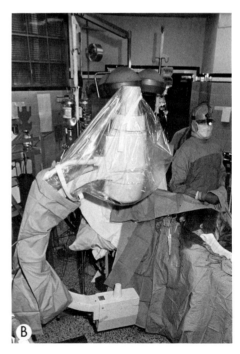

Fig. 4-16A. Draping of portable x-ray unit requires two persons.

Fig. 4-16B. X-ray unit ready to rotate under operating room table.

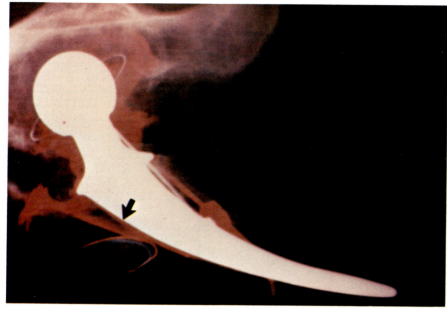

Color Plate I.2. Color subtraction dramatically confirms femoral component loosening (arrow).

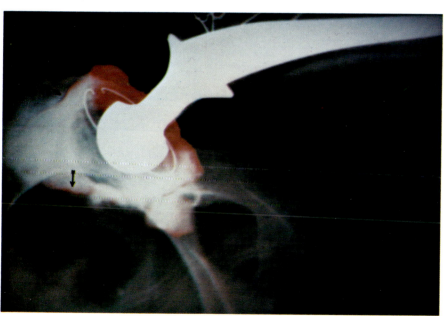

Color Plate I.1. Color subtraction technique applied to this film confirms definite loosening with obvious contrast around acetabular component (arrows).

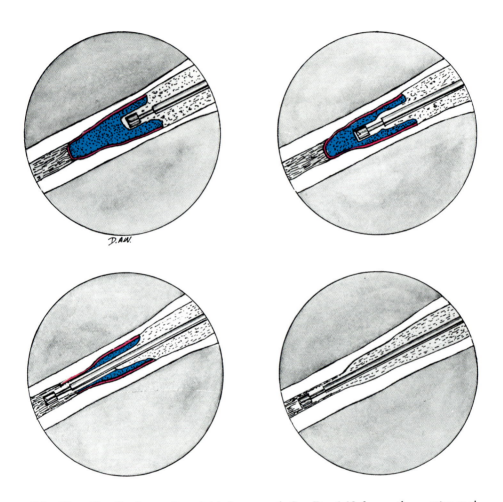

Color Plate II. Cutting tools and debris removal. *See Fig. 4-19 for another cutting tool.*

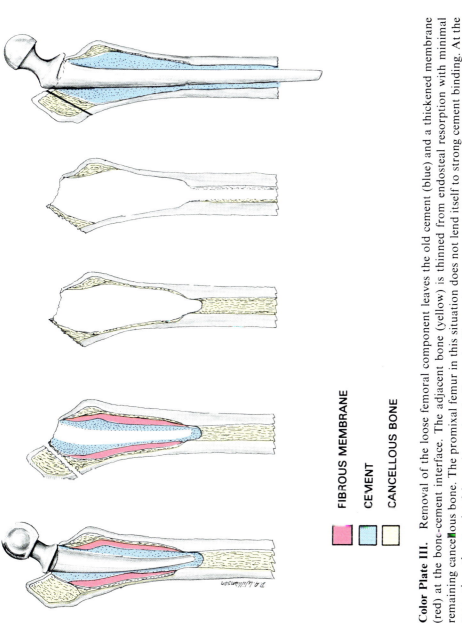

FIBROUS MEMBRANE

CEMENT

CANCELLOUS BONE

Color Plate III. Removal of the loose femoral component leaves the old cement (blue) and a thickened membrane (red) at the bone-cement interface. The adjacent bone (yellow) is thinned from endosteal resorption with minimal remaining cancellous bone. The proximal femur in this situation does not lend itself to strong cement binding. At the same time the proximal bone is mechanically weak. The revision prosthesis should come well below this area of pathologic femur to enhance the revision cementing and protect the weakened proximal bone. *Refer to Chapter 4 for a discussion of this subject.*

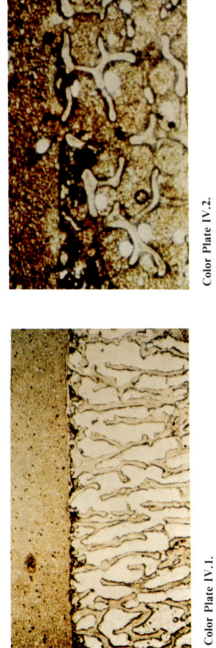

Color Plate IV.1.

Color Plate IV.2.

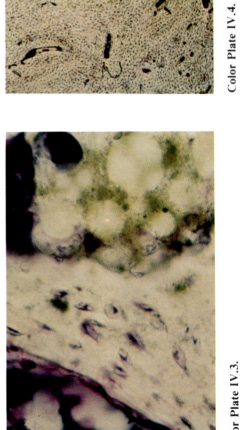

Color Plate IV.3.

Color Plate IV.4.

Color Plate IV.1. Doughy cement applied by hand poorly penetrates into cancellous interstices. The resulting interface is susceptible to micromovement. *See page 186.*

Color Plate IV.2. Cement in a low-viscosity state applied under pressure penetrates into bony interstices, forming good mechanical micro-interlock. *See page 186.*

Color Plate IV.3. Microsection of a cement-bone interface obtained post-mortem. The patient had a spherocentric knee arthroplasty performed 7 years earlier. There was no clinical or radiological evidence of loosening. The micro-interlock appears to be stable and functioning. (Material courtesy of Dr. L. Matthews, Ann Arbor, Michigan.) *See page 186.*

Color Plate IV.4. Microsection of the cement-bone interface from an experimental canine study. There frequently is a gap between cement and bone in the immediate post-operative period. There is evidence that this gap will fill with healing bone if the interface is protected from weight-bearing for 8 to 12 weeks. *See page 195.*

The technique for combining the portable fluoroscopic unit with intermedullar reaming is as follows: The patient is positioned either on a pedestal-type or an extended OR table such that the large receiving end of the fluoroscope is anterior, and the small x-ray generating end is posterior (see Figs. 4-16A through 4-16F). Extreme caution must be exercised when draping and introducing the C-arm to prevent contamination of the operative field. The assistant, on the anterior side of the patient, opposite the side of the surgeon, brings the leg out of the sterile bag (where it has been during the proximal cement removal), and places it on the table, maintaining the leg in approximately 30° of flexion and about 20° of adduction. In this position the leg can be rotated on its own axis a full 90°, thus allowing the fluoroscope to alternatively capture two views of the femur at right angles without any further manipulation of the C-arm (Fig. 4-17). Once positioned, the C-arm fluoroscope is left in place throughout the remainder of the case, and biplane exposure is easily obtained by the simple rotation of the leg.

The 12.5-cm (AM) or 19-cm (TU) sleeves for the Midas Rex are sufficient in most cases for cement removal and femoral canal preparation. Even longer 24-cm (R) and 40-cm (RX) sleeves may be required for some extremely long femurs or for long-stem femoral components. The number 1,4,10,14, and 16 bits (Fig. 4-18) are the most commonly used cutting instruments in femoral cement removal.

A potential complication of power instrumentation for cement removal is perforation of the femoral shaft. It has been our experience that avoiding such perforations is a function of experience with the high-speed drill and the fluoroscopic C-arm unit. The technique of using the cutting tools with the fluoroscope has

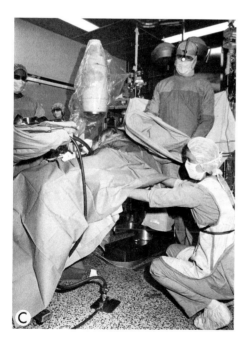

Fig. 4-16C. Care must be taken to avoid contamination of drapes as x-ray unit is positioned.

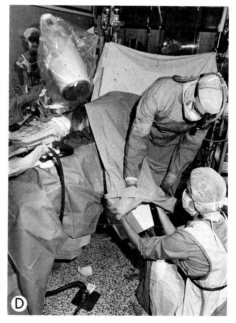

Fig. 4-16D. Mayo stand cover is ideal drape for x-ray unit. The drape is applied as the x-ray unit is rotated.

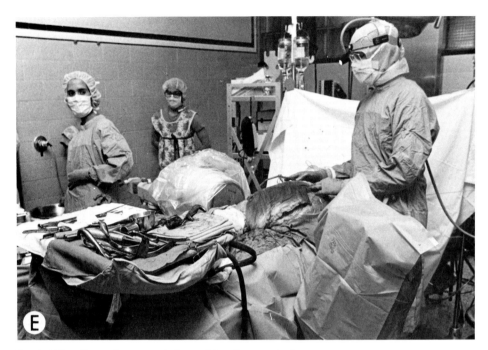

Fig. 4-16E.   Draped x-ray unit in position for use during surgery.

reduced the incidence of performation to approximately 10 percent of cases. The surgeon must slowly and deliberately proceed, with repeated checks on the position of the cutting tool in both planes. The more distal the cement column extends into the isthmus of the meduallary canal, the more technically difficult the cement removal process.

The technique for removing the distal cement includes first breaking centrally through the cement mass, and then widening the canal sufficiently to accept the revision component stem surrounded by an adequate cement mantle. Short, alternating strokes with the Midas Rex tool seems to be the best technique to allow for both cooling of the tip and removal of the accumulated debris (chip clearance), as well as for avoiding penetration of the femoral shaft. The cutting tool cuts on the forward stroke and is cooled while returning debris on the back-stroke (see Fig. 4-19 and Color Plate II). Cooling is further facilitated by repetive flushing with antibiotic irrigation solution. Once a central channel has been established in the cement mass, the cutting tool tends to follow it. If progress seems slow with a particular cutting head, it should be changed, as the tools will become dull on prolonged exposure to cement. Once a pathway has been established through the cement, longer stroking, back-and-forth motions are safe, as long as very little side pressure is exerted on the cutting tool. These cuts widen the canal and also contribute to removal of the adherent membrane on the endosteal surface. Even after a good central canal is established through the cement mass, reaming should continue with repeated reference to biplane fluoroscopic images. A long curette can be intermittently used in the cement removal process to "feel" the inside of the femur for loose cement and to aid in the removal of remaining membrane.

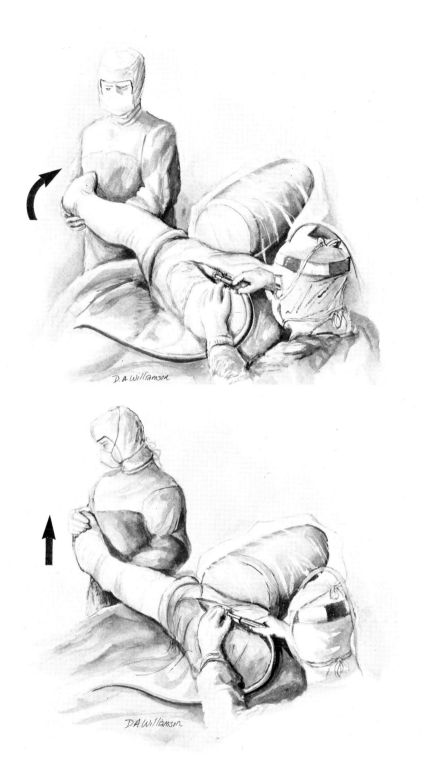

Fig. 4-17. With the leg in approximately 30° of flexion and about 20° of adduction, two views of the femur at right angles can be visualized without C-arm manipulation.

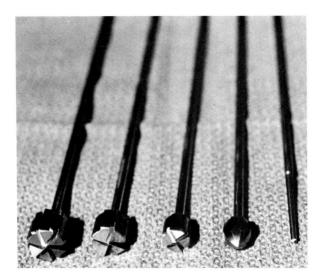

Fig. 4-18. Cutting bits for the Midas Rex high speed drill. Bit numbers (left to right) 16, 14, 4, 1, and 10.

The two most common complications of cement removal are cortical perforation and cortical shaft fracture. Perforations can be anticipated, especially early in one's experience with the cutting tools. Perforations should be recognized, pinpointed, surgically exposed, obturated and, ultimately, bone-grafted.[52] If a perforation of the femoral shaft is suspected, a Foley catheter is placed into the proximal femoral canal and inflated proximal to the level of suspected perforation. Water-soluble, radio-opaque iodine contrast (60 cc) is then injected into the canal through the catheter; the canal then is scanned in both planes with the C-arm fluoroscope. Extrusion of contrast into the soft tissues will reveal both the presence and the localization of any cortical perforation. The perforation should then be exposed so that it can be manually occluded during cement pressurization and during revision component insertion. Bone graft should be packed around the exposed perforation prior to closure of the soft tissues and muscle. If local graft sources (heterotopic or acetabular bone) are not readily available, bone can be obtained either from the ipsilateral ilium or from a bone bank. Cement extrusion into the soft tissues of the thigh resulting in less-than-optimal cement penetration into the femoral endosteal bone is the consequence of unrecognized and unexposed cortical perforations. The revision femoral component should extend well below any perforations of the shaft in order to prevent potential post-operative femoral shaft fracture. If perforation defects are large and/or it is not possible to bring the revision component well beyond any cortical defects in the shaft, the patient should be protected for 6 to 12 months with bilateral axillary crutches, to allow at least preliminary healing of the perforation.[48,52] The larger the perforation, the more important it is to have an autogenous bone graft and to treat the patient as if he or she had a femoral shaft fracture.

Femoral shaft fracture usually is easily recognized; it must be treated as will be presented in Chapter 6. Circlage wiring, followed by the use of a long-stem prosthesis which goes well beyond the area of fracture, is usually sufficient.[29] Care should be taken to avoid the interposition of cement between the femoral fracture surfaces. In most instances, sufficiently secure fixation can be obtained by the cement long-stem prosthesis combination so that the circlage wires can be removed

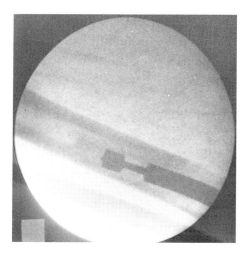

Fig. 4-19. Cutting tool. (See Color Plate II for additional cutting tools and debris removal.)

prior to wound closure. As with significant perforations, the femoral fracture patient should be maintained on bilateral axillary crutches until the fracture has solidly healed, at least 6 and sometimes 12 months, depending on x-ray evidence of solid healing.

FEMORAL COMPONENT SELECTION AND IMPLANTATION

The choice of a femoral component for revision surgery is important. The neck and stem length are usually longer than the femoral component removed. Both varus translation of the femoral component and calcar resorption are frequently found in patients undergoing femoral revision arthroplasty. Therefore, at revision, the new component will almost invariably be seated further down the femoral neck, or even on the lesser trochanter. Accordingly, long-neck prostheses and calcar replacement components should be available when revision surgery is undertaken.[21] Cupic, following up Charnley's original series with an average follow-up of 11 5 years, noted 4 to 5 mm of calcar resorption in 74.7 percent of the cases.[7] Oh and Harris theorized that this is due to stress-shielding of the medial femoral neck with the relatively collarless Charnley design.[41]

We are convinced of the importance of implanting long-stem femoral components when performing revision hip arthroplasty (Fig. 4-20). Long-stem components provide maximum surface area for cement fixation, as well as bypassing areas of weakened femoral cortical bone. A review of post-operative femoral shaft fractures has shown that they are frequently associated with pre-operative violation of the femoral shaft, either by a cortical window or by perforation of the femoral stem.[48,52] At the very least, the femoral component should bypass any areas of weakened proximal femur by 110 mm, as discussed in Chapters 3 and 10. The extra length of distal stem, when cemented in an area of uncompromised cortex with fresh bone surfaces, provides a superior surface for good bone-cement bonding when compared to the permanently damaged proximal femoral medullary canal (Color Plate III). It may be difficult to appreciate very small perforations and other defects involving

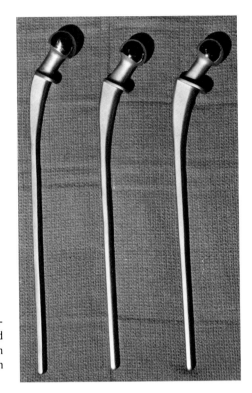

Fig. 4-20. Long-stemmed ATS design revision femoral components. Small, medium, and large stem sizes are seen, each with a 42-mm neck length. Nine combinations of neck length and stem size are available.

the femoral shaft during the cement removal process; a long-stem prosthesis therefore provides the utmost margin of safety from this point of view.

In 1979, 173 cases of long-stem revision femoral arthroplasties for a variety of indications were reviewed by Turner[54] and by Hamati and Stillwell et al.[17] Six of the long-stems were therapeutically inserted after femoral shaft fractures. The remainder were prophylactically used for revisions of either failed total hip replacement, failed femoral endoprostheses, or for hip sepsis. The complications directly attributed to a long-stem prosthesis in these 173 cases included 5 cases of violation of anterior or lateral cortex and 1 case where the knee joint was entered. In 25 cases, it was recognized that the available 300 mm long-stem was overlong for the patient's femur; the stem was accordingly shortened in the hospital machine shop either before or during the operation.

Prior to cementing the prosthesis in place, as with primary total hip arthroplasty, the femoral component should be placed in the shaft and a trial reduction should be performed. Leg lengths should be measured. Both range of motion and stability should be carefully checked. The greater trochanter should be pulled down to its donor bed to determine the ease of later trochanteric reattachment. The position of the revision stem in the shaft should be checked with the C-arm to be sure that it has neither perforated or violated the cortex in either the AP or the medial-lateral (M-L) plane.

If the tip of the prosthesis contacts the anterior femoral cortex distally, more reaming in the area of the proximal femur and the isthmus should be done, to permit better central positioning of the femoral stem. If central positioning is impossible, the component needs to be shortened in order to avoid creating a stress-raiser in the femoral shaft. Depending on the amount of calcar resorption, as much calcar contact as possible should be sought, as advocated by Oh and Harris,[41] in order to maintain a physiologic stress-loading situation on the medial femoral neck. Resorption of the femoral neck noted at revision surgery is frequently irregular; ideal collar-calcar contact is rarely possible in difficult revision cases.

Prior to cementing, the femoral canal should be scanned with the C-arm for any retained pieces of cement and for a final check on femoral component position. Fiberoptic illumination and a sharp curette are used in a final check for residual interface membrane. The endosteal surface of the femur, especially proximally, can also be finished with the power drill. This should be done with a very light hand, as an artist would "air-brush" a final piece of art, as it is intended to remove membrane and cement, and not to remove bone. The wires for later trochanteric reattachment are inserted in the proximal femur prior to the femoral component cementing.

CEMENTING TECHNIQUES

Cementing techniques for revisions are difficult, but do not vary in principle from those used in primary total hip arthroplasty. Extra-long tipped cement-injecting guns are necessary, because of the size of the implants (See Fig. 4-21). There are data that show that the pressurized injection of the cement improves the mechanical properties of the final polymerized cement.[57] It does so by decreasing the number and size of internal defects during the polymerization. As Miller and

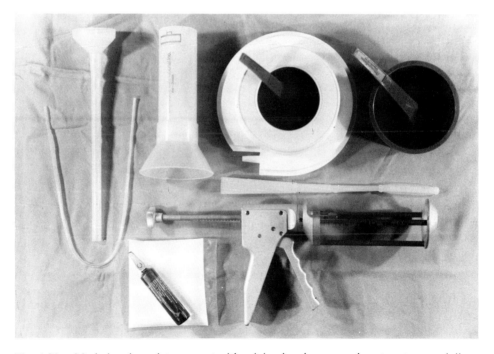

Fig. 4-21. Methylmethacrylate cement with mixing bowl, vapor exhaust system, medullary brush, vent tube, cement gun, and cement syringe with long tip.

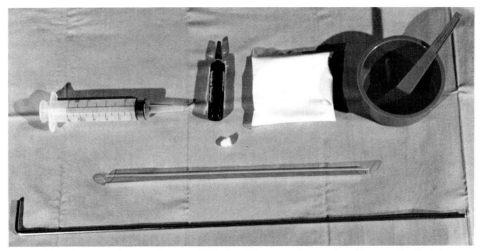

Fig. 4-22. Cement plug equipment: Number 36 gauge chest tube, 10 mm silastic intramedullary plug, metal plunging rod, and methylmethacrylate with catheter-tipped syringe for loading chest tube.

his co-authors stress in Chapter 8, pressurization is essential to obtain strong microinterlocking between cement and bone.

In revision hip surgery, proper cement pressurization is even more vital because of previous failures, the large volume of cement, and the anatomic contour of the medullary canal. The greatest problem lies in achieving a plug effect in the metaphyseal flare of the canal distal to the narrower isthmus. Obviously, prefabricated synthetic or bone plugs narrow enough to pass the isthmus would not be large enough to plug the distal femur.

We have devised a technique to deliver an appropriate amount of methymethacrylate cement to the distal canal without fear of dragging the cement bolus proximal while removing the delivery system.

A 36-gauge chest tube is cut to the appropriate length (depending on stem length). Approximately 10 g of very liquid, low-viscous stage cement are pumped into the chest tube. The tube is passed to the proper depth in the canal; proper position is confirmed by fluoroscopy. The end of the tube is placed approximately 2 to 3 cm past the projected level of the distal end of the femoral prosthesis. A 10 mm silicone silastic plug is driven down the tube by a metal plunging rod, forcing the cement out ahead of the advancing plug. Once the plug is seen by x-ray to exit the tube, the chest tube and plunging rod are removed. The silastic plug prevents cement from adhering to the tube while it is withdrawn. (See Figs. 4-22 and 4-23.)

The prosthesis selected for implantation is then inserted, and the cement plug is checked by x-ray to assure adequate clearance for 2 to 3 cm of cement below the final prosthesis proximal to the plug. If there seems to be insufficient gap between the plug and the prosthesis, a longer stem should be inserted to distally force the cement down the canal.

Once the cement plug has polymerized, the canal is thoroughly cleaned with a medullary femoral endosteal brush as described by Miller.[36] The canal is repeatedly flushed with pulsating irrigation. The canal is now dried and tightly packed with dry sponges. Methacrylate is mixed in two separate aliquots, prepared 3 minutes apart. (This assumes that the room temperature is between 66° and 70° F and that the cement has been refrigerated overnight.)

The aliquot of cement mixed second contains two packages of cement and is injected first, while in a low viscous state. A long-tipped cement delivery system introduces cement into the femoral shaft and a polyethylene vent tube is removed. The first cement aliquot is entering the dough phase at this point, because of the 3-minute earlier mixing time, and the time elapsed during low-viscous-stage cement injection. The first cement aliquot is now hand-packed into the proximal canal in order to prevent the low-viscous cement from running out onto the soft tissue, to permit better distal microinterlock, and to provide proximal bulk filling of the femur as the femoral component is inserted.

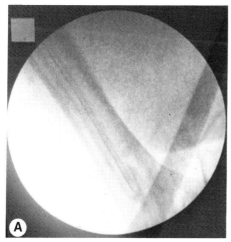

Fig. 4-23A. Chest tube in place on fluoroscopic screen.

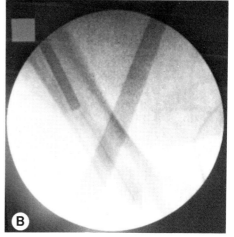

Fig. 4-23B. Plunging rod coming down chest tube.

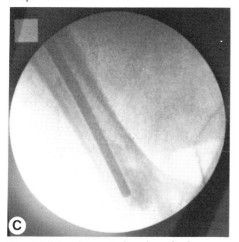

Fig. 4-23C. Cement plug deposited.

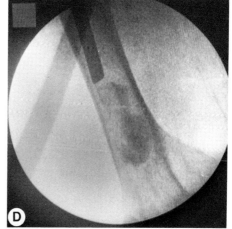

Fig. 4-23D. Chest tube/plunging rod removed with cement plug in place; trial of the long stem implant is checked to be sure that the cement plug is distal to the tip of the prosthesis.

The femoral revision component is now pushed into position with a single steady plunging motion, maintaining 10° of femoral neck antiversion. Because of the long stem, there is minimal ability to vary the varus/valgus positioning. Excess cement is cleared by sharp dissection from around the collar of the prosthesis (Fig. 4-24).

The safety of polymethylmethacrylate has been established with years of clinical experience. Nevertheless, there is a documented incidence of cardiovascular collapse related to the use of methylmethacrylate, especially in the femur.[6] Several studies on laboratory animals have documented a decrease in cardiac output as well as peripheral vasodilatation related to insertion of the methylmethacrylate into the canal.[23,24] It has been our experience that cementing of longer stem prostheses into the femur is associated with increased incidence of cardiovascular compromise, especially in the patient with a history of cardiac arrthymias, congestive heart failure, hypertension, or other cardiac disease. Accordingly, extreme care must be taken during the procedure to maintain adequate circulating blood volume, systolic pressure, and cerebral perfusion. It is for this reason that a central venous line, Foley catheter, and arterial line are routine in the elderly and in other high-risk patients.

We routinely use antibiotics in combination with the cement for revision cases. There are ample data that the addition of powdered antibiotics (e.g., cephamandol, tobramycin, prostaphlin, oxacillin, erythromycin, or colistin), does not significantly alter the mechanical properties of the acrylic cement.[27,32,57] The quantity of antibiotics is usually 1 gram per package of cement; under no conditions should more than 2 grams per package be added. (Experimental and clinical aspects of antibiotic-cement combinations will be discussed in Chapter 13.)

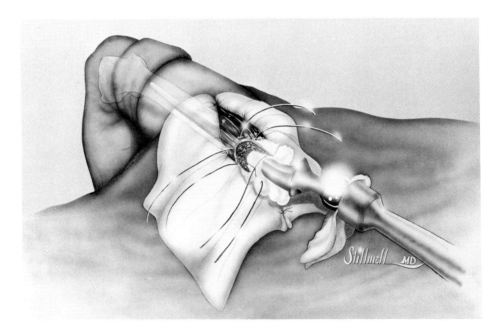

Fig. 4-24. Insertion of revision component. Note wires for trochanteric attachment.

WOUND CLOSURE AND TROCHANTERIC FIXATION

After completion of the femoral cementing, the hip is relocated and the leg-lengths rechecked. Both range of motion and stability should be noted and documented in the operative report. The hip is then placed into abduction and the greater trochanter is brought down onto the femoral trochanteric bed. There are various techniques for fixation of the greater trochanter. Three-wire fixation is recommended, and wire mesh can be added as needed (discussed in Chapter 11). Soft-tissue repair of the vastus lateralis fascia is an important reinforcing layer to supplement wire or bolt fixation and should be done at all times. At the end of the trochanteric reattachment, a judgment must be made as to the quality of bone in the trochanter and the quality of the fixation. When trochanteric fixation is very secure and the bone is firm, the revision patient can be ambulated in a few days, as with a primary total hip replacement. However, fixation is often tenuous and trochanters may be osteopenic in revision surgery. It is our practice, therefore, to keep patients with tenuous trochanteric reattachment in bed in wide abduction for 3 weeks, to provide an optimal environment for fascial healing and for eventual trochanteric union.

Hemostasis is checked at the end of the surgery. The wound is copiously lavaged with pulsating irrigation to remove excess cement and bone debris. Two complete portable suction drainage units (four egress tubes) are used because of the extensive tissue dissection necessitated by revision surgery. The closure is carefully done, with attempts to define the original tissue planes and to close fascial layers with interrupted nonabsorbable sutures. Subcutaneous fat and subcuticular layers are closed with biodegradable sutures. Dressings are applied, taking care to avoid skin pressure by the four drainage tubes. The patient is then moved to a bed and the operated leg is placed in balanced suspension in wide abduction with 5 to 7 pounds of skin traction, depending on the size of the leg. The portable suction drains are removed at 36–48 hours. The patient is maintained on antibiotics until the intraoperative cultures are reported as negative.

SUMMARY

This chapter has presented a rationale and a surgical technique for removing and replacing femoral prosthetic components. Repeated practice and careful attention to surgical detail will reward both surgeon and patient with maximal preservation of existing femoral bone stock. Meticulous attention to cementing techniques and to trochanteric repair are essential to the achievement of an enduring prosthetic-cement-bone composite.

REFERENCES

1. Amstutz HC, Markolf KL, McNeice GM: Loosening of total hip components: Cause and prevention, St. Louis: The Hip: Proceedings of the Fourth Open Scientific Meeting of the Hip Society. St. Louis, CV Mosby, 1976, pp 102–116.

2. Beckenbaugh RD, Ilstrup MS: Total hip arthroplasty. *J Bone and Joint Surg* 60A:306–314, 1978.

3. Charnley J: Fracture of femoral prostheses in total hip replacement. *Clin Orthop* 111:105–120, 1975.

4. Clegg J: The results of the pseudoarthrosis after removal of an infected total hip prosthesis. *J Bone and Joint Surg* 59B:298–301, 1977.

5. Collis DK: Femoral stem failure in total hip replacement. *J Bone and Joint Surg* 59A:1033–1041, 1977.

6. Convery FR, Gunn DR, Hughes JD, et al: The relative safety of polymethylmethacrylate. *J Bone and Joint Surg* 57A:57–74, 1975.

7. Cupic A: Long-term follow-up of Charnley arthroplasty of the hip. *Clin Orthop* 141:28–43, 1979.

8. Dandy DJ, Theodoru BC: The management of local complications of total hip replacement by the McKee-Farrar technique. *J Bone and Joint Surg* 57B:30–35, 1975.

9. Drinker J, Turner RH, McKenzie JD, et al: Color subtraction arthrography in the diagnosis of component loosening in hip arthroplasty. *Orthop* 1:224–229, 1978.

10. Eftakhar NS, Smith DN, Henry JH, et al: Revision arthroplasty using Charnley low-friction arthroplasty technique. *Clin Orthop* 95:48–59, 1973.

11. Eftakhar NS: Re-channelization of cemented femur using a guide and drill system. *Clin Orthop* 123:29–31, 1977.

12. Feith R, Slooff TJH, Kazem I, et al: Strontium 87m bone scanning for the evaluation of total hip replacement. *J Bone and Joint Surg* 58B:79–83, 1976.

13. Fornasier VL, Cameron HU: The femoral stem/cement interface in total hip replacement. *Clin Orthop* 116:248–236, 1975.

14. Galante JO, Rostoker W, Doyle JN: Failed femoral stems in total hip prostheses. *J Bone and Joint Surg* 57A:203–236, 1975.

15. Gruen TA, McNiece GN, Amstutz HC: Modes of failure of cemented stem-type femoral components. *Clin Orthop* 141:17–27, 1979.

16. Hallel T, Salvati EA, Botero PM: Polymethylmethacrylate in the knee. *J Bone and Joint Surg* 58A:556–557, 1976.

17. Hamati J, Stillwell W, Turner RH: Long-stem total hip replacement (unpublished).

18. Harris WH, Jones WN: The use of wire mesh in total hip replacement surgery. *Clin Orthop* 106:117–121, 1975.

19. Harris WH, Schiller AL, Scholler J, et al: Extensive localized bone and resoption in the femur following total hip replacement. *J Bone and Joint Surg* 58A:612–618, 1976.

20. Harris WH, Oh I: A new power tool for removal of methylmethacrylate from the femur. *Clin Orthop* 132:53–53, 1978.

21. Harris WH, Allen JR: The calcar replacement femoral component for total hip arthroplasty: design, uses and surgical technique. *Clin Orthop* 157:215–225, 1981.

22. Johnston RC, Smidt GC: Hip motion measurements for selected activities of daily living. *Clin Orthop* 72:205–215, 1970.

23. Kallos T, Enis JE, Gollan F, et al: Intramedullary pressure and pulmonary embolism of femoral medullary contents in dogs during insertion of bone cement and a prosthesis. *J Bone and Joint Surg* 56A:1363–1367, 1974.

24. Kim KC, Ritter MA: Hypotension associated with methylmethacrylate in total hip arthroplasty. *Clin Orthop* 88:154–160, 1972.

25. Knight WE: Accurate determination of leg-lengths during total hip replacement. *Clin Orthop* 123:27–28, 1977.

26. Lazasky NG: Complications revisited in total hip arthroplasty. *Clin Orthop* 95:96–103, 1973.

27. Levin PD: The affectiveness of various antibiotics in methylmethacrylate. *J Bone and Joint Surg* 57B:234–237, 1975.

28. Ling RSM: Loosening experience at Exeter. Proceedings of the AOA International Hip Symposium. Boston, Massachusetts May, 1981.

29. Lowell JD: Complications of arthroplasty and total joint replacement in the hip, in Epps C (ed): *Complications in Orthopedic Surgery.* Philadelphia, JR Lippincott Co, 1979, pp 915–948.

30. Markolf DC, Amstutz HC: In vitro measurement of bone-acrylic interface pressure during femoral component insertion. *Clin Orthop* 121:60–66, 1976.

31. Markolf KC, Amstutz HC: Penetration and flow of acrylic bone cement. *Clin Orthop* 121:99–102, 1976.

32. Marks KE, Nelson CC, Laufenschlager EP: Antibiotic impregnated acrylic cement. *J Bone and Joint Surg* 58A:358–364, 1976.

33. Marmor L: Femoral loosening in total hip replacement. *Clin Orthop* 121:116–119, 1976.

34. Marmor L: Stress fracture of the pubic remus stimulating a loose total hip replacement. *Clin Orthop* 121:103–104, 1976.

35. McBeath AA, Foltz RN: Femoral component loosening after a total hip replacement. *Clin Orthop* 141:66–70, 1979.

36. Miller J: Proceedings of the American Orthopedic Association International Symposium. Boston, Massachusetts, May, 1981.

37. Müller ME: Total hip prostheses. *Clin Orthop* 72:46–68, 1970.

38. Murray WR, Rodrigo JJ: Arthrography for the assessment of pain after total hip replacement. *J Bone and Joint Surg* 57A:1060–1065, 1975.

39. Nolan DR, Fitzgerald RH, Beckenbaugh RD, et al: Complications of total hip arthroplasty treated by re-operation. *J Bone and Joint Surg* 57A:977–981, 1975.

40. Oh I, Carlson CE, Tomford WW, et al: Improved fixation of the femoral component after total hip replacement with methylmethacrylate intramedullary plug. *J Bone and Joint Surg* 60A:608–613, 1978.

41. Oh I, Harris WH: Proximal strain distribution in the loaded femur. *J Bone and Joint Surg* 60A:75–85, 1978.

42. Razzano CB: Removal of methylmethacrylate in failed total hip arthroplasties. *Clin Orthop* 126:181–182, 1977.

43. Reckling FW, Asher NA, Dillon WC: A longitudinal study of the radiolucent line at the bone cement interface following total joint replacement procedures. *J Bone and Joint Surg* 59A:355–358, 1977.

44. Ritter MA: Dislocation and subluxation of the total hip replacement. *Clin Orthop* 121:92–94, 1976.

45. Salvati EA, Ghelman B, McLuren R, et al: Substraction technique in the arthrography for loosening of total hip replacement fixed with radiopaque cement. *Clin Orthop* 101:105–109, 1974.

46. Salvati EA, Freiberger RH, Wilson PD: Arthrography for complications of total hip replacement. *J Bone and Joint Surg* 53A:701–709, 1971.

47. Salvati EA, Chuen EI, Aglietti P, et al: Radiology of total hip replacement. *Clin Orthop* 121:74–82, 1976.

48. Scott RD, Turner RH, Leitzes SN, et al: Femoral fractures in conjunction with total hip replacement. *J Bone and Joint Surg* 57A:494–501, 1975.

49. Scott RD, Turner RH: Avoiding complications with long-stem total hip replacement arthroplasty. *J Bone and Joint Surg* 57A:722, 1975.

50. Stinson NE: Tissue reaction induced in guinea pigs by particulate polymethylmethacrylate polythene and nylon of the same size. *Br J Exper Pathol* 46:135–146, 1965.

51. Stillwell WT, Hamatti YI, Turner RH: Revision of failed total hip replacements indications and surgical techniques. Howmedica Surgical Techniques Publication, 1979.

52. Talab YA, States JD, Evarts CN: Femoral shaft perforations. *Clin Orthop* 141:158–165, 1979.

53. Thompson RC, Culver JE: The role of trochanteric osteotomy in total hip replacement. *Clin Orthop* 106:102–106, 1975.

54. Turner RH: Revision arthroplasty in the USA, in Caldwell AD, Elson RA, (eds): *Proceedings of the International Revision Arthroplasty Symposium.* Oxford, England, Med Education Services, March, 1979, pp 85–88.

56. Weber FA, Charnley J: A radiological study of fracture of acrylic cement in relation to the stem of a femoral head prosthesis. *J Bone and Joint Surg* 57B:297–301, 1975.

57. Weinstein AM, Bigham DN, Sauer W, et al: The effect of high pressure insertion and antibiotic inclusions upon the mechanical properties of polymethylmethacrylate. *Clin Orthop* 121:67–73, 1976.

58. Weissman NW: Radiologic evaluation of total joint replacement, in Kelly WN, Harris E, Ruddy S, et al (eds): *Textbook of Rheumatology.* Philadelphia, WB Saunders Co., 1981, pp 2020–2054.

59. Weisman HJ, Simon SR, Ewald FC, et al: Total hip replacement with and without osteotomy of the greater trochanter. *J Bone and Joint Surg* 60A:203–210, 1978.

60. Wilde AH, Greenwald AS: Shear strength of self-curing acrylic cement. *Clin Orthop* 106:126–130, 1975.

61. Wilson JN, Scales JT: Loosening of total hip replacements with cement fixation. *Clin Orthop* 72:145–160, 1970.

62. Wroblewski MD: A method of management of the fractured stem in total hip replacement. *Clin Orthop* 141:71–74, 1979.

Benjamin E. Bierbaum

5

Acetabular Revision Arthroplasty

Many of the recent and difficult problems dealing with revision surgery for total hip replacement arthroplasty relate to the acetabulum. Long-term studies analyzing cup loosening suggest that acetabular problems can be expected in increasing numbers. Delee and Charnley, in an early 10-year follow-up of 145 patients, found 69 percent radiolucency about the bone cement interface of the acetabular component.[5] Nine percent of these showed proximal migration of the cup. Eftekar has quoted Müller as experiencing a 10 percent incidence of cup migration.[7] Salvati evaluated the first 100 Charnley hips from the Hospital for Special Surgery in New York City and recorded a radiolucent line at the bone-cement junction in most of them.[24] The Mayo Clinic's 10-year experience indicated a persistent increase in acetabular loosening with length of time from surgery (Figs. 5-1A,B, and C). Insufficient acetabular stock as a presenting problem for first-time total hip replacement is even more threatening as subsequent loosening, erosion of bone stock, and revision debridement further contribute to bone insufficiency. The holistic deficiency of acetabular bone stock eventually may lead to resection arthroplasty in cases of septic or sterile loosening, may require massive pelvic homografts, or even autografts prior to reimplantation of the polyethylene acetabulum.

It is difficult to sort out problems specific to revision acetabular reconstruction from those which apply to deficient acetabulae in primary construction of bony support for the polyethylene acetabulum. This chapter will attempt to define basic concepts and specific examples of acetabular reconstruction as they apply to revision total hip replacement arthroplasty.

TYPES OF ACETABULAR DEFICIENCY

To crystalize planning for revision acetabular construction, various types of bone deficiency are defined (see Table 5-1).

107

REVISION TOTAL HIP ARTHROPLASTY
ISBN 0-8089-1466-9

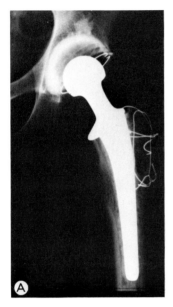 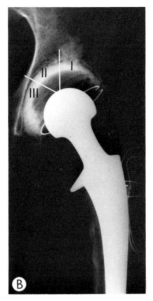 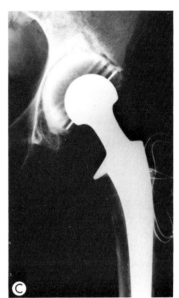

Fig. 5-1A. Six weeks after total hip replacement operation for traumatic arthritis in a 25-year-old male.

Fig. 5-1B. Twelve months post-operative (same patient). Note radiolucent areas throughout zones I, II, and III of the acetabular component.

Fig. 5-1C. Five years post-operative. The patient remains free of symptoms. Note increasing radiolucency of bone-cement interface and increasing calcar resorption.

Each situation presents unique problems in creating bony support for the polyethylene cup.

Superior and Lateral Wall Deficiencies

Superior and lateral wall deficiencies occur by far most commonly in congenital dysplasia. These defects can also occur following trauma, polio, overzealous reaming of acetabular bone, resection of tumor or large cysts, and neuromuscular disease. Principles of a reconstruction involve medialization of the socket to the iliopectineal line, or medialization to the point where the center of the plastic dome is equidistant between the medial and lateral walls of the ilium. A small acetabular component allows greater coverage of the polyethylene by the osseous socket. Superior-lateral bone grafts are frequently required for sufficient bony support (Figs. 5-2A and B). At least two thirds of the superior dome of the polyethylene

Table 5-1
Types of Acetabular Deficiency

Superior and lateral wall deficiency
Protrusio acetabulae
Medial wall deficiency without protrusio
Posterior and inferior wall deficiency

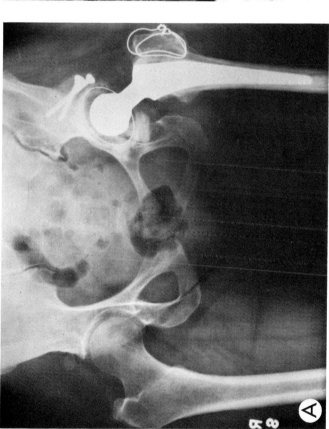

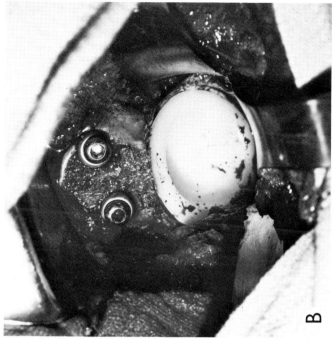

Fig. 5-2A. Lateral bone deficiency managed with autologous bone graft fully incorporated 2 years after surgery.

Fig. 5-2B. Intraoperative photograph showing lateral autologous bone graft with two-screw fixation.

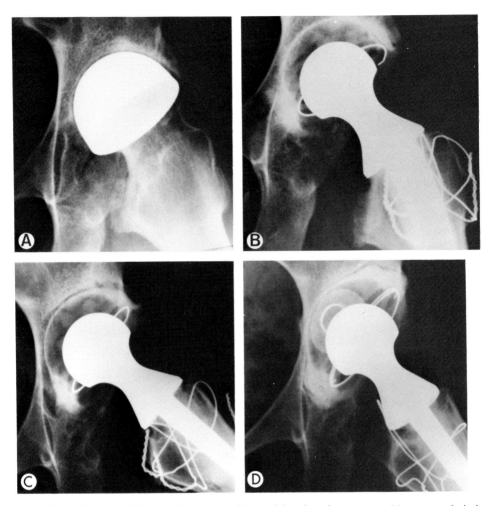

Fig. 5-3A. Congenital hip dysplasia treated by mold arthroplasty at age 16; note cephalad orientation of the acetabulum.

Fig. 5-3B. Three weeks post conversion to total hip replacement. The cephalad position of the acetabulum prevents use of anchoring cement in the ischium and pubis.

Fig. 5-3C. Symptomatic acetabular loosening 5 years following total hip replacement. There is significant erosion of bone stock without evidence of cup migration.

Fig. 5-3D. One year post acetabular revision surgery with recurrence of radiolucent lines in zones I, II, and III.

socket needs to be covered by iliac bone. Although cement is used to fix the acetabular component, support for the component must come from bone in order to prevent socket breakout. Problems unique to congenital hip dysplasia include the choice of using a false or true acetabulum. If the first hip replacement, positioned in the false acetabulum, has failed, then finding and reaming the true socket is usually the best option for revision. Regardless of the choice of use of the false or true acetabulum, augmentation with lateral bone graft is usually required in congenital dysplasia (Figs. 5-3A through 5-3D, and Table 5-2).

Table 5-2
Lateral Wall Deficiency: Principles of Reconstruction

Medialize socket to the iliopectineal line
Bone graft the lateral ilium
Smaller acetabular component

Acetabular Protrusion

Most acetabular failures in protrusio acetabulae are related to failure to lateralize the socket outside the iliopectineal line (Figs. 5-4A through 5-4E).

No accessory medial support is necessary in protrusio surgery if the socket is lateralized to transmit the resultant force vectors through the femoral head to the midline of the iliac bony support (Figs. 5A and B; Fig. 6A and B). Following lateralization of the socket, some medial barrier or reinforcement is necessary to prevent intrapelvic protrusion of cement and to allow for optimum pressurization of the acetabular bone cement. When lateralization has not been accomplished by previous total hip replacement, acetabular loosening and eventual medial migration can be expected in sequential fashion. Schatzker has demonstrated increasing load-bearing stress to the rim of the acetabulum when rings are used to enhance acetabular fixation.[25] Weber (personal communication) recommends screws in the ilium to strengthen fixation in protrusion conditions. McCollum reports satisfactory results using bone grafts in protrusio (Table 5-3).[17]

Table 5-3
Acetabular Protrusio

Lateralize the polyethylene socket outside the iliopectineal line
Large diameter polyethylene socket
Utilize autologous bone graft to augment medial bone stock
Utilize previous acetabular socket for medial stock (if solidly fixed)
Utilize previous bone cement for medial buttress (if solidly fixed)
Accessory support with protrusio rings, screws, mesh, etc.

Medial Wall Deficiency

Medial wall deficiency states are associated with excessive acetabular reaming from prior hemiarthroplasty, Vitallium* mold, or total hip replacement. Medial wall deficiencies can also be seen following sepsis, trauma, and the erosion associated with gross acetabular loosening with medial migration of the acetabular component. Principles in medial wall deficiency are similar to acetabular protrusio;

Table 5-4
Medial Wall Deficiency Principles of Reconstruction

Lateralize acetabular component
Augment medial wall with bone graft
Medial barrier to contain bone cement

* Howmedica Inc.

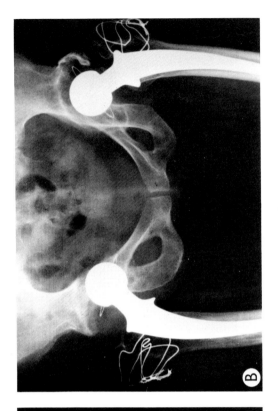

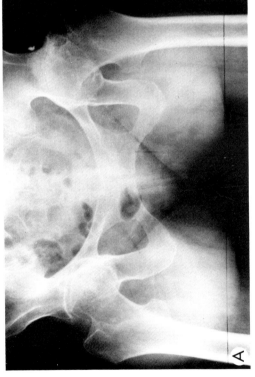

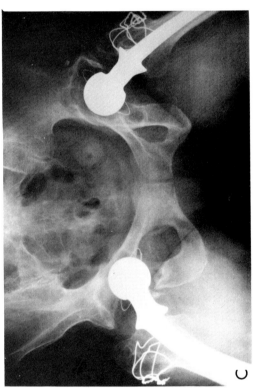

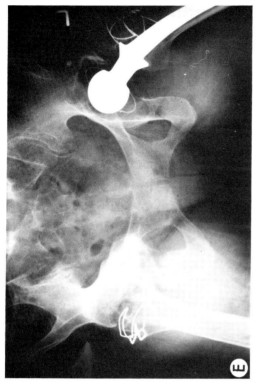

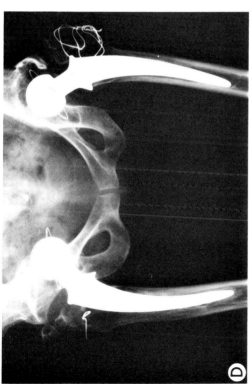

Fig. 5–4A.   B lateral acetabular protrusio with associated osteoporosis.

Fig. 5–4B.   Post-operative bilateral total hip replacements with excessive reaming of medial wall on the right and failure to lateralize acetabular component.

Fig. 5–4C.   Resorption of ischium noted 3 years post-operative.

Fig. 5–4D.   Medial acetabular breakout and medial acetabular migration six years after surgery. Note unchanged position of left acetabulum.

Fig. 5–4E.   One year following resection arthroplasty of right total hip replacement and massive iliac bone graft

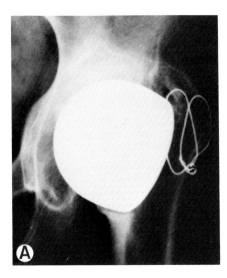 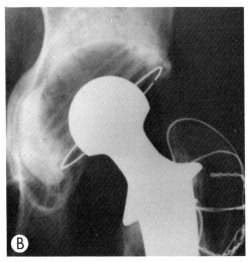

Fig. 5-5A.   Acetabular protrusion treated by mold arthroplasty in 1968. Observe lateral position of the mold in the acetabulum.

Fig. 5-5B.   Six years after conversion to total hip replacement. Note the large acetabular component lateralized in the bony socket.

they include lateralization of the acetabular component using a larger-sized polyethylene component (Table 5-4). Bone cement needs to be contained within the acetabular cavity to prevent intrapelvic protrusion and to allow for optimum pressurization. Building on prior, stable intrapelvic cement and polyethylene is acceptable unless sepsis has been present or the intrapelvic cement is causing pressure symptoms on the urinary bladder, iliac vessels, sciatic nerve, etc. (Figs. 5-7A,B, and C). In fact, erosion of the iliac vessels has occurred from a loose acetabular component with medial migration, as will be discussed in Chapter 14. If no medial wall exists and anchoring holes from pubis to ilium cannot be bridged with synthetic material, bone grafting to the medial wall may be chosen. A staged revision, however, may be more desirable. Stage 1 involves thorough debridement of the prior acetabular component, bone cement, and all membranous tissue, followed by the insertion of bone graft bridging the pillars of the ilium, ischium, and pubis. Stage 2, converting the resection arthroplasty to a total hip replacement, is performed 1 to 2 years later, depending on graft incorporation. Tomograms and computed tomography (CT) scans are especially useful in evaluating graft incorporation (see Chapter 2).

Posterior and Inferior Wall Deficiencies

Posterior and inferior wall deficiencies are infrequently encountered unless associated with severe trauma or excessive acetabular reaming. Both one- and two-stage revision surgical procedures associated with internal fixation and grafting have proven effective. It is important both to recognize the level of nonunion or posterior-inferior wall deformity and to direct the acetabular construction toward osseous union employing sound mechanical principles (Table 5-5).

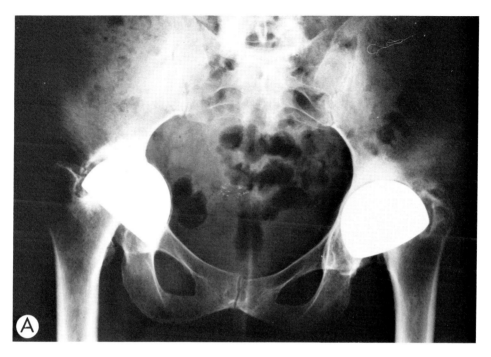

Fig. 5-6A.   Acetabular protrusion following Vitallium model arthroplasty.

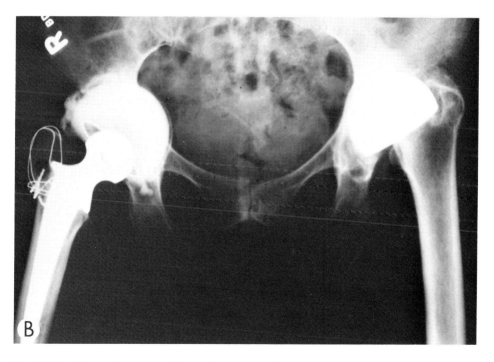

Fig. 5-6B.   Conversion to total hip replacement with lateralization of acetabular component with a large acetabular component and medial cement.

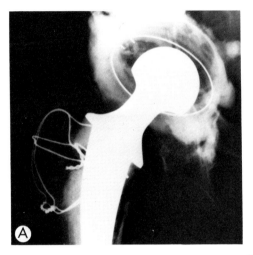
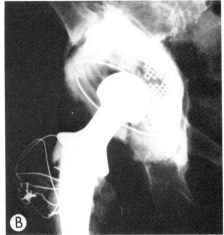
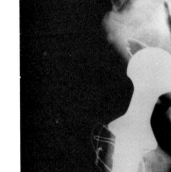

Fig. 5-7A. Loose acetabular component with intrapelvic portion of acetabulum.

Fig. 5-7B. Acetabular revision using wire mesh. Again note medial acetabular position.

Fig. 5-7C. Second revision total hip replacement using old acetabular cup as a medial buttress.

Because variations and combinations of these deficiency states exist, careful assessment of bone stock is a prerequisite to surgical intervention. Specialized x-ray techniques, including CT scanning, Judet and inlet views of the pelvis, arthrography, and tomography, are helpful in defining the areas of bone deficit. Three-dimensional planning in building the new socket aids in understanding the deformity, and assists in deciding which surgical techniques to apply. Use of plate and screws to maintain alignment and stability augmented with bone graft can salvage a potentially disastrous situation (Figs. 5-8A,B, and C).

Table 5-5
Posterior and Inferior Wall Deficiencies: Principles of Reconstruction

Accurate assessment of deficiency
Appropriate bone grafting for deficiency
Stabilization of acetabular ring
Prolonged protective weight-bearing

BIOMECHANICAL ANALYSIS AND
ACETABULAR WEAR

Several mechanical factors are related to acetabular component loosening. Volz has used displacement transducers to study all increments of motion in sockets implanted in cadavers.[28] Data from displacement force analyses indicate that the femoral head tends to be displaced in two directions: medially-superiorly and laterally. The vector displacement of the cup is altered, depending on varus or valgus forces transmitted from the femoral head. Volz proposed a mechanism of aseptic cup loosening commencing as a result of hoop stresses located at the hemispheric rim of the bone-cement composite.[28,29] The cement mantle around the polyethylene cup is more vulnerable to failure because less force is necessary for the deformation of cement than for polyethylene. A cement mantle less than 2 mm in thickness is inadequate for rigid cup fixation. Nelson et al[20] have devised acetabula spacers to ensure an adequate cement mantle.[20] Removal of the acetabular subchondral bone in Volz's study did not weaken cup fixation, presumably due to better interdigitation of cement within cancellous bone. This finding is not borne out by studies from Müller[7] and Delee and Charnley,[5] who postulate that subchondral bone plate is essential for rigid fixation of the polyethylene cup. Acetabular designs with a flange to dissipate weight-bearing forces to the acetabular cortical bone edge may reduce the lateral thrust force transmitted from the femoral head.

Continued study of these mechanical factors is of key importance in revision of failed acetabular sockets if maximum longevity of the new socket is to be achieved.

Wear of the Acetabular Socket

Few acetabular sockets implanted in the USA have "worn out." This differs from the European experience in a 15-year follow-up evaluation. Eftekhar reported

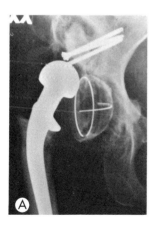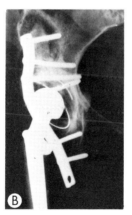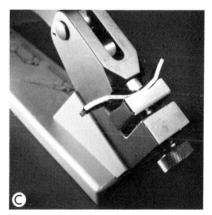

Fig. 5-8A.   Lateral socket breakout in a shallow actabulum with posterior deficiency.

Fig. 5-8B.   One-stage revision total hip replacement using plate and screws to fix posterolateral bone graft.

Fig. 5-8C.   Instrument to bend metal plate to the contour of the posterior acetabulum.

Table 5-6
Indications for Acetabular Revision

Pain
Instability
Migration
Increasing bone resorption
Excessive acetabular wear
Sepsis
Fracture of polyethylene
Fracture of acrylic cement

an average wear rate 9 to 10 years after surgery of 0.05 mm/year.[7] However, 15 percent of patients in his study exceeded 2.50 mm of wear after 10 years. Dowling et al report that the Charnley socket wears predominantly on the superior part, and that wear is a direct consequence of the orientation of the cup within the body and the direction of loading of the hip.[6] The femoral head, in effect, bores out a new socket. Electron microscopy shows that the predominant mechanism is adhesion, but after several years surface cracks can occur, suggesting that surface fatigue also takes place.

Fracture of the polyethylene acetabular cup is an indication for revision surgery; fortunately, it rarely occurs. All reported cases are in small (44 mm) components.[28] Fracture of acrylic cement often occurs in the peripheral non-supporting areas and may be of little significance. Separation fracture of the acrylic on the major weight-bearing areas often leads to mechanical separation and subsequent need for reoperation.

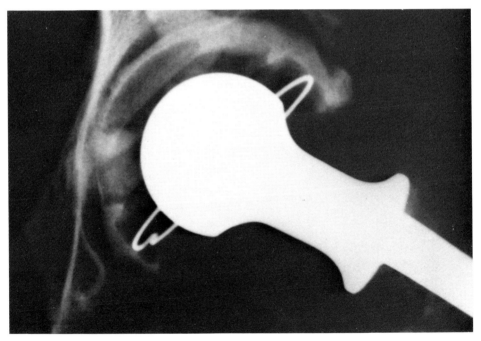

Fig. 5-9. Marked separation at bone-cement interface with loose acetabular component.

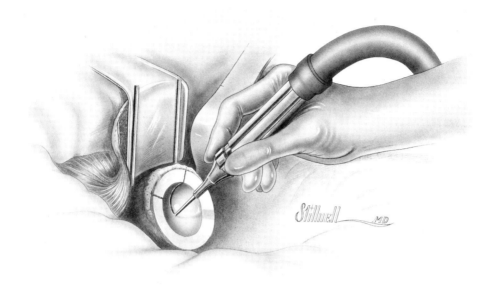

Fig. 5-10. Quartering the polyethylene socket with the high-speed Midas Rex drill.

INDICATIONS FOR ACETABULAR REVISION

Indications for revision surgery based on acetabular problems are listed in Table 5-6. Pain, instability, sepsis, and fracture of the high-density polyethylene cup are absolute indications that the patient is experiencing pain and is totally disabled. Intervention for reasons of increasing bone resorption or increasing polyethylene wear are relative indications, and partially dictate timing for exchange of the component. As a general guide, once a pattern of increasing acetabular bone stock erosion has begun, revision surgery should not be delayed (Fig. 5-9). A thorough preoperative assessment of periacetabular structures is indicated (see Fig. 5-11).

Technique

The technique for removal of an implanted acetabular component is dependent on broad exposure. Greater trochanteric osteotomy is indicated in all cases to obtain this exposure. If there is no indication for femoral component replacement, the polished femoral head should be carefully protected from the retractors and tools used for the revision surgery. Removal of the femoral component from an intact cement column can facilitate the exposure and prevent damage to the femoral component. It can then be reinserted in the same intact cement column, following acetabular reconstruction.

All ectopic bone, pseudocapsule, and synovium must be removed; the overhanging acetabular hypertrophic bone should be excised so that a full-perimeter inspection at the bone-cement-polyethylene interfaces can be obtained. If it is unclear whether the acetabular component is loose, firm pressure on multiple peripheral areas of the polyethylene socket is made with a blunt impactor. Any evidence of motion or egress of fluid at the composite interface indicates acetabular loosening. The use of a tiny curette to more accurately visualize the bone-cement interface may help assess the bond in uncertain cases. Once the decision to proceed with acetabular replacement has been made, extreme care must be exercised to prevent any further acetabular bone stock loss. Curved gouges of the Smith-Petersen type can be used to fracture the acrylic mantle surrounding the polyethylene socket away from the anchoring holes. If the socket cannot be lifted out as a unit, the author recommends quartering the socket with the high-speed Midas Rex drill (Fig. 5-10). Once quartered, the polyethylene can be lifted out in segments and the acrylic removed from anchoring holes. In the absence of sepsis and patient symptoms, intact intrapelvic cement is best left in place rather than to attempt extraction (Fig. 5-11). Preparation of a sclerotic bony bed can be aided with the Midas Rex high-speed drill. Virgin anchoring holes can be made in remaining iliac bone stock; those anchoring holes present in (*existing*) pubic and ischial bone can be enlarged to afford a better interdigitation of cement with cancellous bone. Preserve at all costs the medial wall in cases of protrusio and medial wall deficiencies to prevent intrapelvic migration of cement.

BONE GRAFTING THE DEFICIENT SOCKET

Although the femoral head is the best source of bone graft material, this is not a viable choice in revision surgery unless the contralateral hip is ready for hip replacement and can be salvaged for the revision side. Alternative autologous donor sites include contralateral or ipsilateral full-thickness iliac wings. The bone graft is first harvested through a separate incision and the patient is then repositioned, prepped, and draped for the hip revision surgery. Bone is harvested at surgery during conventional total hip replacement by carefully denuding the remaining articular cartilage, maintaining sterility, and freezing it at $-70°$ C. Frozen bone is thawed at room temperature in warm saline solution during preparation of the socket and may be shaped to fit the bony deficit. Fixation to the patient's ilium can be made successfully with compression screws, technically easier to use than bolts. Two or three compression cancellous screws adequately positioned through both cortices of the ilium give adequate fixation. Once in place, the graft may be gently reamed, allowing bone dust to impact at the graft-host junction. This discourages interposition of methylmethacrylate from interdigitating at the graft-host interface. Union of graft can be expected in 6 to 12 months (see Table 5-7).

Revision surgery is an indication for antibiotic-impregnated cement. The addition of 0.6 g of tobramycin to each 40 g packet of bone cement has given adequate levels of antibiotic in the wound hematoma without signs of toxicity. Preparation of the acetabular bed with pulsating lavage, 10 percent hydrogen

Table 5-7
Ideal Bone Grafts if Femoral Head is not Available

Frozen homologous bone
Contralateral iliac wing
Ipsilateral iliac wing

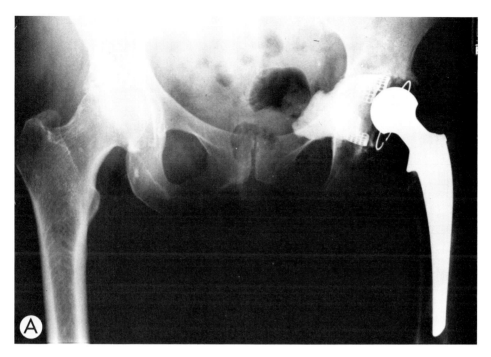

Fig. 5-11A. Large intrapelvic protrusion of acrylic cement associated with cystitis.

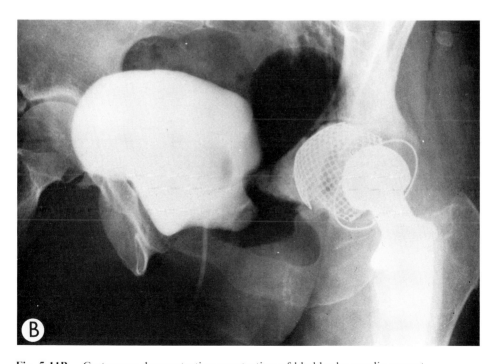

Fig. 5-11B. Cystogram demonstrating penetration of bladder by acrylic cement.

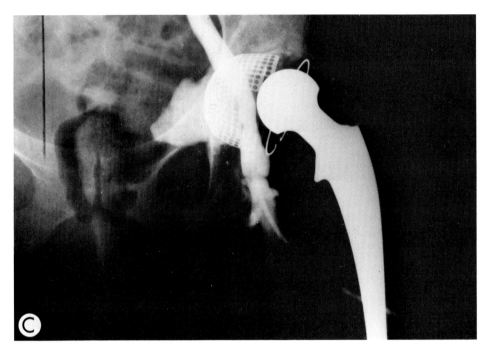

Fig. 5-11C. Femoral venogram demonstrates iliac vessel is not displaced by intrapelvic cement.

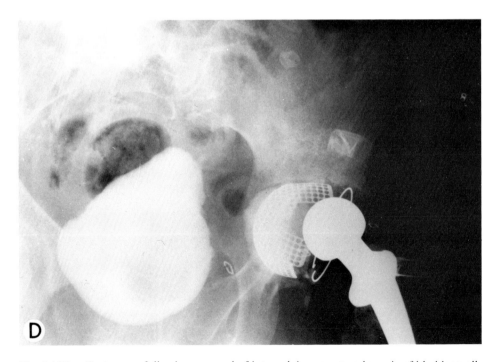

Fig. 5-11D. Cystogram following removal of intrapelvic cement and repair of bladder wall.

122

peroxide solution, thrombin-soaked Gelfoam packing, and firm packing of sponges in anchoring holes all assist in keeping the acetabular bed free of blood. Cement is pressurized into anchoring holes digitally, with a syringe or by using a rubber dam, if low viscosity cement is used. We find pressurization with a ball or similar spherical object covered with a rubber dam to be very effective in forcing acrylic into the subchondral bone. Socket orientation is critical. Thickness of the high-density polyethylene socket is important in determining total limb length. The larger the socket, the thicker the dome, and the longer the limb is lengthened at surgery. Patients with a short limb should have their sockets placed in more abduction as the pelvis will be tilted to that side. Anteversion, fixed lumbar lordosis, fixed flexion deformities, abductor muscle weakness, and ankylosing spondylitis each require consideration in proper socket orientation so the functional use of the hip will allow maximum stability of the implant. For patients with excessive femoral anteversion, the acetabular component needs to have slightly less flexion. This allows for stability in extension and external rotation. The acetabular component is best seated in more flexion, in cases of fixed lumbar lordosis or fixed flexion deformity of the hip or knee. Patients with abductor weakness require a socket in less abduction to enhance stability of the hip. In ankylosing spondylitis where any fixed flexion deformity can limit forward vision, less flexion of the acetabular pocket helps prevent a fixed flexion deformity.

POST-OPERATIVE MANAGEMENT

Because acetabular loosening has a linear relationship with time and increased physical activity, reasonable prudence should be exercised by the patient as far as physical activities are concerned. Ideal post-operative management includes 3 weeks in bed with the leg supported in balance suspension. The patient is instructed in guided muscular activity with gravity eliminated. A partial weight-bearing crutch gait (bearing one half of the patient's body weight) is recommended for 4 months, assuming greater trochanteric fixation is complete. Longer crutch-walking is indicated in cases of non-union or bone grafting. Patients under the age of 30 years who have already experienced one acetabular revision are advised to stay with a single crutch or cane support on an indefinite basis. All patients should avoid impact loading to the hip, including running, jogging, jumping, and racquet and net sports. Obesity is to be avoided; all patients should be encouraged to maintain optimum weight.

SUMMARY

Revision acetabular surgery requires great ingenuity. It tests the mechanical, intuitive, and interpretive skills of even the most experienced hip surgeon. All the principles of primary socket replacement and mechanical realignment (adjusting for leg length inequality, muscle weakness, and distal leg deformities) need be included in the pre-operative assessment of the patient who requires acetabular revision. The particular type and location of bone deficiency need be defined and handled in a sound mechanical fashion. An adequate inventory of prosthetic sizes, graft material, internal fixation equipment, and revision surgical tools are a prerequisite before beginning this arduous task.

REFERENCES

1. Amstutz HC, Markoff KL, McNeice GM, et al: Loosening of total hip components: Cause and prevention. The Hip: Proceedings of the Fourth Open Meeting of the Hip Society, 1976, pp 102–116.
2. Aufranc OE: Personal communications.
3. Bronson JL: Articular interposition of trochanteric wires in a failed total hip replacement. *Clin Orthop* 121:50–52, 1976.
4. Baldursson H, Hansson LI, Olsson TH, et al: Migration of the acetabular socket after total hip replacement determined by roentgen stereophotogram. *Metry Acta Orthop Scand* 51(3):535–540, 1980.
5. Delee JG, Charnley J: Radiological demarcation of cemented sockets in total hip replacement. *Clin Orthop* 121:20–32, 1976.
6. Dowling M, Atkinson JR, Dowson D, et al: The characteristics of acetabular cups worn in the human body. *Brit J Bone and Joint Surg* 60(B)3:375, 1978.
7. Eftekhar NS: *Principles of Total Hip Arthroplasty.* St Louis, CV Mosby, 1978.
8. Griffith MJ, Seidenstein MD, Williams D, et al: Eight year results of Charnley arthroplasties of the hip with special references to the behavior of cement. *Clin Orthop* 137:24–36, 1978.
9. Griffith JJ, Seidenstein MD, Williams D, et al: Socket wear in Charnley low friction arthroplasty of the hip. *Clin Orthop* 137:37–47, 1978.
10. Harris WH: Lateral deficiency of the acetabulum. *Orthop Rev* 9:5, 1980.
11. Harris WH, Jones WN: The use of wire mesh in total hip replacement surgery. *Clin Orthop and Rel Rsch* 106:117, 1975.
12. Harris WH: Loosening in the Hip Proceedings of the Sixth Annual Scientific Meeting of the Hip Society, 1978, pp 162–175.
13. Hastings DE, Parker SM: Protrusion acetabuli in rheumatoid arthritis. *Clin Orthop and Rel Rsch* 108:76, 1975.
14. Heywood AW: Arthroplasty with a solid bone graft for protrusion acetabuli. *Brit J Bone and Joint Surg* 62(3):322, 1980.
15. Johnson RC, Brand RA, Crowninshield RD: Reconstruction of the hip. A mathematical approach to determine optimum geometric relationships. *Amer J Bone and Joint Surg* 61A(5):639, 1979.
16. Johnson JT: Reconstruction of the pelvic ring following tumor resection *Amer J Bone and Joint Surg* 60(6):747, 1978.
17. McCollum DE, Nunley JA, Harrelson JM: Bone grafting in total hip replacement for acetabular protrusion. *Amer J Bone and Joint Surg* 62(7):1065, 1980.
18. Muller ME: Total hip prostheses. *Clin Orthop* 72:46–48, 1970.
19. Murray MP, Gore DR, Brewer BJ, et al: Comparison of functional performance after McKee-Farrar, Charnley, and Müller total hip replacement. A six-month follow-up of one hundred sixty-five cases: *Clin Orthop* 121:33, 1976.
20. Nelson CL, Haynes DW, Weber MJ, et al: Device and method for controlling cement thickness. *Clin Orthop* 151:160, 1980.
21. Pellicci PM, Salvati EA, Robinson HJ: Mechanical failures in total hip replacement requiring reoperation. *Amer J Bone and Joint Surg* 61(1):28, 1979.
22. Salvati EA, Wright TM, Burstein AH, et al: Fracture of polyethylene acetabular cups. Report of two cases. *Amer J Bone and Joint Surg* 61(8):1239, 1979.

23. Salvati EA, Bullough P, Wilson PD Jr: Intrapelvic protrusion of the acetabular component following total hip replacement. *Clin Orthop* 111:212, 1975.
24. Salvati EA, Im VC, Aglietti P, et al: Radiology of total hip replacements. *Clin Orthop* 121:74, 1976.
25. Schatzker J, Hastings DE, McBroom RJ: Acetabular reinforcement in total hip replacement. *Arch Orthop Trauma Surg* 94(2):135, 1979.
26. Satelo-Garza A, Charnley J: The results of Charnley arthroplasty of the hip performed for protrusio acetabuli. *Clin Orthop* 132:12, 1978.
27. Vakili F, Salvati EA, Warren RF: Entrapped foreign body within the acetabular cup in total hip replacement. *Clin Orthop* 150:159, 1980.
28. Volz RG: Fracture of the bony acetabulum following total hip replacement: Significance of broken acetabular wire sign. *Orthop Rev* 9:91, 1980.
29. Volz RG, Karpman RR: Mechanical factors relating to acetabular component loosening in total hip replacement (in press).

Richard D. Scott and
James P. Schilz

6

Femoral Fracture and Revision Arthroplasty

The orthopedic literature is replete with reports concerning total hip arthroplasty and its complications. A few papers directly address the subject of femoral shaft fracture in conjunction with total hip arthroplasty.[5,6,7,10,11,13,14] These reports make it clear that femoral fracture is a severe complication which often compromises the end result of the arthroplasty.

In this chapter, we attempt to develop a systematic approach to this problem by providing a means for its classification, evaluation, treatment and, hopefully, the prevention of those fractures which may be avoided.

HISTORICAL BACKGROUND AND CLASSIFICATION

Numerous papers in the early 1970s describe an occasional fractured femur in association with total hip arthroplasty. It was 1974 when the first definitive report by McElfresh and Coventry described in detail the case reports of six patients.[6] Scott et al, in 1975, discussed 38 patients who had femoral fractures in conjunction with total hip replacement.[11] In that paper, the patients were divided into three groups: (1) pre-operative femoral fractures; (2) intraoperative femoral fractures; and (3) post-operative femoral fractures. Talab et al, in 1979, reported on four femoral fractures in the post-operative period.[13] Schilz and Turner, in 1980, reported on six cases of post-operative fractures;[10] in 1981, Johansson et al reported on 37 femoral fractures in the intraoperative and post-operative period.[5] They further categorized the femoral fractures as to their location with respect to the tip of the femoral prosthesis (Table 6-1).

127

REVISION TOTAL HIP ARTHROPLASTY
ISBN 0-8089-1466-9

Table 6-1
Chronological Case Studies

McElfresh and Coventry[6]	1974	6 cases
Scott, Turner et al[11]	1975	38 cases
Taylor, et al[14]	1978	11 cases
Talab et al[13]	1979	4 cases
Schilz and Turner[10]	1980	6 cases
Johansson et al[5]	1981	37 cases

PREOPERATIVE FRACTURES

Clinical Presentation

This group represents those patients who present with fresh or old nonunited fractures of the proximal femur, and coxarthrosis of the ipsilateral hip joint.

Incidence of this fracture is reported as 0.3 percent in Scott's series in 1975.[11] The etiology is antecedent trauma. Scott et al reported in depth on 13 patients and found 7 intertrochanteric fractures (4 acute and 3 nonunions); 5 subtrochanteric fractures (all old nonunions); and 1 midshaft fracture (acute).

On presentation, the patients with acute fractures had a typical history, and had physical examination results as would be expected. Those patients with nonunion primarily presented with pain at the nonunion site which was increased by weight-bearing. The hip joints were previously diseased, or had degenerated, either secondary to the penetration of devices for fracture fixation or secondary to osteonecrosis.

Treatment

The goal of treatment is restoration of normal hip function with the least risk of complication.

Some would argue against total hip arthroplasty in an acute fracture and would recommend first obtaining fracture healing. If the arthritic hip remained symptomatic, then the arthroplasty could be done as a delayed secondary procedure. We feel that in the elderly patient, if coxarthrosis is already present and symptomatic, a primary total hip arthroplasty is warranted. The hip and the fracture can be treated by one surgical procedure. If two operations are necessary, the chance of infection is enhanced. In a recent report from the Robert Breck Brigham Hospital in Boston, the incidence of deep infection after total hip arthroplasty increased eight-fold in patients with previous hip surgery when compared with patients who had no prior hip surgery.[9]

Definitive surgical treatment depends upon the location of fracture. These fractures have been divided into three zones: (1) proximal to the base of the neck; (2) intertrochanteric; and (3) subtrochanteric.

In fractures proximal to the base of the neck, a standard total hip arthroplasty is recommended (Figs. 6-1 A,B). In the intertrochanteric fractures, the proximal fracture fragment is excised, a long-neck femoral component is utilized, and the greater trochanter is reimplanted on the proximal part of the femoral shaft (Figs.

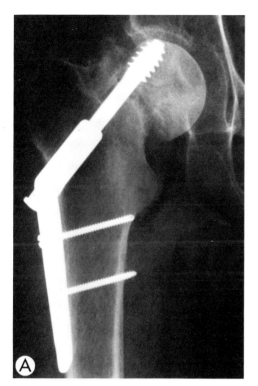
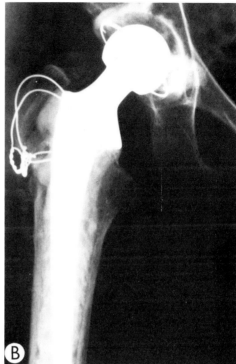

Fig. 6-1A.   Pre-operative fracture proximal to base of neck with fixation device penetration.

Fig. 6-1B.   Post-operative arthroplasty.

6-2 A,B). In subtrochanteric fractures, a long-stem femoral component is used to traverse the fracture site; cerclage wires and bone grafting are utilized when necessary (Figs. 6-3 A,B).

Surgical Technique and Pitfalls

Pre-operatively, adequate radiographic evaluation of the pelvis and entire femur is necessary to accurately assess the fracture, the anterior femoral bow, and the femoral component that will be required. The use of templates is strongly advised. A large selection of femoral components, including long-neck and long-stem prostheses, is mandatory (Fig. 6-4).

As with all complicated hip surgery, wide surgical exposure with trochanteric osteotomy is necessary in order to adequately visualize the hip joint and the proximal femur. Once the fracture is exposed, if the proximal fragment is to be resected, this is done in a routine fashion, preserving the greater trochanter; a femoral component of appropriate neck length is utilized.

If the fracture fragment is to be traversed, the fracture is identified, isolated, and clamped in place. The femur is reamed as needed using flexible Kuntscher reamers. The ideal length of the femoral component is a minimum 6 cm distal to the fracture; we have routinely used a 30 cm femoral component, especially when the proximal femoral bone stock is compromised. This can be cut down in length

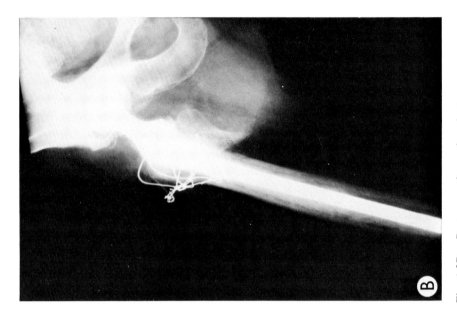

Fig. 6-2B. Post-operative arthroplasty.

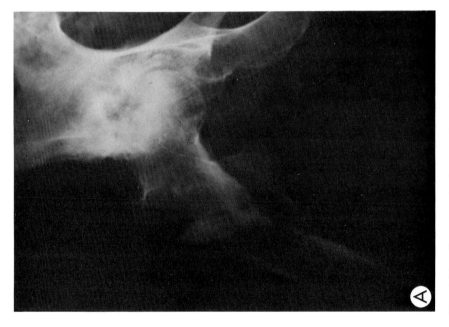

Fig. 6-2A. Pre-operative intertrochanteric fracture.

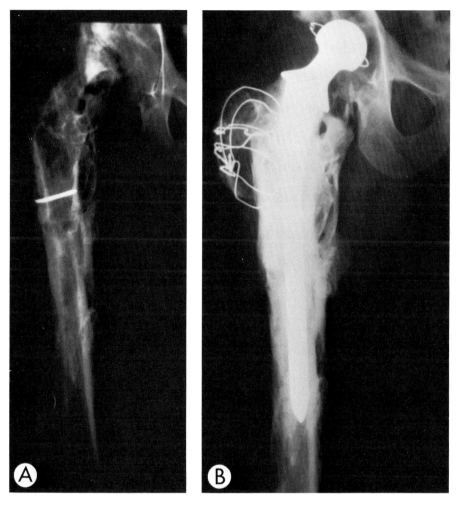

Fig. 6-3A.   Pre-operative subtrochanteric nonunion.
Fig. 6-3B.   Post-operative arthroplasty.

pre- or intraoperatively in a short or bowed femur. In these patients, it is necessary to be certain that the femoral component is within the canal and does not anteriorly or laterally perforate the femur. Routine intraoperative x-rays are thus obtained after the fracture is reduced and the trial femoral component is positioned (Fig. 6-5).

The acetabulum is prepared and the acetabular component is then cemented in place. A trial reduction with the femoral component is performed to check stability. The femoral canal is now prepared for cementing. We use a distal femoral cement plug employing one package of methylmethacrylate inserted either with a routine cement-plug inserter or a chest tube. After the plug has hardened, the femoral component is cemented in place. The technique often requires four packages of refrigerated methylmethacrylate inserted in a low-viscosity state using a cement gun. The femoral component is then seated in place and the methacrylate allowed

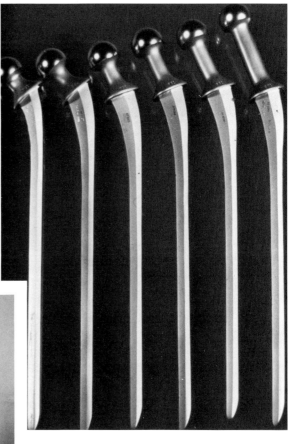

Fig. 6-4. Selection of long-stem (30 cm) and long-neck femoral components. Stem length may be pre-operatively or intraoperatively shortened for short or excessively bowed femurs.

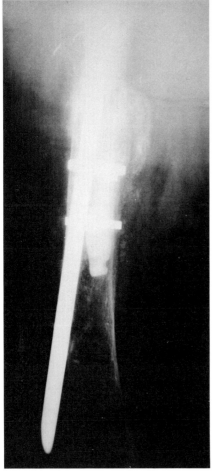

Fig. 6-5. Failure to obtain intraoperative roentgenograms resulted in this distal femoral penetration by the long-stemmed femoral component.

to polymerize. After the cement has hardened, x-rays are repeated if a long stem has been used to assure that there has been no extravasation of methacrylate or component penetration of the cortex.

Post-operatively the patients are placed in balanced suspension, and, depending upon the trochanteric bed, ambulation is started 7 to 21 days post-operatively. If the fracture is subtrochanteric and has been traversed, weight-bearing is protected until fracture healing is evident on x-ray.

The post-operative complication of trochanteric nonunion can be minimized by careful reattachment and prolonged protected weight-bearing. The rare occurrence of heterotopic ossification may be eliminated if fresh fractures are treated early (Fig. 6-6).

INTRAOPERATIVE FRACTURES

Clinical Presentation

The incidence of intraoperative fractures ranges between 0.4 to 3.0 percent, depending upon the report.[14]

The etiology of these fractures relates to the quality of the bone and the handling of the femur during arthroplasty. Fractures were noted to occur at different stages of the operation. These stages are, in order of increasing frequency: (1) during dislocation of the hip; (2) during seating of the new femoral component; and (3) during reaming of the proximal femur, or during the removal of the already

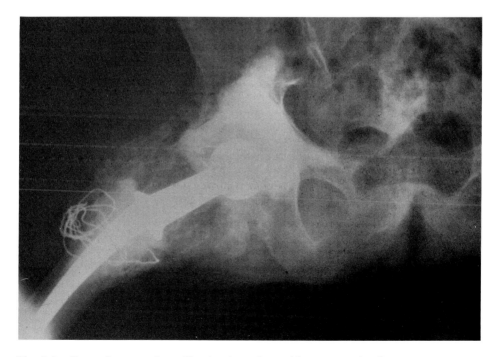

Fig. 6-6. Severe heterotopic ossification in patient with pre-operative fracture.

Table 6-2

Surgical Maneuvers Causing Intraoperative Fracture

	Scott et al[11]	Johansson et al[5]
During hip dislocation	2	3
Seating femoral component	4	2
Reaming femur		
Routine	4	5
During mm removal	3	11

present methacrylate. During removal of methacrylate the femur appears to be at its highest risk for fracture. Johansson et al noted that 50 percent of the fractures in their series occurred during this stage of the operation (Table 6-2).[5]

The location of these fractures is primarily proximal, with the fracture usually at the tip of the femoral component. Scott et al had 88 percent of their fractures in the proximal third,[11] whereas Johansson et al had 90 percent fracture in the proximal third; of these, 75 percent occurred at the prosthesis tip.[5]

Factors which put the patient at risk for intraoperative fractures are consistent in the two larger series of reports. Previous surgery is the most common, followed by femoral bone defects (i.e., cortical windows or defects from previous internal fixation devices), and osteoporosis, especially noted in rheumatoids.[12] All of the 22 patients in the Johansson et al series had undergone previous surgery (20 patients had a previous total hip replacement).[5] In the series by Scott et al, 75 percent of the 18 patients had previous surgery (Table 6-3).[11] In Taylor's series, 73 percent of the 11 patients had a failed total hip arthroplasty.[14]

Treatment

The goal of treatment is recognition of fracture, adequate internal fixation with fracture healing, and a functional hip arthroplasty.

Methods of treatment for these proximal fractures have been multiple. Various authors have detailed the results using traction, cerclage wiring around a standard length femoral component, and the use of long-stem femoral components with and without additional internal fixation. The success of the modes of treatment is seen in Table 6-4. Traction was used but once. The data suggest that long-stem femoral components with or without cerclage fixation and bone grafting is the method of choice. Though fracture healing will usually occur with the other methods outlined, the long-term incidence of component loosening is minimized with the use of long stem femoral components and bone grafting. In the series by Scott et al, there was

Table 6-3

Risk Factors For Intraoperative Femoral Fracture

	Scott et al[11] (18 patients)		Johansson et al[5] (22 patients)	
Previous surgery	12	(66%)	22	(100%)
Previous total hip arthroplasty	3	(16%)	20	(90%)
Cortical defects	2	(11%)	8	(36%)
Osteopenia	2	(11%)	3	(14%)

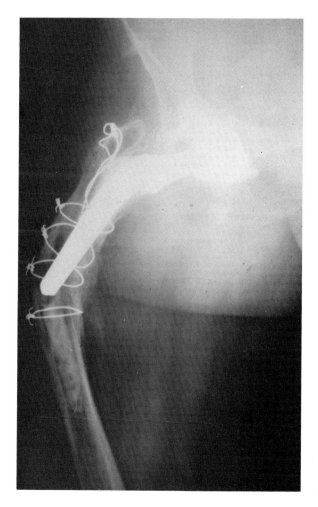

Fig. 6-7. Intraoperative fracture treated with standard stem femoral component and cerclage wiring, with poor result.

a 33 percent failure rate secondary to loosening of the femoral component in 12 proximal fractures when long-stem components were not used (Fig. 6-7);[11] when a long-stem femoral component was used in 4 cases, there was healing in all four fractures and no evidence of loosening. Additional circlage fixation had been used in two of these four cases. Johansson et al found that if a long-stem femoral

Table 6-4
Treatment Success of Proximal Third Intraoperative Fractures

	Scott et al[11]		Johansson et al[5]	
Traction	0/1	(0%)	Not reported	
Short Stem				
With fixation	4/7	(64%)	2/6	(33%)
Without fixation	3/4	(75%)	Not reported	
Long Stem				
With fixation	2/2	(100%)	7/8	(88%)
Without fixation	2/2	(100%)	2/5	(40%)

component with additional internal fixation was used, healing occurred uniformly with no evidence of late loosening in most cases.[5] In contrast, when they used a long-stem femoral component without additional internal fixation, only two out of five cases healed without loosening. Of the three remaining, two became symptomatically loose and one had a nonunion.

In those few fractures distal to the tip of the stem there was uniform healing in both series using internal fixation with plates, without any evidence of loosening (Fig. 6-8).

Surgical Technique and Pitfalls

Prevention is the key to success in these fractures. If one is aware of the risk factors, such as previous surgery, cortical defects, and osteopenia, in conjunction

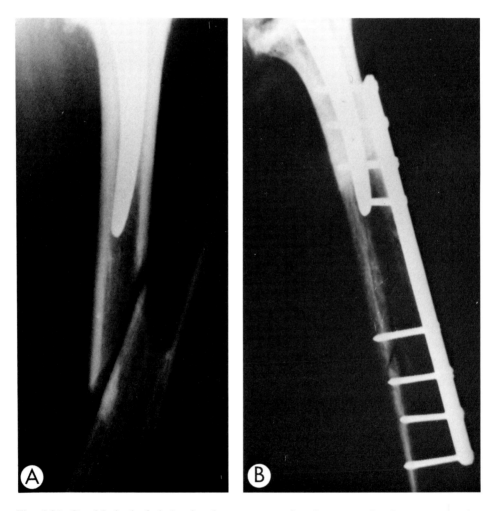

Fig. 6-8A, B.   Method of choice for the treatment of an intraoperative fracture occurring below a femoral component. (A). Pre-operative; (B) Post-operative.

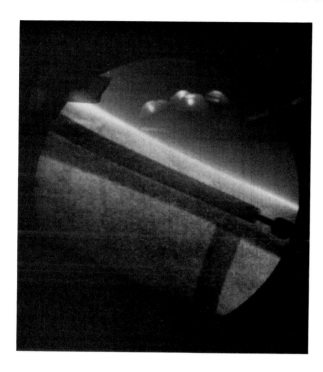

Fig. 6-9. Intraoperative use of the image intensifier during cement removal employing the high-speed drill.

with the knowledge of the surgical maneuvers which may cause a fracture, then the likelihood of fracture occurring will be minimized.

To decrease the chance of fracture during revision surgery, wide exposure is necessary; a transtrochanteric approach is used. On approaching the hip joint, a complete and thorough capsulectomy is performed. The psoas tendon is identified anteriorly and the bony acetabular margins superiorly and posteriorly. This is performed prior to any attempts at dislocation of the hip. Gentle handling of the tissues is mandatory. If an internal fixation device is present, it should not be removed until the hip has been dislocated. Dislocation of the hip should be done gently and without undue tortional stress upon the femur, which may lead to fracture.

Once the hip is adequately exposed, the problems of methacrylate removal from the prior total hip must be addressed. Cement removal in revision arthroplasty can be difficult and hazardous. Recently, more surgeons use a high-speed drill for cement removal rather than making a distal cortical window [4] Though the absence of the cortical window decreases the chances for post-operative fracture, the high-speed drill can still produce cortical defects which can lead either to immediate or late femoral fractures. The technique for removing the cement is to employ cement osteotomes to remove the proximally located cement. After this is completed, the high-speed drill is used to remove the distal portion of the cement column. It is important that during this time a biplane image intensifier is used to monitor the advancing drill bit and prevent cortical penetration (Fig. 6-9). When the femoral canal is fully prepared, seating of the trial femoral component should be attempted. If it does not adequately seat, the canal can be further reamed using flexible Kuntscher reamers.

If, despite all precautions, an intraoperative fracture does occur, it is first

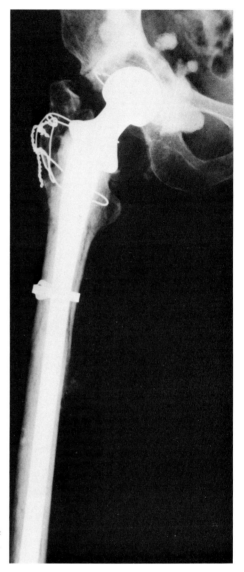

Fig. 6-10. Correctly treated intraoperative fracture using long-stemmed femoral component and cerclage fixation.

necessary to recognize the fracture, as nine percent were unrecognized in series by Johansson et al.[5] Adequate radiographic examination in the operating room is important for determining the extent of the fracture. When the fracture is identified it must be fully exposed. It is then reduced and held with bone clamps. At this time, a long-stem femoral component with cerclage wires and bone grafting is the method of choice. Immediate access to long-stem femoral components is critical. Once the fracture is reduced and held, the femoral shaft is prepared to accept the long-stem femoral component. If the shaft is too tight, reaming should be done using flexible Kuntscher reamers. Once the canal had been prepared, trial reduction with the real component in place is done, and x-rays are taken of the entire femur. If satisfactory, the long-stem femoral component is cemented in place, using refrigerated methylmethacrylate, again with a distal plug of cement, and retrograde filling, using the cement gun. After the cement has polymerized, the area of the fracture can then be cerclage-wired and bone grafted (Fig. 6-10). Post-operatively, prolonged protected weight-bearing is indicated, because clinical and radiographic proof of fracture healing is often impossible to obtain. The complications of trochanteric nonunion may be minimized by using prolonged protective weight-bearing; the problem of fracture nonunion may again be minimized by using good surgical technique, i.e., using a long-stem femoral component with additional internal fixation, bone grafting, and protected weight-bearing (Fig. 6-11).

POSTOPERATIVE FRACTURES

Clinical Presentation

This group represents a small but relatively increasing patient population. Reported incidence ranges between 0.1 and 0.8 percent. The etiologic factors that characterized these fractures, as defined by McElfresh and Coventry,[6] are divided into three categories: (1) stress fractures due to increased use of the leg after hip arthroplasty; (2) fractures caused by stress-raisers in the femoral shaft, including defects in the cortex and insufficient cement around the tip of the prosthesis; and (3) fractures caused by trauma sufficient to produce a fracture in a normal limb. Of

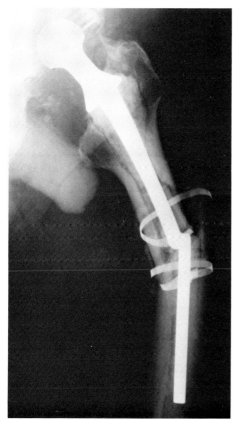

Fig. 6-11. Intraoperative fracture correctly treated, but without protected weight-bearing post-operatively, led to this fractured femur and stem 14 months post-operatively.

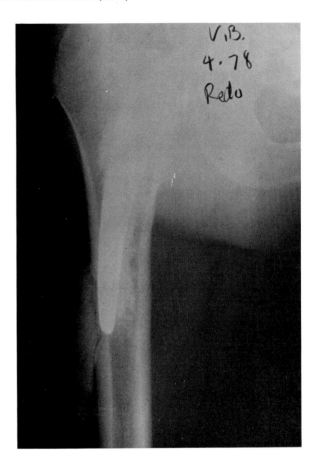

Fig. 6-12. Stress-raiser which occurred during revision surgery and was unrecognized.

these three factors, the presence of cortical defects appears to be the major, preventable etiology.

The location of the fractures is usually at or above the femoral stem tip. Scott et al[11] reported that 72 percent of the fractures were located proximally, while Johansson et al[5] noted 86 percent were proximal.

The time interval between total hip arthroplasty and fracture ranged between 4 and 24 months, depending upon the series. In patients who had a cortical defect present without stem perforation prior to fracture, however, the interval between hip arthroplasty and fracture averaged 5.1 months, with a range 1 to 12 months post-operatively. It appears, therefore, that a cortical defect is a major factor responsible in these post-operative fractures. Frankel has shown that a single drill hole in an experimental femur model would reduce energy absorption, equivalent to bone strength, by an average of 55.2 percent.[1,2] This decreased bone strength is persistent regardless of the hole size, as long as the hole involves less than 30 percent of the bone surface area. Oh and Harris showed that the forces acting on the lateral proximal femur are increased over the normal value for the intact femora when a cemented femoral component is in place.[7]

Consequently, those patients with cortical defects in conjunction with their total hip arthroplasty have two factors producing a disposition toward fracture. First, the defect causes a stress-raiser which will decrease bone strength by at least

50 percent, and second, the abnormal amount of energy focused on the lateral cortex is inherent in the design of the total hip components.

Charnley has noted that methylmetacrylate does not interfere with bone healing when there is good bone-to-bone opposition,[3] yet Yablon has shown, in an experimental model, that if methylmethacrylate is placed endosteally and periosteally, bone healing is histologically absent at 9 weeks.[15] Thus, those cases with cortical defects where there is periosteal extravasation of methylmethacrylate have a permanent stress-raiser and are predisposed to femoral fracture. Stress-raisers should be avoided if possible, but if inadvertently produced, they must be recognized and treated (Fig. 6-12).

Treatment

The goal of treatment is fracture healing and a functional, painless hip arthroplasty. The modes of treatment of these fractures varies from skeletal traction to the use of open reduction and internal fixation.

Traction has been attempted by various authors, from McElfresh and Coventry[6] in 1974 to Johansson et al[5] in 1981. In the six-patient series from the Mayo Clinic,[6] all six were initially treated with skeletal traction, but it was abandoned in two patients, one of whom developed a malunion at 8 weeks. Another additional patient healed his fracture but a loosened femoral component required revision surgery at 3 years post-fracture. The other three patients healed in traction without any problems related to fracture healing or late evidence of loosening (Fig. 6-13). Johansson et al[5] had 10 patients with post-operative fracture who were treated with traction; 90 percent healed. More significantly, 80 percent of the femoral components became loose and required (or will require) revision (Table 6-5).

In light of the above statistics, early surgical intervention appears to be the treatment of choice. The surgical techniques employed have varied; some surgeons tried open reduction with internal fixation using plates, others used long-stem femoral components with or without cerclage wires. Limited data regarding the use of compression plates are available. Scott et al[11] and Johansson et al[5] each reported one case using plates. Though the fracture healed in both patients, each patient subsequently refractured the femur at the end of the plate. The use of cerclage wires alone with the previous standard femoral components in place has been tried without good success. Scott et al had but one case that went on to nonunion;[11] Johansson et al[5] reported a 75 percent failure rate with this mode of treatment, with respect to loosening, though the fractures had healed.[5] The best results in all series reported were in the use of a long-stem femoral component, in which the fracture was bypassed, along with cerclage wiring and bone grafting. Scott et al had one case where this method of treatment was used and had a good result of fracture

Table 6-5

Results of Traction Treatment for Postoperative Fractures

	Healed (%)	Malunion (%)	Loosening (%)
McElfresh and Coventry[6]	66% (4/6)	16% (1/6)	16% (1/6)
Scott and Turner[11]	100% (2/2)	50% (1/2)	Not reported
Johansson et al[5]	90% (9/10)	20% (2/10)	80% (8/10)

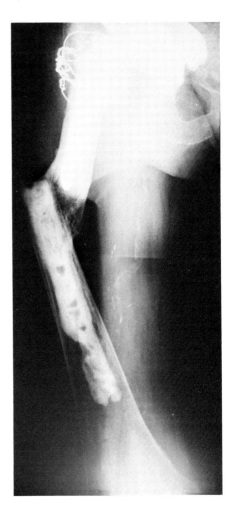

Fig. 6-13. Post-operative fracture treated with traction with resultant malunion.

healing and no evidence of late loosening.[11] Schilz and Turner reported two cases using this technique with good results,[10] and Johansson et al[5] reported that if post-operative infection can be avoided, the best results are obtained with this method.[5] Though all these numbers are small, it appears that the use of long-stem femoral components with internal fixation and grafting is recommended (Fig. 6-14). Occasionally, electrical stimulation might also be employed.

Surgical Technique and Pitfalls

In post-operative femoral fractures, the use of a long-stem femoral component with cerclage wiring is a major surgical procedure with potential for multiple complications. Diligent pre-operative evaluation of the patient, including roentgenographs of the entire femur in both anteroposterior (AP) and lateral planes, is essential. Immediate access to a variety of long-stem femoral components during surgery is mandatory.

Wide exposure is employed using the transtrochanteric approach. After the trochanter is osteotomized, a complete capsulectomy is performed, the hip dislocated, and the previous femoral component removed. The incision is then distally extended and the fracture site exposed. The fracture is identified and isolated. The proximal cement column is now removed. Cement removal technique usually involves removing the methacrylate in a retrograde fashion, through the proximally exposed hip joint. The distal cement can then be removed either with cement osteotomes or when under direct visualization with the high-speed drill. Next, the fracture is reduced and held in place with bone-holding clamps.

The femur is reamed to accept the long-stem femoral component, preferably a 30-cm-length stem, appropriately shortened in the small or bowed femur. The long-stem femoral component is seated, and a trial reduction is done with the utmost care. Using the image intensifier, the entire femur is scanned in AP and lateral planes to assure proper component placement. If the trial reduction is satisfactory then the femoral component can be cemented in place.

The cementing technique involves pulsatile lavage of the femoral canal, sponge-drying, and introducing a distal cement plug. Any defects in the femoral shaft cortex at the fracture are occluded with bone graft in attempts to restrict cement

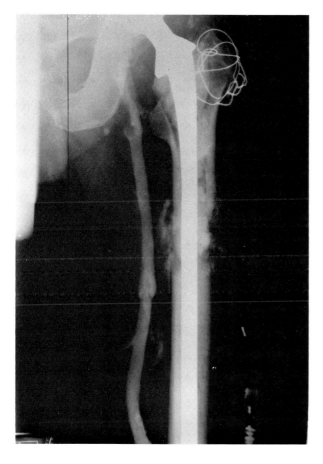

Fig. 6-14. Successfully treated post-operative fracture with long stem, bone grafting, and electrical stimulator.

extrusion. Low viscous refrigerated methylmethacrylate, usually four packets, is now inserted into the femur with a cement gun. In those cases where the patient is felt to be at risk for post-operative infection, antibiotics are routinely put into the cement, using either a cephalosporin or an aminoglycoside. After the cement has polymerized, the clamps are removed, the fracture site is bone grafted, and optional cerclage wires are placed.

DISCUSSION

Prevention of fracture should be the surgeon's prime goal. The majority of intraoperative and post-operative cases are preventable if the principles of revision hip surgery are not violated.

Intraoperative fractures can be minimized by an awareness of those factors which put a patient at risk and of those surgical maneuvers which are associated with fractures.

Furthermore, prophylaxis against fractures during revision surgery should encompass both the intraoperative and post-operative periods. It is recommended that any cortical defects produced during revision surgery be given immediate attention, as they appear to predispose to post-operative fractures. Though cortical defects do not impair immediate results, they can definitely be associated with femoral fractures within 1 year,[5,6,7,8,10,11,13] severely compromising the long-term result of the hip arthroplasty.

We have developed an aggressive attitude toward the recognition and treatment of these defects. During any revision hip procedure we employ biplane image scanning of the femoral shaft during cement removal, canal reaming, prosthetic component seating, and after cementing. If, during revision surgery, a defect is produced and recognized prior to cementing in the femoral component, it is advisable to have the tip of the new femoral component a distance of two-and-one-half times the diameter of the bone distal to the defect. After the femoral component is cemented in place the defect should be bone grafted. If the component is already cemented in place with cement extravasation, and then recognized intraoperatively, the bolus of extravasated cement should be surgically exposed, the methylmethacrylate removed, and the defect bone grafted. Postoperatively, the patient should be protected from full weight-bearing until the area of the stress-raiser is healed radiographically, thereby returning normal strength to the bone.

SUMMARY

Three categories of femoral fractures have been outlined. Pre-operative evaluation, surgical techniques, and post-operative management have been discussed. The basic premises regarding these fractures are: (1) prevention is the prime objective with adequate knowledge and preoperative planning; (2) necessary availability to long-stem prostheses; (3) the surgical technique is demanding; (4) wide exposure is mandatory and the key to elimination of the majority of intraoperative fractures; (5) long-stem femoral components with cerclage wiring and bone grafting is the treatment of choice in those intraoperative and post-operative fractures of the proximal femur at or above the tip of the femoral component; and (6) those fractures in the femur distal to the femoral component can be treated as if no arthroplasty is present, and appear to have no direct effect upon the long-term result of the hip arthroplasty.

REFERENCES

1. Brooks DB, Frankel VM: Biomechanics of torsional fractures. *J Bone and Joint Surg* 52(A):507–514, 1970.
2. Burstein AH, Frankel VM, Currey J: Bone strength, the effects of screw holes. *J Bone and Joint Surg* 54(A):1143–1156, 1972.
3. Charnley JA: The healing of human fractures in contact with self-curing cement. *Clin Orthop* 47:157–164, 1966.
4. Harris WH, Oh I: A new power tool for removal of methylmethacrylate for the femur. *Clin Orthop* 132:53–54, 1978.
5. Johansson JE, McBroom R, Barrington TW, et al: Fracture of the ipsilateral femur in patients with total hip replacement. *J Bone and Joint Surg* 63(A):1435–1442, 1981.
6. McElfresh, EC, Coventry MB: Femoral and pelvic fracture after a total hip arthroplasty. *J Bone and Joint Surg* 56(A):583–492, 1974.
7. Oh I, Harris, WH: Proximal strain distribution in a loaded femur. *J Bone and Joint Surg* 60(A):75–85, 1978.
8. Pellicci PM, Inglis AE, Salvati EA: Perforation of the femoral shaft during total hip replacement. *J Bone and Joint Surg* 62(A):234–240, 1980.
9. Poss R, Ewald FC, Thomas WH, et al: Factors influencing the risk of infection following total joint replacement. Paper presented at the American Academy of Orthopaedic Surgery Convention, Las Vegas, March 1981.
10. Schilz JP, Turner RH: Proximal femur fractures after total hip arthroplasty. (Unpublished data.)
11. Scott RD, Turner RH, Leitzes S, et al: Femoral fractures in conjunction with total hip replacement. *J Bone and Joint Surg* 57(A):494–501, 1975.
12. Singh M: Changes in the trabecular pattern of the upper end of the femur as an index to osteoporosis. *J Bone and Joint Surg* 52(A):457–462, 1970.
13. Talab YA, States JD, Evarts CM: Femoral Shaft Perforation. *Clin Orthop* 141:158–165, 1979.
14. Taylor MM, Meyers MH, Harvey JP: Intraoperative femur fractures during total hip replacement. *Clin Orthop* 137:96–103, 1978.
15. Yablon I: The effects of methylmethacrylate on fracture healing. *Clin Orthop* 114:358–360, 1976.

Arnold D. Scheller, Jr.,
Susan B. Mitchell, and
Forest C. Barber

7

Femoral Component Fracture in Revision Hip Arthroplasty

The fractured femoral stem presents one of the most challenging problems to the surgeon attempting revision of a failed total hip arthroplasty. The incidence of stem fracture in the literature ranges from 0.23 to 0.67 percent.[3,9,11,14,17,19,21] The largest study by Chao and Coventry of the Mayo Clinic quotes an incidence of 0.6 percent.[11]

Although Chao and Coventry attempted to develop a risk index for prospective analysis of stem fracture,[11] few studies have concentrated on the inter-relationship of a multitude of variables connected with this complex problem.

The composite structure formed by femoral bone, methylmethacrylate, and metal endoprosthesis is acted upon by numerous basic forces. Muscle and joint reaction forces apply tensile stresses along the lateral cortex and compressive stresses medially. Shear forces occur between the conjoint surfaces of those three materials. Failure of one or more of these highly stressed materials may occur between their conjoint surfaces. Failure of one or more of these highly stressed materials may occur due to the applied forces. Resultant forces on the composite depend on clinical and technical factors (Table 7-1).

Certain clinical parameters—age, height, weight, activity level, and osseous quality—are among factors that usually lead to stem loosening and bone resorption.[4,20,24,35] Technical parameters include: endoprosthetic design configurations;[3,6,15,17,21,38,44,48,51] metals;[3,6,5,17,21,38,44,48,51] cement quality and distribution about the stem; relative component position; the surgical technique of bone preparation;[1,2,3,9,14,17,18,24,30,33,37,38,48,51,55] and cement insertion.

147

Table 7-1
Factors in Fatigue Fracture of Femoral Stem

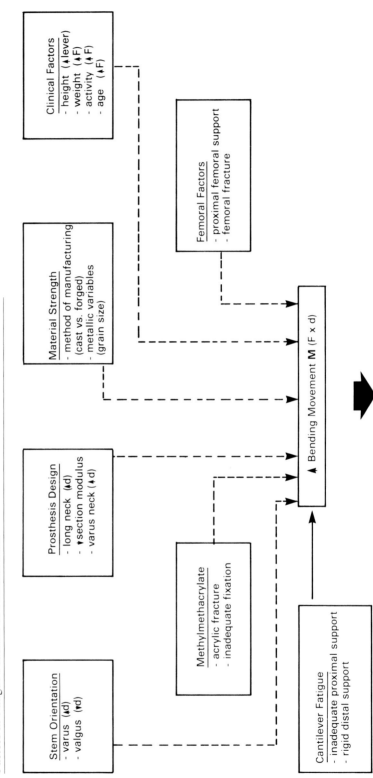

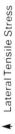

Lateral Tensile Stress

Fatigue Failure
- slow crack laterally
- fast fracture

To develop a logical pattern of pre-operative analysis and surgical treatment we have drawn upon an extensive review of the literature and on our review of 29 stem fracture revisions at the New England Baptist Hospital, including 21 cases with greater than 3-year follow-up.

CLINICAL EVALUATION

Of the 29 patients who underwent stem fracture revisions at the New England Baptist Hospital, 80 percent of the femoral endoprosthetic failures in total hip replacement occurred in males. The average age was 64 years, height 178 cm, and weight 94 kg. All of the patients had uncomplicated wound healing post-operatively, and had been managed with a 3-month course of progressive weight-bearing and physical therapy after their initial total hip replacement.

After the initial arthroplasty, the majority of the patients in this study had an excellent functional range of motion. Only three patients had flexion of less than 90°, with difficulty in putting on their stockings or shoes. All other patients exhibited flexion to 90° or greater, with good rotation and no impediment in their routine activities. The patient with an excellent range of motion is generally more apt to apply stress to the femoral endoprosthesis than the patient with a restricted range of motion. The problems with the contralateral hip or adjacent joints, such as the back and the knee, were minimal in this study.

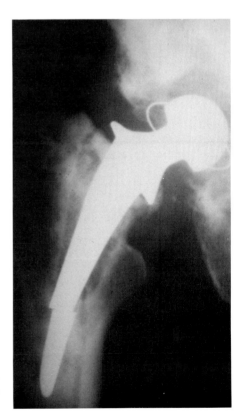

Figure 7-1. Stem fracture in a varus implanted prosthesis. Note gross failure of cement fixation about the proximal stem.

The activity level reported in our study was variable, but concurred with the findings in the literature. Approximately 83 percent of our patients were either very active or moderately active. Only 17 percent were minimally active; none of our patients used ambulatory aids when the endoprosthesis failed.

The onset of symptoms in these patients is interesting. Twenty-one patients noted a gradual increase in hip pain with weight-bearing. The pain insidiously progressed in intensity for a period of 4 to 6 months before fracture of the endoprosthesis was noted. Eight patients reported an acute onset of symptoms associated in all cases with a traumatic episode, ranging from a fall on an icy surface to an automobile accident. We feel that this gradual progression of pain on weight-bearing is consistent with the evolution of loosening of the femoral prosthesis which precedes the final climactic failure of the implant. Probably, some component of stem loosening, whether symptomatic or asymptomatic, always precedes stem fracture.

Clinical factors which contribute to the failure of the endoprosthesis have been outlined by Charnley,[14] He notes a three-fold increase in fractures of the femoral stem in patients weighing more than 90 kg. Collis concurred with Charnley's observations,[17] and added that a patient's height is a factor in femoral stem failure. Similarly, the taller, heavier patient was a likely candidate for failure in our study as well. Both authors also pointed out that young, active patients were at significant risk for femoral stem fracture. The average age of 64 years in our study suggests that the older patient may also be at risk. We believe, therefore, the femoral stem failure can occur at any age and is dependent on a number of clinical variables (Table 7-1).

RADIOGRAPHIC EVALUATION

It is important to analyze numerous variables in evaluating roentgenographs for patients with asymptomatic total hip replacement to determine if stem fracture is imminent. If, after analysis, stem fracture seems imminent, then prophylactic revision prior to stem fracture is in order.

In analyzing the anteroposterior (AP) view of the pelvis, it is important to evaluate femoral head placement. The incidence of stem fracture increases if the superior-to-inferior or the medial-to-lateral difference is greater than 1.0 cm. Leg-length discrepancy greater than 2.0 cm also increases stress on the femoral component. In analyzing the proximal femur, stem-to-canal ratios of less than 50 percent have a markedly increased incidence of loosening and predisposition to stem fracture.[11] Evaluation of metal implant trauma or varus stem placement is also crucial (Fig. 7-1).

Trochanteric integrity is important, since avulsion or nonunion seriously compromises the lateral buttress to the femoral hip composite and decreases the stability of the component (Fig. 7-2). Proximal femoral osseous resorption of excessive unremoved cancellous calcar bone stock during initial stem insertion also increases the likelihood of femoral stem fracture (Fig. 7-3).

Analysis of the bone-cement and metal-cement interface is crucial. Excessive cement thickness (especially in the areas of the femoral neck), voids, and fractures are predisposing factors to implant failure (Fig. 7-4). The bone-cement interface is

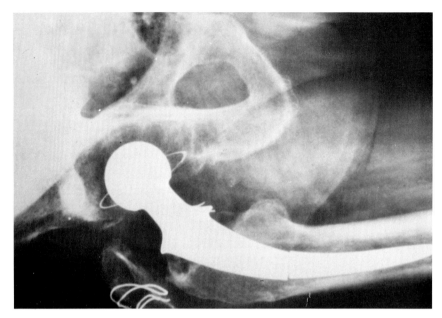

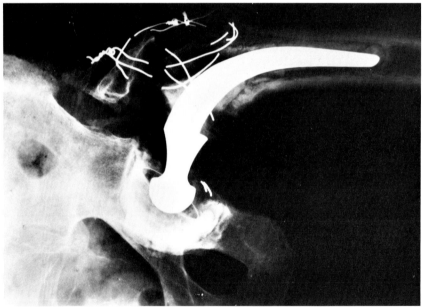

Figure 7-2 *(left)*. Acrylic fracture, especially laterally and proximomedially, is noted with severe proximal femoral resorption, a bent stem, and avulsed greater trochanter. These findings are precipitating factors in fatigue fracture of the stem.

Figure 7-3 *(right)*. Stem fracture in prosthesis with proximal femoral resorption.

seriously compromised when radiolucent lines of greater than 2.0 mm are noted. Radiolucent lines at the metal-cement interface are consistent with a migrating femoral stem.

Intermedullary position of the femoral stems have a significant effect on the stresses within the stem. Varus positioned stems have a higher stem stress than neutral or valgus positioned stems, because of the increased moment arm. The bending moment and the lateral tensile stresses are both increased, making the varus positioned stem more susceptible to fatigue failure. Interestingly, roentgeno-graphic analysis in our series revealed 50 percent of the failed femoral components had been positioned in varus with respect to the longitudinal axis of the femur. Thirty percent were in neutral alignment; only 11 percent were in valgus. Although neutral and valgus stems have lower stresses, they can also undergo fatigue failure. Utilizing an analysis of the respective mode of loosening in association with stem position gives one an intimate knowledge of the potential for stem fracture.

Gruen et al did a particularly detailed analysis of femoral stem loosening and developed four specific modes of failure of the stems.[24] (Refer to Chapter 3, on biomechanics, and Chapter 4, on femoral stem revision, for a more critical perusal of these modes of failure.) Twenty-four of 26 of the femoral stems that fractured failed by the cantilever mode of loosening, as described by Gruen. Two patients, or

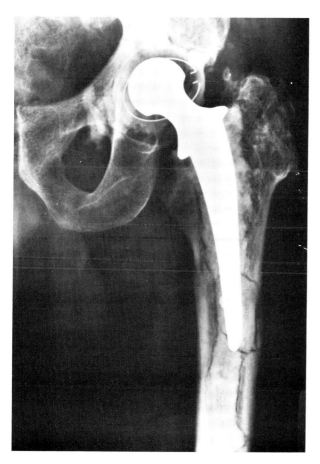

Figure 7-4. Failure of cement fixation to the stem.

seven percent of the patients that failed in the stem area, failed by a midstem pivot mode. Another three patients had fractures through the head-neck junction but no fracture through the stem. If one simultaneously analyzes the mode of loosening with respect to stem position, 60 percent of our patients that failed from a cantilever mechanism were in varus, 24 percent were in neutral, and 13 percent were in valgus. The two patients that failed by the midstem pivot mode were in varus. Fig. 7-5A through F demonstrates examples of each mode of loosening and the respective percentages in our study. Progressive moderate-to-severe proximal femoral resorption was noted in all cases, which developed into stem fracture; this was not true in those prostheses that failed in the head-neck area (Fig. 7-6). Defects in cement or cement interface lucencies, initially absent post-operatively at 3 months, were noted in radiographs initially taken to evaluate pain on weight-bearing before stem fracture. Moderate-to-severe proximal transverse fractures of the acrylic cement were seen in 25 cases. Minor fractures were observed in four cases.

Pre-operative arthrograms were positive for loosening in all eight cases in which they were done. Temporal analysis of roentgenograms revealed no evidence of cement failure on the initial post-operative film nor on the 3-month post-operative studies. Cement fracture initially noted on x-rays taken for pain on weight-bearing probably evolved from an initial failure of the bone-cement interface. In 25 of 29 patients, a linear radiolucency of greater than 1.0 mm at the interface was found, usually in the proximal medial region. Transverse fractures in the acrylic

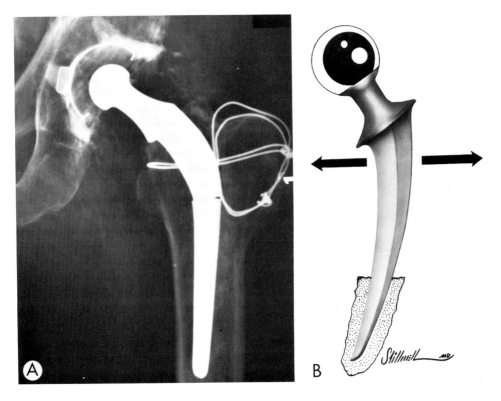

Figure 7-5A, B. (cantilever, 8290).

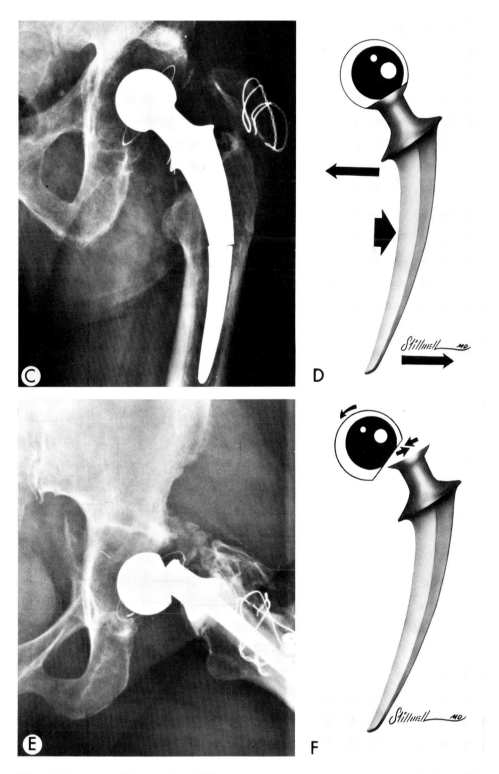

Figure 7-5C, D.   (midstem, pivot, 9%).   **Figure 7-5E, F.**   (head-neck shear, 9%).

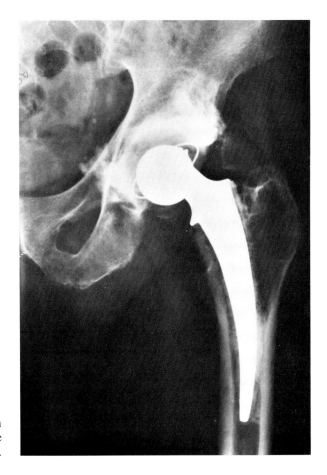

Figure 7-6. AP view from a case of fracture through the weld at the head-neck junction.

were found in subsequent radiographs. Failure at the cement-stem interface defined by lucency of greater than 1.0 mm, most often seen laterally in the proximal femur (Fig. 7-7), was found in 19 patients, usually with varus component tilt. It should be noted that in two patients, in whom failures occurred in the head-neck junction, there was no evidence of acrylic fracture (Fig. 7-6).

METALLURGY AND FATIGUE FAILURE

All structures, if repetitively stressed at a sufficiently high level for a sufficient number of cycles, will ultimately fail by the mechanism referred to as fatigue failure. The process of fatigue essentially has three stages: (1) initial fatigue damage leading to crack initiation; (2) crack propagation until the remaining uncracked cross-section becomes too weak to sustain the loads which are imposed; and (3) final sudden fracture of the remaining intact cross-section.

Fatigue testing is usually performed on selected specimen types either with uniform axial loading or in uniform bending which produce only tensile and compressive stresses. The stress can be cycled: (1) between zero stress and a maximum tensile stress; (2) between a maximum tensile stress and a maximum compressive stress; or (3) between a minimum tensile stress and a maximum tensile stress.

Testing of specimens provides information relative to the stress below which failure will not occur after a selected number of cycles, usually 10 to 100 million for metallic materials used in orthopaedic appliances. This value of stress is referred to as the fatigue strength or endurance limit of the material. The higher the value, the more satisfactorily a device of a specific design should perform when made from a material having such characteristics (Table 7-2).

A number of factors are significant to fatigue resistance behavior of an orthopaedic implant device. These are: the geometrical configuration; the magnitude of stress; the frequency of stress application; the method of stress application; and the physiologic environment.

The actual size and geometry of a device plays a significant role in how such a device behaves under specific conditions of loading in a patient's body. It is important to recognize the different functions of fixation appliances and prosthetic bone replacements. Fixation appliances, such as bone plates, intertrochanteric nail-plate devices, and intramedullary rods, are used primarily to hold the bone sections in proper apposition and alignment during bone healing. If stress of a sufficient magnitude is repetitively applied over time in the presence of bone nonunion, the

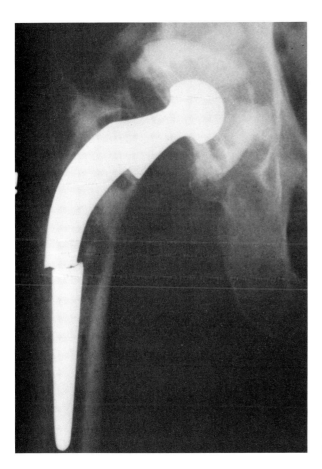

Figure 7-7. Bone-cement radiolucency associated with stem fracture.

Table 7-2
Typical Mechanical Properties of Implant Materials

Alloy	Tensile strength (psi)*	0.2% Offset yield strength (psi)	Reduction of Area (%)	Elongation (%)	Fatigue strength (psi) (10^7 cycles)
Cast Vitallium® heat treated	115,000	70,000	15	45,000	
Vitallium® FHS® Forged	219,000	149,000	28	29	140,000
Vitallium® FHS® Swaged-forged	245,000	198,000	26	18	115,000
MP-35 Solution annealed	145,000	95,000	65	50	—
MP-35 Forged	175,000	140,000	65	28	85,000
MP-35 cold-Worked and aged	260,000	230,000	35	8	108,000
Micrograin®	192,000	116,000	15	14.5	115,000
Stainless steel Annealed	80,000	35,000	65	55	35,000
Stainless steel Cold-worked	140,000	115,000	55	22	55,000
Ti-6Al-4V Forged and annealed	140,000	130,000	40	15	80,000
Ti-6Al-4V Cold-worked and aged	160,000	150,000	25	10	100,000

*psi = per square inch

appliance will be prone to fatigue failure. In the case of hip prostheses, the use of configurations having a greater section modulus with rounded lateral and medial edges has resulted in prostheses designs which, when produced in forged high-strength cobalt-chrome (CoCr) and titanium (Ti) alloy, displayed superior fatigue-resistant characteristics in vitro and in vivo. Proper design must be coupled with higher fatigue-strength materials in order to ensure prostheses which will serve without breakage in those areas where high stresses are expected (Chapter 3).

If the stress magnitude applied by the patient on a prosthesis is below that which would be required to initiate fatigue cracking mechanism, it is reasonable to expect that the integrity of the device will endure. However, there are occasions when an incrementally high stress is applied which could initiate a crack that progresses if a sufficiently large number of stress cycles are applied. The material and design must anticipate such overload so that the prosthesis will serve the patient without danger of fatigue breakage. Orthopaedic appliance endurance is increased with proper instruction to the patient; this instruction is a fundamental and significant factor in the implant's ultimate success or failure.

The stresses applied to an implant are dependent on the activity level of the patient; they could reach significant values which might have an adverse effect.

Such would be the case in the patient skiing, engaging in intensive tennis play, or mountain-climbing. These are cases where particular stresses of sufficiently high value could be applied to initiate the beginning of a fatigue crack.

It is generally recognized that when a material is exposed to a corrosive environment, such as a human implant, the endurance limit or fatigue strength of the material will be lower than when tested in an air environment. It is imperative that materials be corrosion-fatigue resistant to the environment to obviate corrosion induced fatigue failure. The materials used today for hip prostheses have displayed adequate corrosion resistance and biocompatibility characteristics for successful implant performance.

MICROSCOPIC EVALUATION OF FATIGUE FRACTURE

A fatigue fracture is examined initially with a relatively low magnification microscope or binoculars to determine if specific characteristics of fatigue failure actually exist. One should focus on the lateral area, as it is more highly stressed in tension. Fatigue breakage in metal structures originates from and is caused by the imposition of repetitive tensile stresses of sufficiently high magnitude and for a sufficient number of cycles.

In many cases, fatigue striations or "tide marks" are the characteristic features found on fatigue-fracture surfaces; they usually center around a common point that corresponds to the fatigue-crack origin. Such markings are colloquially called clamshell, conchoidal, and arrest marks. These markings occur as a result of loading and frequency, or by oxidation of the fracture surface during the period when there is crack arrest due to intermittent application of stress on the part or component. The photomicrograph in Figure 7-8 shows portions of the fracture surfaces of a broken prosthesis stem illustrating the corresponding positions of the fatigue rings on each section at a magnification of 8×. On closer analysis (magnification of 20), in Figure 7-9, the rings are followed to the point of origin; this point is usually at or near the lateral surface. At times, it is important to study the characteristics of a fatigue-fracture surface with an electron microscope to ascertain the integrity of the material as well as to observe the characteristic shape of the surface which has resulted from the propagation of a fatigue crack.

Figures 7-10A and B are photographs taken on the electron microscope at a magnification of 1700×, showing the many striations which occurred during the propagation of the fatigue crack across the prosthesis stem illustrated in Figures 7-8 and 7-9. The arrows point in the direction of the approximate location of the fatigue origin.

In order to observe the characteristics of the fracture surface and fatigue rings at still higher magnification, a photograph was made at a magnification of approximately 5700×, Figure 7-12. Here one can clearly see many striations which resulted from successive application of stress and periods of resting by the patient.

Once the crack has progressed to a point where the remaining uncracked cross-section becomes too weak to sustain the loads imposed by the patient, cracking may occur in a rapid manner across the remainder of the structure through a "tearing" or acute type process (Fig. 7-5), rather than the successive crack

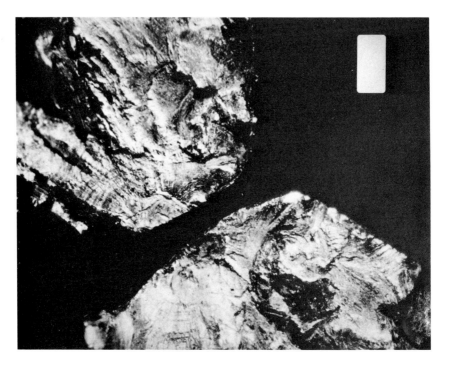

Figure 7-8. Cross-section of fractured stem (8×).

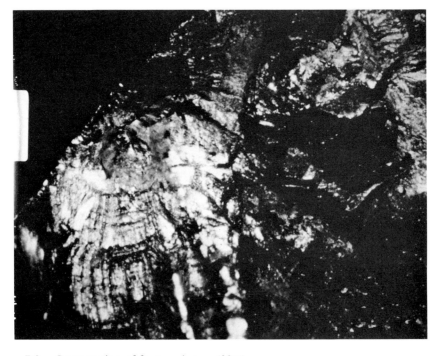

Figure 7-9. Cross-section of fractured stem (20×).

160

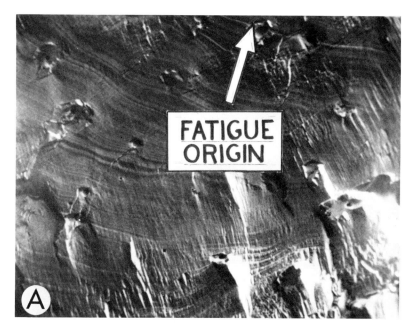

Figure 7-10A. Cross-section of fractured stem (1700×).

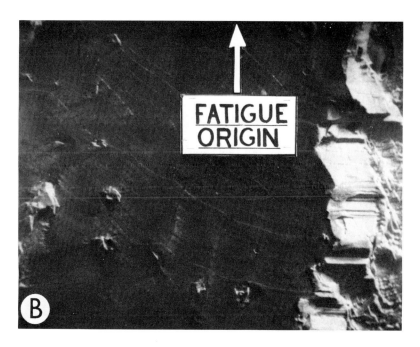

Figure 7-10B. Cross-section of fractured stem (1700×).

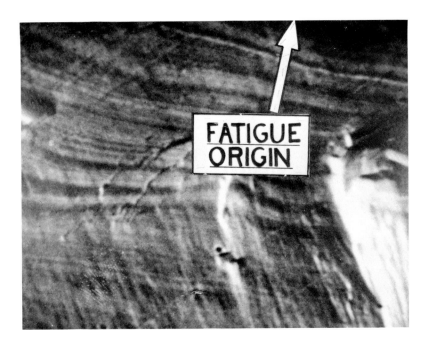

Figure 7-11. Cross-section of fractured stem (5700×).

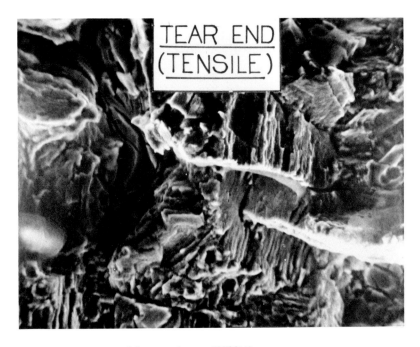

Figure 7-12. Cross-section of fractured stem (5700×).

162

propagation as indicated by the fatigue rings shown in Figures 7-8 to 7-11. There is a significantly different appearance and characteristic to this area as compared to the example shown in Figures 7-8 through 7-11. There are times when a prosthesis breaks in a fatigue mode but the identification possibility is lost because the two portions of the prosthesis repetitively contact each other after total breakage, thus obliterating many of the original surface characteristics. In such cases, it is difficult to establish whether the breakage occurred through fatigue.

EVOLUTION OF SURGICAL TECHNIQUES

The fractured femoral stem presents one of the most challenging problems to the surgeon attempting revision of a failed total hip arthroplasty. Removal of a retained stem fragment without inadvertant perforation or fracture of the femoral shaft is difficult and technically demanding. Specific techniques for stem extraction have evolved in the treatment of 29 patients who presented with fractured femoral stems at the New England Baptist Hospital. The general technique of femoral revision arthroplasty is well described in Chapter 4, but certain points in the surgical technique deserve repetition with additional emphasis on those specific techniques which relate to stem extraction.

Each patient undergoes a thorough pre-operative medical and surgical evaluation, as outlined in Chapter 1. Even if the cause of failure appears to be fracture of the endoprosthesis, there is no reason to assume that it is the sole cause of failure. Indeed, bony resorption, with or without infection, can easily result in sufficient motion at the bone-cement interface to cause failure of the acrylic, followed by stem fracture. For this reason, we advocate a full diagnostic work-up to fully assess this complex problem.

A thorough analysis of the component position is mandatory when planning a revision of the broken prosthesis. It should be noted that extraction of the proximal fragment of a varus-placed stem leaves a laterally directed path within the cement column which may guide a drill or osteotomy out of the lateral cortex. Awareness of femoral component position relative to the long axis of the femur can help the surgeon compensate for an eccentric path in the acrylic and avoid inadvertant violation of the shaft.

We use the lateral decubitus position for revision surgery. A modified posterolateral incision is made through the old scar with the distal limb straight, allowing extension of the wound if necessary. Subcutaneous dissection is carried from normal tissue planes distally and carried proximally through the dense subcutaneous scar, re establishing tissue planes for closure. Trochanteric osteotomy is performed after release of the origin of the vastus lateralis about 5.0 mm distal to the vastus tubercle. The capsule is incised, and specimens of joint fluid are sent for Gram stain and culture; sections of the capsule are sent for pathological examination as well. A complete capsulectomy is then performed, providing complete visualization of the joint.

The femoral component is disarticulated from the acetabular cup with the hip in flexion, external rotation, and adduction, and the leg is placed in a sterile bag anteriorly. The femoral component is disimpacted and extracted. This will leave the retained distal fragment of the stem imbedded in acrylic. The residual proximal

Table 7-3

Prosthesis*	Metal†	Position	Fracture Site§	Window	TU-10
CM	C-CoCr	varus	7.0 cm	+	
CM	C-CoCr	varus	7.0 cm	+	
CM	C-CoCr	varus	12.5 cm	:pl	
CM	C-CoCr	varus	7.7 cm	+	
CM	C-CoCr	varus	9.4 cm	+	
CM	C-CoCr	valgus	3.8 cm	+	
C	W-SS	neutral	8.4 cm	+	
CM	C-CoCr	neutral	7.0 cm	+	
CM	C-CoCr	neutral	7.6 cm	+	
CM	C-CoCr	neutral	5.0 cm	+	
B	C-SS	varus	6.5 cm	+	
B	C-SS	varus	2.6cm	+	
CM	C-CoCr	varus	7.0 cm	+	+
B	C-SS	varus	10.7 cm		+
CM	C-CoCr	neutral	H-N		+
C	W-SS	valgus	11.1 cm		+
CM	C-CoCr	neutral	H-N		+
CM	C-CoCr	varus	8.6 cm		+
CM	C-CoCr	varus	6.8 cm		+
B	C-SS	varus	10.2 cm		+
CM	C-CoCr	neutral	6.5 cm		+
CM	C-CoCr	varus	7.5 cm		+
CM	C-CoCr	varus	8.2 cm		
CM	C-CoCr	varus	7.5 cm		
C	W-SS	neutral	8.0 cm		
CM	C-CoCr	varus	4.0 cm		
CM	C-CoCr	varus	3.5 cm		
C	W-SS	varus	7.2 cm		
C	W-SS	neutral	7.6 cm		

*CM = Charnley-Mueller
C   = Charnley
B   = Becktol
AT   = Aufranc-Turner
†C = cast
W = wrought
SS = stainless steel
CoCr = cobalt chrome
§Fracture site = distance along lateral edge from the distal tip to the
   site of fracture.
**12″ = 300 mm
11″ = 275 mm
10″ = 250 mm
 9″ = 225 mm
Reg = 110 mm
NEBH = 150 cm

164

Extraction Device	Intraoperative Complication	Exchange component**	EBL	Operating Time (min)
		AT12″	3120 cc	300
		AT reg	2000 cc	270
		AT 12″	4200 cc	300
		AT 12″	3150 cc	310
		AT 12″	1275 cc	240
		AT reg	1600 cc	270
		AT 10″	3350 cc	300
	Cortical Perforation	AT 9″	700 cc	270
		AT 10″	4000 cc	240
		AT 12″	2200 cc	360
		AT reg	2000 cc	300
		NEBH 15 cm	1500 cc	240
		AT 11″	2400 cc	330
		AT 12″	1800 cc	270
	Cortical Perforation	AT 10″	2725 cc	255
		CAD 12″	3412 cc	360
		AT 12″	2250 cc	285
		AT 10″	2900 cc	330
		AT 12″	1380 cc	360
		B reg	2700 cc	300
		AT 12″	1800 cc	270
		AT 10″	1800 cc	270
+		AT 12″	2400 cc	300
+		AT 10″	2300 cc	300
+		AT 9″	2000 cc	250
+		AT 10″	2100 cc	300
+		AT 11″	2300 cc	270
+		AT 10″	2250 cc	240
+		AT 10″	2600 cc	300

column of cement is fragmented with long, thin osteotomes under the direct vision afforded by a fiberoptic headlamp. Care is taken to avoid following the track left by the removed proximal fragment if that track is laterally directed. When further use of osteotomy endangers the cortex or becomes too difficult, a high-speed, low-torque pneumatic drill is used to remove the last traces of cement and to debride the layer of fibrous granulation tissue resident at the bone-cement interface. At this point, the surgeon must address the problem of the retained femoral stem.

PRIOR TECHNIQUE

"Window" or "Gutter" in Cortical Bone

Prior to the advent of the intramedullary drilling technique, removal of cement and fractured stems was effected through a cortical window or gutter cut into the femoral shaft. This technique was used in 13 of our cases (Table 7-3). The stress-raiser created in the femoral cortex by this procedure was exacerbated if the window was placed laterally where tensile stresses are highest (Fig. 7-13). Because this technique required the exposure of the distal shaft, the potential incidence of

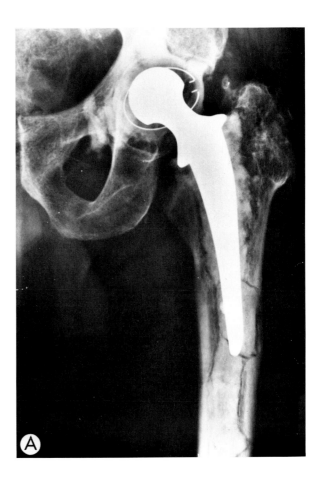

Figure 7-13A. Laterally placed window with evidence of underlying cement fracture.

nonunion was excessive.[43] With modern techniques (to be discussed below), cortical windows should rarely be required. If a window becomes necessary, however, it should be made in the anterior cortex where tensile stresses are less severe.

With the introduction of the high-speed drill, proximal extraction of the retained femoral stem without a cortical window became feasible. Several techniques have developed which have revolutionized the treatment of the retained stem.

Intramedullary Cement Removal with Long, High-speed Power Tools

The development of the Midas Rex TU-10 dissecting tool (Fig. 7-14) for the high-speed drill permitted the surgeon to incise the cement column surrounding the retained stem. This technique alone was used in 10 of our cases. The thin end of this dissecting tool, which can be extended deep into the femoral shaft by means of specially matched equipment combinations, allowed some maneuvering within the narrow confines of the shaft, thereby bringing the previously untouchable cement within the reach of the power drill. Careful monitoring of the dissecting tool with a C-arm fluoroscope was routinely performed to prevent cortical perforation by the

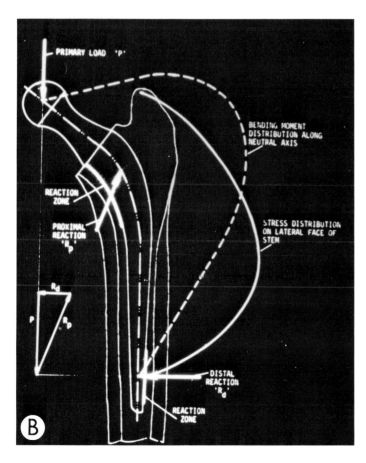

Figure 7-13B. Analytical stress model demonstrating the stress distribution on the lateral stem and cortex.

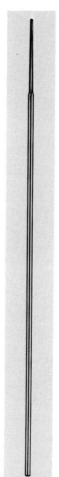

Figure 7-14.   TU-10 Cutting tool.

drill. In this matter, the surgeon could erode the acrylic away from the stem fragment until the stem was free and it could be grasped and extracted.

Although this technique of incising the cement around the broken stem was a significant advance over the prior window or gutter techniques, peripheral cement removal was difficult in certain instances. Extremely narrow canal diameters could frustrate the surgeon's attempts to circumscribe the stem with the slender dissecting tool, and twice led to inadvertent cortical perforation in which the defects were obturated by cancellous bone grafting. Clearly the problem to be solved was how to directly extract the metal stem without jeopardizing the femoral cortex.

PRESENT TECHNIQUE

Intramedullary Drilling and Extracting of the Stem Fragment

The latest technique in the armamentarium of revision surgery for broken stem extraction, briefly summarized (Fig. 7-15 and 7-16), includes a Midas Rex WH-3 dissecting tool for drilling into the presenting metal of the broken stem, and the WH-4 dissecting tool for creating an undercut inside the bottom of the drilled home. Both are effective and efficient when used as designed with the high-speed drill.[27] After the undercut hole is completed, a congruently shaped extractor device is locked into the hole, and a slap-hammer is attached so that the stem fragment may be removed by retrograde impaction. This procedure for removing broken stems may be accomplished without damage to the cortical bone.

A closer look at the procedure begins when the proximal portion of the broken stem is removed and the retained distal stem fragment is exposed. Using the long dissection tool under direct vision, peripheral cement is cleared from around the proximal end of the stem fragment for about a centimeter's depth (Fig. 7-17). If there is unusual geometrical design in the broken stem which creates cement barriers, these should be removed by dissection with the long TU-10 tool. Should the proximal cement in the canal limit the desired angle of drilling into the metal stem fragment, enough cement must be removed to allow the desired drilling angle.

At this point a special drill guide is inserted over the retained stem (Fig. 7-16). The various shapes of the presenting broken stems sometimes allow the guide to settle over the stem like a cap; in other cases the guide can only rest against the metal fragment. The drill guide must be held so as to prevent the end cutting tool from wandering from the center of the broken surface of the stem during the initial stem drilling. Attention to this detail is crucial at this point, because excess side motion of the drill creates a hole too large to obtain firm fixation with the extraction device. The handled attachment is fitted with the WH-3 tool and inserted into the

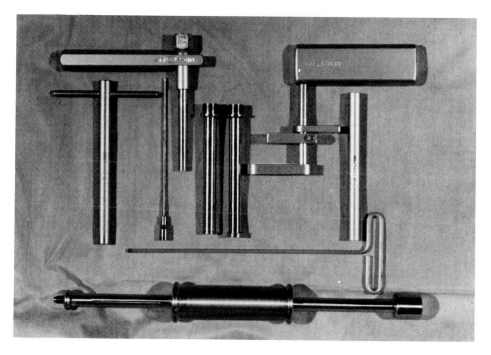

Figure 7-15. Equipment for intermedullary drilling and extraction of the distal fractured stem.

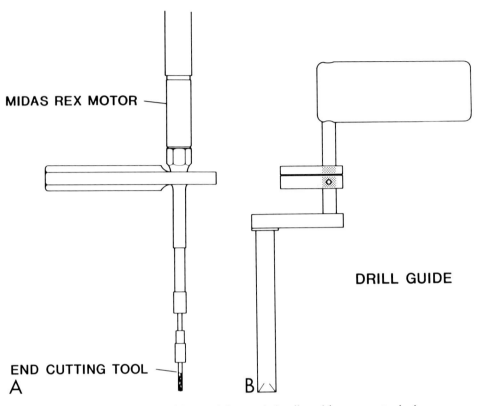

MIDAS REX MOTOR

DRILL GUIDE

END CUTTING TOOL

A

B

Figure 7-16A. WH3 cutting tool in special extended collet with motor attached.
Figure 7-16B. Drill guide in which apparatus in which cutting tool (Fig. 7-16A) is inserted.

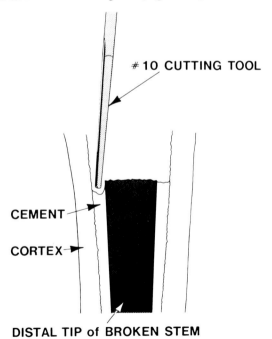

#10 CUTTING TOOL

CEMENT

CORTEX

Figure 7-17. TU-10 dissecting tool is used to expose the proximal portion of the retained distal stem.

DISTAL TIP of BROKEN STEM

drill guide; the special ¼" depth control measurement is set (Fig. 7-18); and the hole is drilled to the preset depth of ¼" (Figs. 7-19 and 7-20). A continuous, copious flow of irrigation is required to remove metallic debris and to dissipate heat.

Once the hole has been drilled, the initial drilling tool is removed and the WH-4 is utilized to effect an undercut at the bottom of the hole (Fig. 7-21). The attachment drilling mechanism is held perpendicular to the bottom of the hole; only lateral pressure is required to effect the undercut, which has two requirements: (1) the undercut spot must enter into a good body of metal; and (2) at 180° opposite, there must exist enough metal to buttress the wedge when it is later extended to lock in the extractor device.

The stem extractor tool, threaded into a cannulated T-handle, is then inserted into the prepared hole in the stem so that its protruding "toe" fits into the undercut at the bottom of the hole (Fig. 7-22). With a hex-wrench insert holding the toe in place in the undercut, the cannulated T-handle is rotated so as to travel distally down the threaded extractor, causing a metal flange to emerge laterally from a groove of the extractor device (Fig. 7-23). This flange acts as a wedge to firmly lock the shaped extractor into the shaped hole. The slap-hammer is then screwed onto the locked extractor and T-handle, and the entire unit is disimpacted proximally, neatly extracting the broken stem without cortical damage (Fig. 7-24).

This procedure is not without its problems, and attention to detail is crucial. Should the extractor slip out without pulling the broken stem, the surgeon should make sure that the undercut is sufficient, that the wedge is sufficiently tightened, and that the geometrical shape of the broken stem is not creating cement barriers requiring further dissection at the metal-cement interface. Residual cement is then fragmented, drilled, and removed in the usual manner. This drilling technique is

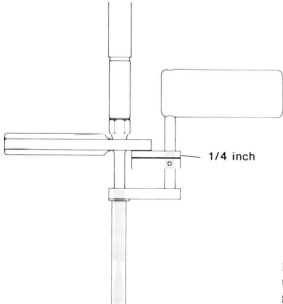

1/4 inch

Figure 7-18. The motor and cutting tool have been installed into the drill guide and the depth guide is adjusted to allow ¼" penetration into the retained distal stem.

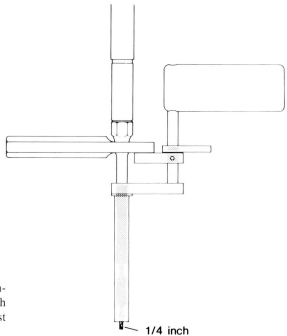

Figure 7-19. Drilling tool has penetrated broken stem ¼″; note depth guide has been set aside to allow just ½″ penetration.

1/4 inch

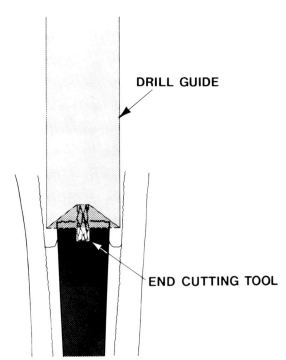

DRILL GUIDE

END CUTTING TOOL

Figure 7-20. Schematic of hole-drilling process.

172

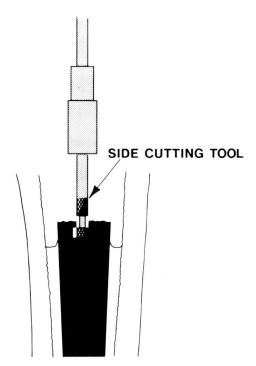

SIDE CUTTING TOOL

Figure 7-21. Side cutting tool. Use lateral pressure to undercut at a place offering a goody body of metal.

successful in all metals, including the superalloys. Reconstruction of the femoral side of the arthroplasty is then performed, in the technique described in Chapter 4.

Fractured stem revision surgery is one of the technically more difficult types of revision arthroplasty. This difficulty has stimulated much thought toward improving the methods for extracting the fragment with minimal trauma to the patient. Operative time was not significantly different for each method, and the blood loss for each method was statistically equivalent (Table 7-4). The average operative time when utilizing the cortical window was approximately 20 minutes less than the other procedure, but equivalent experience with the newer procedures is lacking. As a new technique becomes more familiar and is thoroughly mastered, stem extraction will be greatly facilitated and blood loss and operative time should decrease.

Utilization of the cortical window establishes a structural defect in the cortex. The potential incidence of nonunion is high, because of complete violation of both the endosteal and periosteal blood supplies to the window. A femoral hip prosthesis functions as a composite of three materials: bone, cement, and metal. When the bone is compromised by a cortical window, higher stresses are subsequently

Table 7-4

Method	No. of patients	Average EBL	Operating time Average (in minutes)
Window	13	2422.6	286.9
TU-10	10	2316.7	303
WH-3	7	2278.5	280

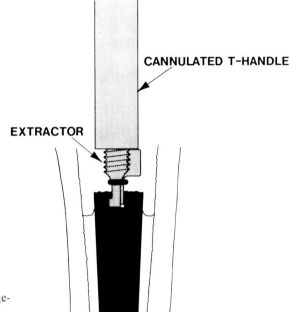

Figure 7-22. Extractor with wedge-locking toe into undercut hole.

transmitted to the other two phases of the composite, increasing their potential for failure.

In order to bypass the pathologic cortical tube created by removal of the fractured implant and the surrounding cement, reach the area in the femur where the stresses become more normal, and reach adequate cancellous bone for rigid fixation of the femoral stem, we have utilized the longer stemmed Aufranc-Turner femoral components in our revision hip arthroplasty, as outlined in Chapter 3. In the present study, the maximum length of the prosthetic stem was limited by the anatomic anterior lateral bow of the femur.

We have utilized three different techniques for removal of the distal fractured stem over the past 6 years and presently recommend direct proximal extraction of the distal fractured stem by center-drilling of the stem and utilizing the extraction device for removal through intermedullary dissection.[27]

The clinical results of revision arthroplasty for a fractured femoral stem are comparable with revision arthroplasty for loosening. Direct proximal extraction of the fractured stem can be expected to improve the clinical results.

We have analyzed the functional results of revision surgery on our 29 patients. These patients were evaluated for residual pain, active range of motion, and activity level; results are summarized in Table 7-5.

SUMMARY

Femoral stem fracture is a complex problem. A multitude of clinical and technical factors integrate to cause a fracture in a femoral stem. The clinical and radiographic experience with this problem at the New England Baptist Hospital is

Table 7-5
Functional Results

No. of Patients	Pain	ROM	Activity
18	None	Equal to Preoperative	Equal to pre-operative
6	None	F < 90°	Mild ↓
3	Yes	F < 90°	Sedentary level
2	—	Unassociated expiration	—

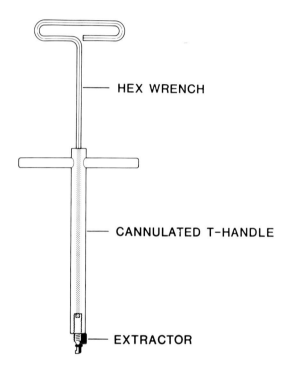

HEX WRENCH

CANNULATED T-HANDLE

EXTRACTOR

Figure 7-23. Clockwise rotation of T-handle drives wedge of extractor downward to lock toe into undercut hole. Note extractor with wedge driven down.

presented to aid the surgeon in identifying symptomatic arthroplasties that are at risk for stem fracture. When these patients are identified, protection of the hip or prophylactic revision is indicated. The mechanics of fatigue failure and relevant metallurgy are discussed to give one an increased awareness and deeper insight into the problem of stem fracture.

When a patient presents with a fractured femoral stem as an etiology to the symptomatic arthroplasty, then revision surgery is indicated. Pre-operative evaluation and specific techniques for extraction of the retained distal stem fragment are discussed. The basic premises regarding revision surgery in stem fracture are (1) thorough pre-operative analysis, (2) wide surgical exposure with trochanteric osteotomy, (3) intramedullary drilling and extraction of the distal stem fragment, and (4) reconstruction with a longer femoral stem of a modern design fabricated from a high-strength superalloy.

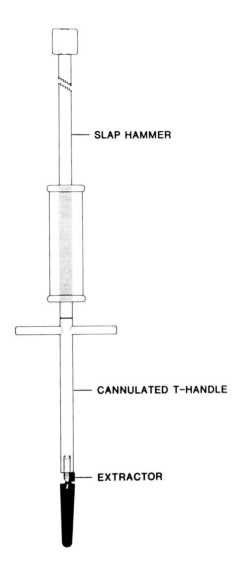

Figure 7-24. Slap-hammer attached to cannulated T-handle; broken stem has been extracted from cement with repetitive taps.

REFERENCES

1. Amstutz HC: Loosening of total hip femoral components: cause and prevention, in *The Hip: Proceedings of the Fourth Open Scientific Meeting of the Hip Society.* St Louis, CV Mosby, 1976.

2. Andriacchi TP, Galante JO, Belytschko TB, et al: A stress analysis of the femoral stem in total hip prosthesis. *J Bone and Joint Surg* 58(A):618–623, 1976.

3. Bechtol CO: Failure of femoral implant components in total hip replacement operations. *Orthop Rev* 4:23–29, 1975.

4. Bechenbaugh RD, Ilstrup DM: Looking back at total hip arthroplasty. A review of thirty-three hips four to seven years after surgery with special emphasis on loosening and wear. Paper presented at the 45th Annual Meeting of the American Academy of Orthopaedic Surgery, Dallas, February 1978.

5. Blacker GJ, Charnley J: Long-term study of changes in the upper femur after low-

friction arthroplasty. Paper presented at the 44th Annual Meeting of the American Academy of Orthopaedic Surgery, Las Vegas, February, 1977.

6. Blackwell RS, Pilliar RM: Fatigue in a hostile environment. *Industr Rsch.* March 1977, pp 89–93.

7. Bocco F, Langan P, Charnley J: Changes in the calcar femoria in relation to cement technology in total hip replacement. *Clin Orthop* 128:287–295, 1977.

8. Brockhurts PJ, Svensson NL: Design of total hip prosthesis—the femoral stem. *Med Prog Technol* 5:83–102, 1977.

9. Carlsson AS, Gentz CF, Stenport J: Fracture of the femoral prosthesis in total hip replacement according to Charnley. *Acta Orthop Scand* 48:650–655, 1977.

10. Chao EYS, Coventry MD, Rostoker W, et al: Biomechanical analysis of fractured femoral components. Paper presented at the First International Hip Society Meeting, Kyoto, Japan, October 1978.

11. Chao EYS, Coventry MD: Fracture of the femoral component after total hip replacement: An analysis of fifty-eight cases. *J Bone and Joint Surg* 63A:1078–1093, 1981.

12. Charnley J: *Low-Friction Arthroplasty of the Hip.* Springer-Verlag, Berlin Heidelberg NY 1st Ed 1979.

13. Charnley J: A biomechanical analysis of the use of cement to anchor the femoral head prosthesis. *J Bone and Joint Surg* 47(B):354–363, 1965.

14. Charnley J: Fracture of femoral prostheses in total hip replacement. A clinical study. *Clin Orthop* 111:150, 1975.

15. Charnley J, Follacci FM, Hammond BT: The long-term reaction of bone to self-curing acrylic cement. *J Bone and Joint Surg* 50(B):822–827, 1968.

16. Clarke IC, Gruen T, Matos M, et al: Improved methods for quantitative radiographic evaluation with particular reference to total hip arthroplasty. *Clin Orthop* 121:83–89, 1976.

17. Collis DK: Femoral stem fracture in total hip replacement. *J Bone and Joint Surg* 59(A):1033–1039, 1977.

18. Crowninshield RD, Brand RA, Johnston RC, et al: An analysis of femoral component stem design in total hip arthroplasty. *J Bone and Joint Surg* 62(A):68–78, 1980.

19. Ducheyne P, Aernoudt E, Martens M, et al: Fatigue fractures of the femoral component of Charnley and Charnley-Müller type total hip prostheses. *J Biomed Mat Res* 9:199–219, 1975.

20. Fornasier VL, Cameron HU: The femoral stem-cement interface in total hip replacement. *Clin Orthop* 116:249–255, 1976.

21 Galante JO, Rostoker W, Doyle JM: Failed femoral stems in total hip prostheses. A report of six cases. *J Bone and Joint Surg* 57(A):230–236, 1975.

22. Greenwald SA, Nelson CA: Biomechanics of the reconstructed hip. *Orthop Clin N Amer* 4:2, 1973.

23. Goel VK, Svensson NL: The finite element stress analysis of a human femur fitted with Charnley prosthesis. Paper presented at the Sixth Australian Conference on the Mechanics and Materials, Christ Church, New Zealand, August 1977.

24. Gruen TA, McNeice GM, Amstutz HC: Modes of failure of cemented stem type femoral components—a radiographic analysis of loosening. *Clin Orthop* 141:17–27, 1979.

25. Hamati YI, Scott R, Stillwell WR, et al: Long-term follow-up on long stem total hip replacement. (Submitted for publication to *J Bone and Joint Surg.* 1980.)

26. Harris WH, Schiller AL, Scholler JM, et al: Extensive localized bone resorption in the femur following total hip replacement. *J Bone and Joint Surg* 58(A): 612–617, 1976.

27. Harris WH, White RE, Mitchell S, et al: A new technique for removal of broken femoral stems in total hip replacement. *J Bone and Joint Surg* 63A:843–845, 1981.

28. CAD Total Hip Presentation, Howmedica, Inc, 1976.

29. Huiskes R, Elangovan PT, Banens JPA, et al: Finite element computer methods for

design and fixation problems of orthopaedic implants. *Lab of Exp Orthop*, Dept of Orthopaedics, The Netherlands, University of Nijmegan, 1978.

30. Jaeger JH, Gaesener R, Briot B, et al: Fracture of total hip arthroplasties at the level of the femoral component. *Acta Orthop Belg* 40:861–876, 1974.

31. Kwak BM, Lim OK, Kim YY, et al: Study on the effect of cement thickness in an implant by finite element stress analysis. *Internat Orthop* 2:315–319, 1978.

32. Markolf KL, Amstutz HC: A comparative experimental study of stresses in femoral total hip replacement components: the effects of prostheses orientation and acrylic fixation. *J Biomech* 9:73–80, 1976.

33. Markolf KL, Amstutz HC: Stem fracture in total hip replacement. AAOS Committee of Biomechanical Engineering Exhibit, New Orleans, Academy Meeting, February 1977.

34. Markolf KL, Amstutz HC, Hirchowitz DL: The effect of calcar content on femoral compartment micromovement. A mechanical study. *J Bone and Joint Surg* 62(A):1315–1320, 1980.

35. Marmor L: Femoral loosening in total hip replacement. *Clin Orthop* 121:116–122, 1976.

36. Martens M, Aernoudt E, DeMeester P, et al: Factors in the mechanical failure of the femoral component in total hip prosthesis. *Acta Orthop Scand* 45:693–710, 1974.

37. McNeice GM, Amstutz EC: Finite element studies in hip reconstruction. Biomechanics V-A Proceedings of the Fifth International Congress of Biomechanics, Jyvaskyla, *Finland 1975*, Komi PV, ed. Baltimore, Maryland, Baltimore University Park Press, p 394, 1976.

38. Nicholson OR: Failed femoral stems in total hip prostheses. Proceedings of the New Zealand Orthopaedic Association. *J Bone and Joint Surg* 58(B):262, 1976.

39. Oh I, Harris WH: Proximal strain distribution in the loaded femur. An in vitro comparison of the distributions in the intact femur and after insertion of different hip replacement femoral components. *J Bone and Joint Surg* 60(A):75–85, 1978.

40. Park HW, Scheller AD, Harris JM: Mechanical analysis of femoral hip arthroplasty composites as a function of stem length. (Submitted for publication to *Clin Orthop* 1980.)

41. Paul JP: Load actions on the human femur during walking and some stress resultants. *Exper Mechan* 121–125, 1971.

42. Paul JP: Force actions transmitted by joints in the human body. *Prox R Soc Lond* 192(B):163–172, 1976.

43. Rhinelander FW: Tibial blood supply in relation to fracture healing. *Clin Orthop* 105:34–81, 1974.

44. Rostoker W, Chao EY, Galante JO: Defects in failed stems of hip prostheses. *J Biomed Mat Res* 12:635–651, 1978.

45. Rybick EF, Simoner FA, Weis EB Jr: On the mathematical analysis of stress in the human femur. *J Biomech* 5:203–215, 1972.

46. Rydell N: Intravital measurements of forces acting on the Hip Joint, in Evans FG (ed): *Studies on the Anatomy and Function of Bone and Joints.* New York, Springer-Verlag, pp 52–68, 1966.

47. Salvati EA, Im VC, Aglieti P, et al: Radiology of total hip replacements. *Clin Orthop* 121:74–80, 1976.

48. Scales JT: Fractures of the femoral component—the need for fatigue studies. Paper presented at the 42nd Annual Meeting of the American Academy of Orthopaedic Surgeons, San Francisco, 1975.

49. Scheller AD, Hamati YI, Stillwell WT, et al: Femoral component fracture in total hip replacement. (Submitted for publication to *J Bone and Joint Surg*, September 1979.)

50. Svensson NL, Valliappan S, Wood RD: Stress analysis of human femur with implanted Charnley prosthesis. *J Biomech* 10:581–588, 1977.

51. Teuber E, Kottmann B: Vergleichende analyse der schaft-geometrie haufig verwendeter endoprosthesen fur das huftgelenk. *Chirurg* 47:674–681, 1976.

52. Walker PS: The optimum use of materials in total hip design, in The Hip: Proceedings of the Fifth Open Scientific Meeting of the Hip Society. St Louis, CV Mosby Co, 1973, pp 46–66.

53. Weber FA, Charnley J: A radiological study of fracture of acrylic cement in relation to the stem of a femoral head prosthesis. *J Bone and Joint Surg* 58(B):297–303, 1975.

54. Weightman B: The stress in total hip prosthesis femoral stems: a comparative experimental study, in Schaldach M, Hohmann D (eds): *Advances in Artificial Hip and Knee Joint Technology.* New York, Springer-Verlag, 1976.

55. Williams JF, Svensson NL: A force analysis of the hip joint. *Biomed Engin* 365–370, 1968.

56. Wroblewski BM: The mechanisms of fracture of the femoral prosthesis in total hip replacement. *Internat Orthop (SICOT)* 3:137–139, 1979.

57. Zeide MS, Pugh J, Jaffee WL: Failure of femoral component in total hip replacement arthroplasty: a case study failure analysis. *Orthop* 1:291–293, 1978.

58. Zickel RE, Amstutz HC: Metal and orthopaedic surgery. Committee on Biomedical Engineering Exhibit, AAOS Annual Meeting, San Francisco, 1978.

Jo Miller, William R. Krause,
William H. Krug, and Lydia C. Kalaby

8

Implant Fixation

Secure and enduring fixation of implant components is fundamental to the entire concept of total joint arthroplasty. This objective may seem unreachable for the surgeon undertaking revision surgery for the failed hip. The setting is usually less than ideal; trabecular bone has disappeared as a result of movement, granuloma formation, and/or sepsis. Calcar loss is common. The canal has become enlarged and the cortex has thinned, and perhaps perforated. The bony acetabulum may have been damaged or almost destroyed by cup migration.

The surgeon, in undertaking a revision, suggests by implication at least that this second (or third) procedure will not be complicated by loosening even though the operation utilizes components identical to those used in the first procedure (a metallic femoral component, a polyethylene acetabular component, and polymethylmethacrylate cement)

It is obvious, therefore, that the surgeon, operating "in the face of previous failure" must employ all possible skills to achieve fixation of implants to such a degree that loosening will be resisted for an indefinite period of time.

GENERAL CONCEPTS OF FIXATION

Polymethylmethacrylate cement has been used in the large majority of joint replacements and is virtually the only acceptable material in revision arthroplasty. Implant fixation with acrylic cement is accomplished at the time of surgery, and the quality of this fixation is dependent on a large number of variables, many under the direct control of the surgeon.

181

REVISION TOTAL HIP ARTHROPLASTY
ISBN 0-8089-1466-9

It is fashionable to blame the acrylic cement for the high incidence of loosening currently being reported. The cement is "weak in tension," "brittle," and "only a grouting material"[16,20] It has been said to cause "thermal necrosis of bone," "toxic necrosis of bone," and even "an allergic reaction."[3,4,18] The view that "all implants are doomed to loosening" is currently popular.

In contrast to these pessimistic ideas, cement is capable of transmitting load from prosthesis to bone for prolonged periods without failure, as is evident from the significant incidence of cases with no loosening or cement fracture many years after surgery. This clearly implies that if joint arthroplasty with acrylic cement can be carried out in an ideal fashion, then firm and enduring fixation can be expected. Careful reviews have shown that the majority of loosenings can be explained on the basis of technical error, poor implant design, poor patient selection, or sepsis.[1,18,19] In any clinical review, three sites of loosening are apparent.[1] The system may loosen at the cement-bone interface, the cement may fracture, or there may be loosening between cement and prosthesis. It is increasingly apparent, however, that the cement-bone interface is of paramount importance; if this interface remains intact, then failure at the other sites is highly unlikely.

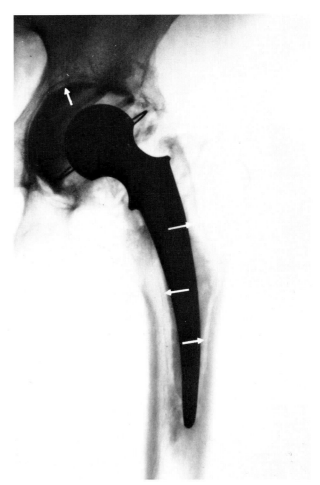

Fig. 8-1. Radiolucent line represents suboptimum cement-bone interface.

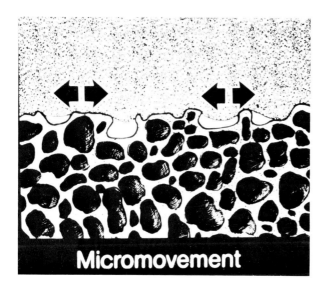

Fig. 8-2. The critical factor which provokes bone resorption at the cement-bone interface is micromovement.

A suboptimum cement-bone interface will probably begin to show signs of loosening in the early postoperative months. This interface is not static; the bone to which the cement is apposed is capable of rapid resorption and replacement by a fibrous membrane which is apparent on x-ray as the radiolucent line (Fig. 8-1). Increasing evidence from clinical and experimental studies suggests that the critical factor which provokes bone resorption in the absence of sepsis is inadequate fixation, at the microscopic level, allowing micromovement (Fig. 8-2).[13,17]

REQUIREMENTS FOR FIXATION

Bone cement as a glue is a concept which has long been discarded. Fixation depends entirely on mechanical considerations. The interface must be mechanically secure with respect to both gross movement and micro-movement; to accomplish this there are two specific requirements, bulk filling and micro-interlock.

Bulk Filling

Bulk filling is a term coined by Ling,[14] which describes complete filling by cement of the bone cavity to which it is apposed. The expression infers that cement is carefully applied to the bone surface and conforms exactly to the irregular shape or surface of the bone. The cement mass, in the femoral canal for example, is of a shape and size that precisely corresponds with that of the medullary canal. The cement is then grossly immobilized in relation to the bone, with a so-called interference fit. Load transfer tends to be evenly distributed over the interface, rather than to concentrate at a few sites of point contact which results from irregular or incomplete filling.

There are several requirements, at surgery, for ideal filling.

Clean bone surface is essential. It must be free of all traces of blood clot, fat,

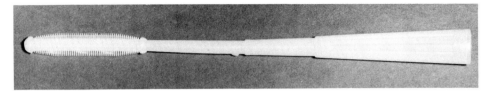

Fig. 8-3.   The intermedullary brush is used to prepare the femoral canal for cementing.

surgical debris, old cement and fibrous membrane which would result in poor cement-bone apposition. In the acetabulum, a clean bone surface can best be achieved by careful irrigation with a pulsating water jet. In the femoral canal, where the bone surfaces are less easily visualized, pulsating water-jet irrigation is supplemented by an intramedullary brush (Fig. 8-3). The brush should be used first as an extractor of debris, by inserting it to the prescribed depth, twisting, and withdrawing (Fig. 8-4). Large amounts of marrow, clot, and bone reamings are brought out, and can be disengaged from the bristles by tapping the brush in a kidney basin or by rinsing with a pulsating water jet. The canal is filled with irrigating saline and the brush used in a reciprocating fashion.

It may be useful to point out that the medullary canal, 6 inches distal to the

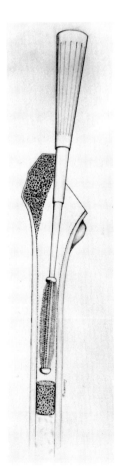

Fig. 8-4.   The brush is inserted into the plugged canal, twisted, and withdrawn. This step is repeated several times to remove clot and bone cuttings. The canal is then filled with irrigating saline, and the brush is used in a reciprocating fashion.

calcar, is often as wide as 16 to 20 mm. The use of a rasp with a tip only 4 mm wide is unlikely to completely remove all soft tissue. More recently, there has been a tendency to use a series of curettes, sizer-awls, or stiff-shafted reamers, *by hand,* simply to remove loose material. Care must be taken not to enlarge the canal or to destroy the bone interstices which are important for fixation.

Bleeding must be minimized.   It is well-recognized that blood clot on the bone surface results in a cement-bone defect. Active oozing after cement has been positioned will either displace the cement or dissect between cement and bone before polymerization occurs.

This problem can be minimized in a number of ways. Hypotensive anaesthesia reduces the magnitude of the problem.[15] Packing the femoral canal with a sponge or a tampon has been suggested as a possible means of reducing oozing.[2] Bleeding from marrow, distal to the site of the rasping, may be controlled in part by plugging of the canal. The plug has the additional advantage of containing the cement mass and of converting the proximal femur into a closed space suitable for pressurization. Application of pressure to the unpolymerized cement results in a tamponade, which further controls oozing.

In the acetabulum, hydrogen-peroxide-soaked sponges applied to cancellous surfaces for a few moments before cement application have been reported to reduce bleeding.[14]

Complete filling.   Cement must be applied in such a way that it is apposed as perfectly as possible to bone. Generally, the poorest apposition of cement to bone results from manual or digital insertion of acrylic into the femoral canal in a proximal to distal direction. This technique may also trap significant amounts of air in the canal. As the cement is forced in a distal direction and the prosthesis inserted, the air can, under certain circumstances, be forced into the venous circulation and may be responsible for some of the cases of hypotension seen during hip replacement surgery.[6]

Acrylic cement should be introduced into the femoral canal with a cement-delivery system beginning distally and filling in a progressively more proximal direction (Fig. 8-5). Intermingling of blood is reduced, air locks are eliminated, and gaps at the cement-bone interface are avoided. In summary, filling should be carried out in such a way that the canal contains nothing but acrylic cement.

Containment of cement before polymerization is essential. Unpolymerized cement "running out" of the femur or acetabulum, or movement of the implant has a deleterious effect on the cement-bone interface and subsequent fixation. Cement in a low-viscosity state is more likely to run out from the site where it has been placed than is doughy cement. In the femoral canal, containment may be enhanced by the use of a large prosthetic collar,[8] or by special stem configurations which render the lateral portion of the stem significantly wider than the medial portion. Containment may be achieved at the same time as cement pressurization with a delivery system and a cement restrictor tip (Fig. 8-6). In this situation, the cement is pressurized for a period varying from 60 to 90 seconds, until a considerable increase in viscosity has occurred, at which time the cement restrictor tip is removed and the prosthesis is inserted. This step will be discussed in more detail in another section.

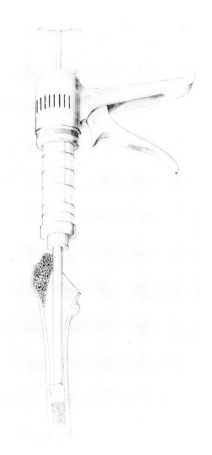

Fig. 8-5. A cement delivery system is essential to insure complete distal to proximal filling of the canal.

Micro-interlock

Acrylic cement does not adhere to bone, and there is no evidence that a biological bond can be established by ingrowth of bone into irregularities on the surface of the acrylic. There is increasing evidence, however, that fixation can best be obtained by forcing the cement to penetrate into the interstices and irregularities of the bone surface at the time of implantation. These mechanical interdigitations have been termed *micro-interlock*.

Doughy cement applied by hand cannot be induced to penetrate and form interlocks in a uniform and predictable fashion (Color Plate IV.1). Cement in a low-viscosity state, applied under pressure, will penetrate displacing marrow and form good mechanical interdigitations (Color Plate IV.2). Experimental studies indicate that these interdigitations should be at intervals of about ½ mm or less, in order to effectively prevent micromovement.[17] Mechanical studies reveal that the cement-bone interface produced by pressure penetration of low viscosity cement is two to four times stronger than that which results from the hand application of doughy cement. (Fig. 8-7).[10]

Microscopic examination of human post-mortem material and experimental animal studies indicate that micro-interlocks can endure for many years in a stable and unchanging fashion (Color Plate IV.3).

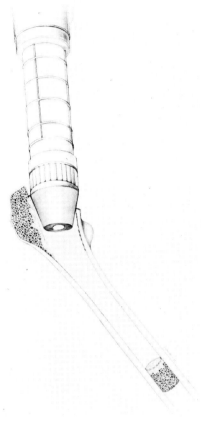

Fig. 8-6. The cement in the canal is pressurized to induce penetration into cancellous interstices.

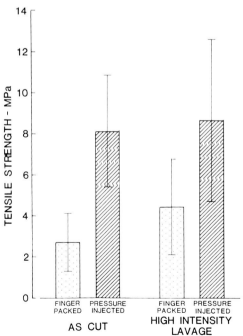

Fig. 8-7. Experimental studies have been carried out comparing the strength of cement-bone interface produced under various conditions. The pressure-injection of low-viscosity cement is clearly superior to finger-packing of doughy cement.

In the absence of micro-interlock, the interface is subject to micromovement and associated resorption of bone and replacement by a fibrous membrane (Fig. 8-8), appreciable on x-ray as a radiolucent line. The radiolucent line is not indicative of gross loosening, but simply indicates a loss of cement-bone contact at this site. There is considerable evidence to suggest that in any specific implant, bone resorption will eventually occur at sites where there are no micro-interlocks, and will not occur at sites where interlocks are present, thus explaining the phenomena of a partial radiolucent line. Incomplete microfixation may be sufficient to prevent gross loosening of the entire implant. In other situations, these interlocks may fail because of excessive loads, with the development of a "complete" radiolucent line.

To recapitulate: micro-interlock produces microfixation, which in turn prevents micromovement, bone resorption, and perhaps eventual gross loosening. Dominating this concept is the idea of a balance between the quality of fixation at the interface and the magnitude of load applied to it. A small individual or a person with multiple joint disease places fewer demands on his or her total hip, so that fixation of marginal quality will be effective. In contrast, the heavy or very active individual places large demands on his or her implant, so that even the most perfect micro-interlock may be subject to stress, great enough to produce micromovement, followed by bone resorption and its consequences.

To achieve micro-interlock, the following requirements must be met:

Bone interstices must be available for micro-interlock. The prepared femoral canal has extensive cancellous surfaces in the trochanteric region, and endosteal

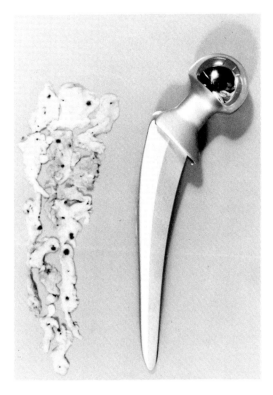

Fig. 8-8. Femoral component removed at revision arthroplasty. The extensive fibrous membrane obtained from the bone surface is typical.

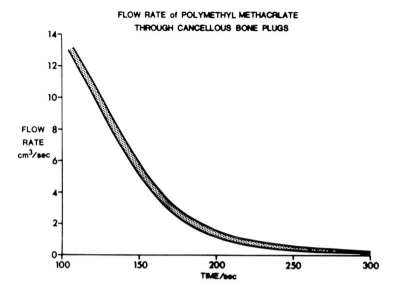

Fig. 8-9. The ability of acrylic cement to penetrate cancellous bone decreases as the viscosity of the cement increases. In an experimental setting, the flow rate of regular cement at 300 seconds after mixing is only a fraction of that rate at 100 seconds.

irregularities more distally suitable for cement intrusion. These interstices must be scrupulously cleaned for optimum fixation.

In the acetabulum, subchondral bone provides minimal opportunity for micro-interlock. In the early days of total hip replacement, some surgeons advocated removal of all subchondral bone; today it is generally agreed that preservation of a major portion (at least half) of the subchondral bone is a positive contribution to the structural integrity of the acetabular bone-cement-polyethylene composite. Micro-interlock must be produced at as many sites as possible, using drill or anchoring holes. These holes need be 1 cm deep or less, as the strongest cancellous bone is found just beneath the subchondral surface. It has been our practise to produce five to seven holes, ⅜ inch in diameter, and to intersperse a multitude of smaller-diameter holes.

Low-viscosity cement.   Cement, during the course of polymerization, progresses from liquid, low-viscosity material into higher viscosity doughy material, and then becomes rubbery material. The ability of cement to intrude into bone decreases as the viscosity values increase. Figure 8-9 indicates the rate of flow of acrylic cement through cancellous bone under constant pressure. The rate of flow, at 100 seconds after mixing, is approximately 13 cc/second; at 300 seconds, it is less than 1 cc/second. This study clearly indicates that the surgeon is less likely to be successful in achieving micro-interlock as he or she uses cement of increasing doughiness. Figure 8-10 indicates the viscosity characteristics of a number of commercially available cements intended for use during reconstructive joint surgery. Ideally, cement, at the time of its application to bone, should have a viscosity of 100 N sec/m² or less.

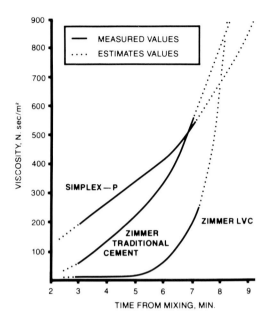

Fig. 8-10. The viscosity characteristics of several commercially available cements is indicated in this graph. For ideal penetration into bony interstices the cement should have a viscosity of 100 N sec/m² or less.

Pressure application. Cement in a low-viscosity state cannot be managed in a suitable fashion by the surgeon's gloved hand. Containment and pressure application of the cement is literally impossible. Cement must be applied to the bone surface under pressure if it is to penetrate and produce micro-interlock; this is best done with a cement delivery system. The delivery system should, in the ideal situation, be powerful and modular, with a variety of attachments for the various demands met during total joint reconstruction (Fig. 8-11).

Pressure measurements during the course of experimental total hip arthroplasty have shown that pressures of between 100 and 200 kPa (15–30 psi) can be maintained throughout the plugged femoral canal, using a delivery system and

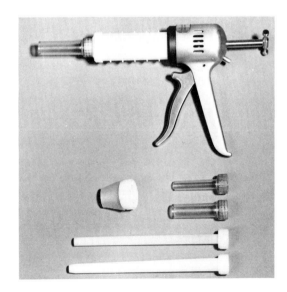

Fig. 8-11. The cement delivery system used in hip reconstruction should be powerful and modular, with a variety of attachments available to meet special demands. A very long flexible nozzle (not illustrated) facilitates complete filling of the middle and distal femoral canal.

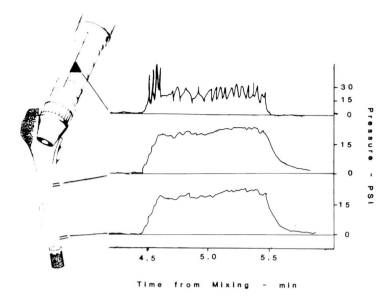

Fig. 8-12.   Using the cement delivery system, pressure in the femoral canal can be sustained without difficulty. This step induces cement penetration and, by creating a tamponade, diminishes blood oozing in the femoral canal.

cement-restrictor attachment (Fig. 8-12). This pressure is sufficient to induce cement, in a low-viscosity state, to intrude into bone interstices.

Pressurization in the acetabulum is considerably more difficult, but can be accomplished in a number of ways. Ling, in the early 1970s, introduced the concept of pressurization of the entire acetabulum,[12] and continues to use the method with success. More recently, other authors have advocated a silicone rubber cement restrictor device to apply pressure to the entire bolus of cement in the acetabulum. These devices all must utilize cement which is relatively doughy, since low-viscosity cement is prone to escape from the cement restrictor. Cement tends to penetrate along the path of least resistance and may establish micro-interlock at one site only. The system cannot be used if there is an unplugged perforation in the acetabulum floor.

A technique has been utilized since 1979; each fixation hole is separately pressurized, using the delivery system, together with a long, stiff, tapered nozzle (Fig. 8-13). The tip of the nozzle is forced into each hole in turn, and one or two squeezes of the gun trigger expresses a few ml of cement, achieving micro-interlock. The extent of penetration can be seen where tinted cement has been used in an experimental setting (Fig. 8-14).

FIXATION IN REVISION ARTHROPLASTY

The problems which present themselves to the surgeon at the time of revision arthroplasty are many. All have a bearing on the success of the procedure. There may be a serious depletion of bone stock in the proximal femur as a result of

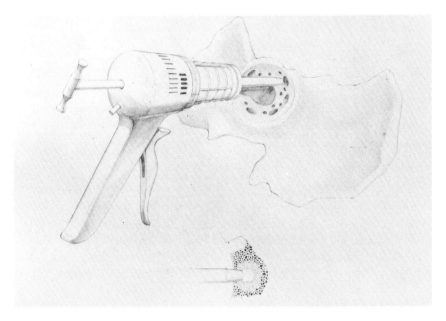

Fig. 8-13. Multiple shallow drill holes (3/8 inch in diameter), are pressurized using the cement delivery system and low-viscosity cement. The acetabulum is then cleared of excess cement and blood, dried, and filled with a bolus of doughy cement; the acetabular implant is then seated.

resorption due to movement, sepsis, massive osteolysis, perforation, or actual fracture. There is often considerable calcar loss. The femoral canal usually is enlarged as a result of bone resorption, thus increasing the size disparity between stem and canal. Loose cement fragments may be present.

The acetabulum may have been damaged in a variety of ways, including resorption of bone due to movement and progressive protrusio, occasionally so severe that the polyethylene cup lies free within the pelvis. The bone surfaces are unsuitable for new cement fixation because of the presence of a fibrous membrane. Anchoring holes, previously made to expose cancellous bone, are often recorticated and filled with cement and/or fibrous tissue.

The proximal femoral canal is lined with fibrous membrane, but the most serious deficiency is the almost complete disappearance of interstices or cancellous bone, providing little or no opportunity for micro-interlock. The femur has been converted, to a greater or lesser degree, into a cortical tube, suitable for fixation only by bulk filling. There is a high prospect for micromovement to develop at the cement-bone interface almost immediately after revision, with the early development of a major radiolucent line. Whatever small opportunities remain for micro-interlock must be utilized, but if the revision is to succeed, flawless bulk filling is essential.

The Proximal Femur

A number of decisions must be made regarding the management of the proximal femur. Removing a loose component, adding a little additional cement, and inserting a new component is not acceptable. Many of the questions which might come to the surgeon's mind regarding the proximal femur were well-answered in Chapter 4. Several additional points need to be made about the following: cement removal, membrane removal, osteolysis, and specific cementing techniques.

Removal of cement.   All loose fragments of cement should be removed. A number of authors have suggested leaving any well-fixed fragments,[5,7] as they are often difficult to remove and persisting efforts to remove them may cause damage to the contiguous cancellous bone, or even a perforation of the cortex.

A good case can be made for complete removal. The presence of old cement may prevent the proper orientation of a new stem in a neutral position. Remaining fragments may obstruct visualization of the canal distally, and may increase the difficulty of removing fibrous membrane from adjacent parts of the endosteal surface. New cement, inserted into the canal at the time of revision, is said to bond to old cement under optimum conditions,[7,11] but the concept is not dependable in practice, where surfaces are contaminated with blood, fat, and remnants of fibrous membrane.

In cases of sepsis, there is no choice, all cement must be removed, with rare exceptions as discussed in Chapter 13.

The fibrous membrane.   This is a constant finding at any site where cement fixation has failed (it may be as thick as 20 mm). The membrane is easily separated from the underlying cortex with a periosteal elevator, and with careful dissection can be cleanly removed in large pieces. A rasp or reamer tends to fray the membrane, and the remaining long strands result in multiple cement-bone interface defects.

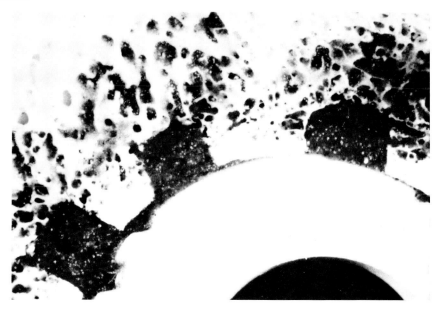

Fig. 8-14. Cross-section of a cadaver acetabulum in which methylene blue-tinted cement has been used. Note the extent of cement penetration. The drill holes are only about 1 cm deep.

Massive Osteolysis.   First described by Harris, et. al,[9] it is thought to be the result of a histiocytic granulomatous process, either in response to particles either from polyethylene wear or from fragmented arcylic cement.[21] The cortex is always very thin as a result of the proliferation of cellular soft tissue, and the canal invariably has been widened. The presence of a pathological fracture through one of these sites presents a particularly difficult problem. At revision, all traces of this granulomatous soft tissue must be removed before cement insertion.[9]

Low-viscosity cement vs doughy cement-pressurization.   Low-viscosity cement and doughy cement both have advantages and disadvantages in revision arthroplasty. Low-viscosity cement has superior intrusion characteristics, but this is of little value if there are no interstices available for interlock. In such cases, the fixation will depend almost entirely on bulk filling, which can be achieved in a satisfactory fashion with doughy cement. In a revision where a very long-stemmed femoral component is to be used, doughy cement may be difficult to express from a delivery system with a long nozzle; low-viscosity cement has a distinct advantage in this regard.

Low-viscosity cement should ideally be used in conjunction with pressurization; it is highly desirable to have the femoral canal plugged. Pressurization with the unplugged canal has a number of disadvantages. Cement may be forced distally beyond that point where it is useful. In the unplugged canal, marrow and fat might conceivably be embolized into the venous circulation. Pressurization with low-viscosity cement is obviously contraindicated in a situation where there may be an unidentified hole or breach in the shaft of the femur, since an unacceptable amount of cement would then be extruded into the soft tissue of the thigh. Wherever possible, shaft defects should be identified and blocked, either manually or with a carefully fashioned bone graft, before cementing.

"Short Stem" Fixation—Surgical Technique

Short stem prostheses are used only in selected cases of revision surgery. The short stem is satisfactory when the proximal femoral bone is very good and the femoral cortex is unviolated. Revision for femoral components malpositioned or femoral component breakage without gross loosening might represent situations where a short stem is acceptable.

The femoral canal is prepared by removal of all cement and all traces of fibrous membrane. The canal should be plugged at a point 1 in distal to the site of the stem tip (5½ to 6 in distal to the calcar), using one of the established methods. A cancellous bone plug has a number of advantages, and can be obtained from a bone bank femoral head. If bone is not available, polyethylene or silicone plugs can be used with comparable results, but represent an additional expense and an additional foreign body.

The canal is irrigated and repeatedly rinsed with sterile saline. The use of a polyethylene brush is essential, as is a pulsating irrigation system. All excess saline is suctioned out, and an attempt is made to dry the canal by repeated packing. Acrylic cement is introduced into the canal from distally to proximally, using a delivery system. Containment is important in order to prevent the cement from running out of the canal, particularly when low-viscosity cement is employed. This is accomplished in combination with pressurization.

It is strongly recommended that the patient be kept on minimal weight-bearing for a period of at least 8 weeks, and on protective weight-bearing for 4 to 6 months following surgery. There is some histological evidence to suggest that as a result of cement shrinkage, a gap forms between cement and bone at the time of polymerization; this is even more likely to occur in the absence of micro-interlock (Color Plate IV.4), or in a situation where there is a large disparity between stem and canal size. It has also been shown in experimental animals that this gap will fill with proliferating bone if the interface is protected from weight-bearing for a period of 8 to 12 weeks.[17] There is no clear evidence that this "filling-in" process will occur in humans, and the recommendation to delay full weight-bearing, although empirical, seems logical.

"Long Stem" Fixation—Surgical Technique

The long stem has the advantage of extending the fixation over a longer interfacial area into a part of the femur where the bone has not previously been disturbed. The stem bypasses sites of weakening from osteolysis or a surgical breach in the femur, and appears to maximize femoral component fixation following revision surgery.

The canal, which must be prepared to a depth of 7 to 10 in distal to the calcar, becomes increasingly less accessible to the surgeon with respect to cleaning, control of bleeding, and completeness of filling. Effective plugging of the metaphyseal flare of the femur is difficult and can be accomplished only by special techniques, as will be discussed later in this chapter. Accidental holes made in the femoral cortex may be difficult to detect. The reader is referred to Chapter 4 for special contrast radiographic techniques for detecting femoral perforations. The choice of low-viscosity vs regular cement has associated advantages and disadvantages. Low-viscosity cement is easier to deliver through the long nozzle of the cement delivery system. A longer working time for cement is desirable and can be accomplished by storing the cement in a refrigerator overnight before surgery. Pressurization of the canal insures better filling and produces a temporary tamponade, but in the unplugged canal the possibility of embolization of the canal contents must not be forgotten (this can also occur at the time of stem insertion). It is quite clear, however, that attempting to fill the canal by hand with doughy cement from the proximal end is ill-advised and should not be considered.

The canal is carefully prepared, using a pulsating irrigating system and a brush. If available, a long-handled brush will facilitate cleaning of the middle and distal portions of the canal.

Rationale for stem length in long stem revision arthroplasty is discussed in Chapters 3, 4, and 10. Once the stem length has been selected, the position of the distal stem should be documented by radiologic reference, if possible with the C-arm fluoroscope. The position of the distal stem can be marked by a hemostat on the drape, which in turn is visible on the x-ray image. An intramedullary cement plug is now established at the hemostat-marked level of the end of the femoral prosthesis by the technique described in Chapter 4. Plugging can also be achieved using a cement delivery system with a very long nozzle. Ten grams of low viscosity cement are introduced into the distal canal at the level previously identified.

Once the distal cement plug has polymerized, the long stem femoral component can be cemented with effective cement pressurization. Three to four mixes of cement will usually be required, depending on the length of the stem and the diameter of the canal. Careful planning and timing are essential.

It should be emphasized that cement formulated specifically to be used in a low-viscosity state has handling and setting characteristics which dramatically differ from those of traditional doughy cement. All cements are exceedingly sensitive to ambient temperature and humidity; under certain circumstances, they might thicken or even set deep within the canal before the prosthesis has been positioned. The surgeon and the operative team should familiarize themselves with the handling characteristics of cement and should practice its use in the operating room at temperatures and humidities which may be expected at the time of actual surgery. The operating room temperatures ideally should be in the range from 66 to 68°F. Temperatures above 70°F are undesirable.

The Acetabulum

The requirements for acetabular reconstruction, and the indications for acetabular rings, wire mesh, bone-grafting, and other augmentation procedures have been established by other authors.

It should be the aim of the surgeon to utilize exposed cancellous bone for micro-interlock wherever possible. When the acetabular component has been grossly loose, the bone surface will be covered with a fibrous membrane which must be removed. The old anchor holes can be utilized, but must be redrilled or curetted to remove recortication and expose cancellous bone. Additional shallow (3/8 in) anchoring holes can be produced for cement pressure penetration if undamaged portions of the acetabular wall are available. Numerous shallow small diameter drill holes should also be made.

Doughy cement is technically easier to use in the acetabulum, but it has inferior intrusion characteristics. Low-viscosity cement, in contrast, is difficult to use and tends to run out of the acetabulum or be displaced by oozing blood, but has superior intrusion characteristics. The most satisfactory technique employs two separate mixes of cement, one used in the doughy state and the other in the low-viscosity state. The low-viscosity cement is pressure-penetrated into fixation holes, achieving micro-interlock; the remainder of the acetabulum is filled with doughy cement to provide bulk filling. This technique takes advantage of the best qualities of the two cements.

Two-cement technique. Doughy cement is mixed in one bowl, and about 2 minutes later, low-viscosity cement is started in a second bowl. The low viscosity cement is poured into the cartridge of the cement delivery system which is used with a nozzle, suitable for pressurization of anchor holes.

The tip of the nozzle is forced into each anchor hole in turn (Fig. 8-13), and the gun trigger squeezed once or twice. Some cement will leak out from around the nozzle, and fat and bone marrow will be expressed from adjacent fixation holes onto the acetabulum floor. After all holes have been pressurized, the blood, fat, and cement spill is removed with a large curette, and the acetabulum is sponged and dried. The doughy cement is now introduced by hand as a bolus into the acetabulum, slightly spread out, and the prosthesis is positioned and seated. The doughy cement, with its easier handling characteristics, provides optimum bulk filling and fuses to the low-viscosity cement, which has been pressure penetrated into the anchoring holes.

SUMMARY

Revision arthroplasty of the hip presents numerous unique problems. The need for such secure fixation is more difficult to satisfy at the time of revision than at the time of original surgery. Fixation will, in the femoral canal, depend less on micro-interlock and more on complete filling of the canal with excellent cement-to-bone apposition. The major problem in the acetabulum is to achieve suitable fixation in the presence of deformity and loss of bone stock. Micro-interlock is an essential requirement in the acetabulum and can be produced by pressure-penetrating low-viscosity cement into drill holes.

REFERENCES

1. Amstutz HC, Markolf KL, McNeice GM et al: Loosening of total hip components: cause and prevention. In *The Hip* (Proceedings of the Hip Society), St. Louis, CV Mosby, 1976, p 102.
2. Amstutz HC: Personal communication, 1981.
3. Charnley J: A biomechanical analysis of the use of cement to anchor the femoral head prosthesis. *J Bone and Joint Surg* 47(B): 354–363, 1965.
4. DiPisa JA, Sih GS, Berman AT: The temperature problem at the bone-acrylic-cement interface of the total hip replacement. *Clin Orthop* 121:95–98, 1976.
5. Eftekhar NS: Principles of Total Hip Arthroplasty. St. Louis, CV Mosby Co, 1978, pp 519.
6. Gilbertson AA, Hoffman A, Kelebay LC et al: Hypotension during total hip arthroplasty. (Submitted for publication.)
7. Greenwald AS, Narten NC, Wilde AH: Points in the technique of recementing in the revision of an implant arthroplasty. *J Bone and Joint Surg* 60(B): 107–110, 1978.
8. Harris WH: Personal communication, 1981.
9. Harris WH, Schiller AL, Scholler J: Extensive localized bone and resorption in the femur following total hip replacement. *J Bone and Joint Surg* 58(A): 612–618, 1976.
10. Krause WR, Krug WH, Miller J: Cement-bone interface—effect of cement technique and surface preparation. *Trans Ortho Res Soc* 5: 76, 1980.
11. Latta L, Cohen J, Sarmiento A: The chemical bonding methylmethacrylate. *Trans Ortho Res Soc* 2: 237, 1977.
12. Lee AJC, Ling RSM: A device to improve the extrusion of bone cement into the bone of the acetabulum in the replacement of the hip joint. *Biomed Eng* 9:522–224, 1974.
13. Lee AJ, Ling RSM, Vangala SS: Some clinically relevant variables affecting the mechanical behavior of bone cement. *Arch Orthop Traumat Surg* 92:1–18, 1978.
14. Ling RSM: Total hip replacement using the collarless femoral prosthesis. Paper presented at the Eighth Open Scientific Meeting of the Hip Society, Atlanta, 1980.
15. Mallory TH: Hypotensive anaesthesian total hip replacement. *Orthop Rev* 4:21–30, 1975.

16. Markolf KL, Amstutz HC: In vitro measurement of bone-acrylic interface pressure during femoral component insertion. *Clin Orthop* 121:60–66, 1976.

17. Miller J, Krause WR, Drug WH, et al: Unpublished data.

18. Mueller ME: Late complications of total hip replacement. In *The Hip* (Proceeding of the Hip Society), St. Louis, CV Mosby, 1974, pp 319.

19. Oh I, Carlson CE, Tomford WW et al: Improvement fixation of the femoral component after total hip replacement using a methacrylate intramedullary plug. *J Bone and Joint Surg* 60(A): 608–613, 1978.

20. Walker PS: Human joints and their artificial replacements. Springfield, Ill, Charles C Thomas, 1977, pp 424.

21. Willert HG: The pathology of the bone-cement interface. Paper presented at the Second American Orthopaedic Association International Symposium, Boston, May 1981.

Michael A. R. Freeman, and
Gary W. Bradley

9

Surface Replacement Revision Arthroplasty

Surface replacement arthroplasty of the hip is a relatively recent innovation. Both the operative approaches and the prostheses vary significantly. The exposure required and most techniques of bone preparation demand methods subtly different from those used for conventional stemmed arthroplasty. In the few years during which hip resurfacing prostheses have been available, several prostheses have undergone design modifications to one or both of the components. Wagner, for example, no longer advocates a metallic femoral component; he now predicts increased longevity from the allegedly more desirable wear characteristics of ceramic.[22]

Because of the changes in prosthetic design, the small number of resurfaced hips available for review, and the short duration of actual implantation, the exact types and rates of failure for resurfacing procedures about the hip are not currently defined. The type and rate of failure now beginning to be appreciated may not necessarily be universally applicable to future generations of implant design and technique. The discussion in this chapter will be directed towards the most commonly employed design configuration today: a metallic femoral component without a centering stem, and a hemispherical, relatively thin-walled acetabular component. Allusions will be made when appropriate toward other implant types. Although the long-term or ultimate rate of failure is indefinable at present, it is apparent that, compared to the current generation of conventional, stemmed hip replacements, the early failure rate for hip surface replacement is high. Figures vary, but reported failure rates of over 30 percent are not rare.[12,14] Our personal experience substantiates these observations.

Generally, the principles of implant revision surgery developed for conventional arthroplasty also apply to surface replacements. There are, however, certain aspects of diagnosis and treatment unique to resurfacing. It is to these differences that this chapter is directed. Specifically, one of the alleged advantages of a resurfacing

199

REVISION TOTAL HIP ARTHROPLASTY
ISBN 0-8089-1466-9

procedure is that bone stock may be preserved. This is certainly the case on the femoral side of a hip resurfacing procedure, and it has certain implications regarding revisability with and without the presence of sepsis. The acetabular side of a hip resurfacing may also be different; the acetabulum may have been largely destroyed by some techniques of resurfacing. Finally, the exact mode of failure and the precise underlying disease process may have more influence on the revision of a failed resurfacing than on the revision of a conventional, stemmed hip arthroplasty.

THE DIAGNOSIS OF PROSTHETIC FAILURE

There are several considerations which, while present in conventional revision surgery, may be accentuated in revision for failed resurfacing procedures. First among these is the fact that if one component is loose the other either is, or very soon will be, loose. Thus, if an attempt to revise only one component is to be made, it must be undertaken very soon after diagnosis. If symptoms or signs have been present for a long period of time, it should be anticipated that both components will require revision. Also, if it has been appreciated for some time that the position of one of the prosthetic components has changed but the patient has only recently become symptomatic, it is a virtual certainty that both components are loose.

The reasons for this are several: Loosening itself, even of only one of the components may cause bone erosion. The ensuing malalignment between components probably leads to an increased production of wear debris, which in turn causes three-body wear and increases the histiocytic response, causing still more bone erosion or resorption.

Certain design features are imposed upon both components of a double-cup prosthesis which might be thought to increase the chance of loosening. Thus, it is difficult to envisage a femoral component design of a purely resurfacing prosthesis which would have much intrinsic stability to torsional loads. A component having a spherical internal configuration would offer the least resistance to load applied in any direction. In addition to the bone resorption to be "normally" expected at the interface if a femoral component is loose, mechanical erosion of the femoral stump by the rough inside cement surface is generally significant; in most instances the femoral stump is eroded beyond the point where reimplantation of a resurfacing prosthesis is possible.

The acetabular side presents its own problems; indeed the acetabulum has been predicted to be the weak link in resurfacing procedures. Charnley has pointed out two important factors: the unfavorable frictional forces and subsequent torsional loads incurred with such a relatively large interface diameter, and, as demonstrated by photoelastic studies, a thin polyethylene layer tends to distribute loads to the pelvis in an undesirable manner.[8] Additionally, thin polyethylene deforms, causing stress concentrations at the interface with the relatively brittle polymethylmethacrylate (PMMA).

Because of the wide exposure required, the desire to conserve pelvic bone, and the widespread use of a hemispherical or nearly hemispherical component, cement techniques may be less than desirable. Cement layers have often been relatively thin, leading to fracture of the PMMA and subsequent prosthesis loosening.

Large-size acetabular components (ie, large in outside diameter) have been employed in order to accomodate the large resurfaced femoral head. This has in turn necessitated the preparation of a very large cavity in the pelvis, in order to insert the acetabular component.

Related both to a large femoral neck (as compared with that of any available stemmed prosthesis) and the use of a large, approximately hemispherical acetabulum is the problem of impingement between the bony femoral neck and the protruding polyethylene. This is a further and, we believe, important cause of acetabular loosening in hip resurfacing arthroplasties.

Finally, the diagnosis of loosening of the acetabulum is confused in our experience by the relatively high incidence of "benign" radiolucent lines. The precise etiology for these lines remains unexplained, but even when apparently benign (ie, nonprogressive), they should be regarded with suspicion.

On the femoral side, the diagnosis of loosening in the current generation of implants is complicated by the fact that all interfaces are obscured by overlying radio-opaque metal. Hence, the main criterion for loosening—bone-cement lucency—is not available. Substantial bone resorption, suggesting gross prosthetic loosening or even sepsis, is likewise obscured, as are the usual signs of osteitis. Criteria that are available for observation include changes in orientation (or angle) of the femoral cup, and settling of the cup on the femoral neck. Even these signs, however, must be interpreted with caution unless strictly standardized roentgen evaluations have been performed. Even small changes in rotation or flexion can greatly distort apparent relationships between the prosthesis and the femoral neck and shaft.

A useful sign on the femoral side is narrowing of the bony femoral neck at its junction with the prosthesis. Actual measurements can be calculated, using the relative magnification of the femoral prosthesis as a reference. Progressive narrowing is suggestive of sepsis. The base of the femoral neck tends to be oval rather than round, so that changes in orientation, especially in flexion—extension, will compromise this measurement.

Notching of the femoral neck is a technical error made at the time of implantation. Initially, it is a worrisome prognostic indictor. Notching of the actual neck must be distinguished from notching of an osteophyte, an occurrence which is not at all ominous. Progression in size of a notch suggests loosening, or, strictly, migration.

Since standardized roentgen views are of paramount importance it is appropriate to mention the methods described to obtain standardized, repeatable x-rays. One technique for a repeatable anteroposterior (AP) x-ray of the hip or pelvis is for the patient to lie supine with knees flexed over the end of an x-ray table. (Unfortunately, many x-ray tables are constructed so that in this position the film cassette will not slide far enough to be placed underneath the patient's pelvis.)

Bone scans have been employed with some success by certain investigators,[5] but we have not been able to obtain much useful information ourselves. Laboratory evaluations further suggest that so much definition is lost in scanning through a

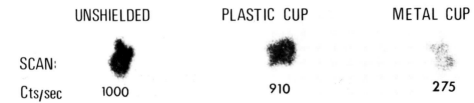

Fig. 9-1. Three standard doses of free Tc[99]: unshielded, shielded by plastic resurfacing femoral component, and shielded by metallic resurfacing femoral component. As in scans performed on patients, this composite scan was standardized. In this instance, the standard or reference is the unshielded Tc[99] at 1000 CTS/sec. Thus, compared to the standard, plastic shields 9% of countable radiation, and metal 72.5%.

metallic femoral component as to render this form of evaluation virtually meaningless (Fig. 9-1).[11] We cannot therefore recommend bone scans for aid in diagnosis of failure on the femoral side when a metallic component has been implanted.

Indications for Revision

The indications for revision of a failed resurfacing arthroplasty are similar to those for a conventional arthroplasty. A combination of symptoms causing the patient to seek revision, accepting the possible risks and complications, and rejecting nonoperative alternatives, plus objective signs of failure are, of course, grounds for revision.

Some patients present with extreme symptoms and an absence of signs. We do not recommend revision surgery for any patient having no objective signs within an absolute limit of 6 months following implantation. One reason for this is that ectopic ossification may cause significant pain in the early post-operative period, although it will not necessarily be roentgenographically visible until 6 months have transpired. We are reluctant to advise revision of a resurfacing arthroplasty at any time with tolerable symptoms but no signs.

Generally, asymptomatic mechanical failure as evidenced on roentgenograms can be treated conservatively, or expectantly. Septic loosening is invariably symptomatic; the decision to revise is obvious. Any type of revision becomes increasingly difficult if significant fibrosis has occurred in the capsule; occasionally, we have found this fibrosis to be severe.

TECHNICAL CONSIDERATIONS AT REVISION SURGERY

Surface replacement arthroplasty failures can generally be related to mechanical failure or sepsis. The type of revision surgery is largely determined by the type of failure with certain special considerations causing intraoperative modifications.

Mechanical failure (i.e., loosening, femoral neck fracture, or prosthetic dislocations) can usually be related to a specific technical or design error, or to an error in diagnosis—for example, performing the initial operation on a patient whose bone does not suit the hip to this type of arthroplasty. Technical errors include inadequate bone preparation; poor cementing technique; notching of the femoral neck; and inaccurate prosthesis orientation.

Adequate operative exposure is the first concern in revising a resurfacing arthroplasty. Experience with the initial implantation of resurfacing devices has demonstrated the hazards of inadequate exposure; many of the techniques of orientation used without full visualization for placement of conventional components (especially the acetabulum) are simply unacceptable for placement of double-cup prostheses. The same is true for revision of double-cups.

An understanding of the approach initially utilized is important if the distortion of the local anatomy is to be understood. An originally wide exposure may have caused a significant modification of local anatomy, which will be accentuated by fibrosis around a failed joint. Different types of implants can fairly consistently be associated with specific approaches. Hence, a Wagner prosthesis is usually inserted via an anterior, iliofemoral approach; a THARIES via a trochanteric osteotomy; an Indiana Conservative by a lateral approach, with or without trochanteric osteotomy; and an ICLH (Imperial College London Hospital) through an antero-lateral approach, similar to a Watson-Jones or a Gibson, but with a complete (anterior and posterior) capsulotomy. Other approaches have been described for resurfacing arthroplasty of the hip; some of these include the lateral "U" approach described by Ollier, and the Harris lateral approach. Regardless of which approach has been used, a trochanteric osteotomy and reflection of the abductors is recommended for exposure in the presence of extreme fibrosis. However, our experience suggests that trochanteric osteotomy *may* compromise reimplantation of another double-cup, a subject discussed below.

The most commonly indicated revision procedure for a failed resurfacing replacement is exchange for a conventional, stemmed implant. If this is to be accomplished, it is obvious that in all instances both components will require revision. There are several technical considerations relevant to the exchange of a resurfacing for a stemmed arthroplasty. The acetabulum should always be revised before the femoral stump is removed, or the femoral canal is violated: unexpected infection may be encountered on the acetabular side. On the acetabular side, the surgeon may be faced with a formidable reconstructive task; depending on the original prosthetic design and implantation technique, a significant pelvic defect may exist. This may be compounded by periacetabular erosion from debris and resorption from a histiocytic and osteoclastic response. As a consequence, revision of the acetabulum may require the use of mesh, metallic support strips, support rings, and bone grafts. We have made use of custom HMWPE (high molecular weight polyethylene) components with centering pegs. Buchholz advocates oversized HMWPE acetabular components in the presence of significant bone loss.[3]

These problems are, however, not peculiar to failed resurfacing prostheses; specific details and the use of custom implants are discussed elsewhere in this book. As with the placement of an acetabular component in the presence of any bone defect, the importance of restoring the load-bearing axis must be emphasized. Thus, if a large lateral defect exists, the acetabular component must be placed in a seemingly medial and distal position. In the case of protrusio (ie, a medial defect), the component must be located relatively laterally and, again, seemingly distal.

The femoral side also presents specific problems. One of the obvious advantages of a resurfacing procedure is that the femoral canal has not been violated; bone loss beyond the femoral neck is theoretically impossible. Even in the instance of sepsis, the femoral side remains relatively unscathed. Conversion to a stemmed prosthesis should therefore be relatively simple, and results on the femoral side might be predicted to be identical to those for a previously performed stemmed arthroplasty. In many situations, however, the remnant of femoral neck itself may be of more importance than the inviolate femoral canal.

The fundamental principle in revision arthroplasty for a failed resurfacing hip procedure is to avoid the initial temptation to amputate the femoral neck until it has been determined that infection is not present, and the acetabulum has been completely reconstructed.

If the femoral component is loose, it should, of course, be removed prior to reconstruction of the acetabulum. Superficial debridement of fibrous tissue is sometimes required (in order to obtain specimens for Gram stain, frozen section, etc, as well as for further visualization); no further removal of bone should be undertaken until the above two considerations have been met. If the femoral component is not loose, removal will probably be impossible without damage to underlying bone. Prosthetic failure secondary to a femoral neck fracture is another circumstance where bone is lost, but even in these instances, the femoral canal should remain inviolate until there is no evidence of sepsis and the acetabulum has been reconstructed. The reason for leaving the femoral side intact is that, in the event of sepsis, the option of performing a relatively functional iliofemoral coaptation or removal arthroplasty remains (see below).

If revision of a failed resurfacing arthroplasty to another resurfacing arthroplasty (in other words, simple exchange of one resurfacing prosthesis for another) is contemplated, it must be borne in mind that some bone loss is likely. In this instance, either a different-sized component must be used or extra cement must be employed. If the size of one component is changed, the other component must also change to a comparable size (a smaller femur requires a smaller acetabulum, etc). Thus, a situation exists where, regardless of technical feasibility, component design considerations are such that revision to another double-cup may be impossible unless a wide range of implants are available, with various inside and outside diameters. Regardless of size considerations, an eroded femoral stump provides poor fixation.

It is apparent from this discussion that it is unusual for a simple exchange of resurfacing prostheses to be possible or indicated; most often, conversion to a stemmed implant will be required. This should be considered during pre-operative planning, including during discussion with the patient and the patient's family.

Femoral neck fracture is related to technical error. In our experience, a generous trochanteric osteotomy often led to neck fracture. Others, using a more conservative osteotomy, have not had this problem. Trochanteric osteotomy is part of the recommended operation for implantation of the THARIES replacement, for example. Furthermore, our implant type, the ICLH, has been used in significant numbers by other surgeons via an approach utilizing a laterally placed trochanteric osteotomy, without the femoral neck fractures of our early experience.[1] Thus, this complication is not related to prosthetic design.

Another technical error leading to femoral neck fracture is inadvertent notching of the femoral neck during implantation. This weakens the femoral neck and, perhaps more importantly, compromises the intraosseous blood supply.[10,16] Mechanical weakening of the femoral cortex, as well as the potential for avascular necrosis, both occur; fracture may follow. If the neck is left too long, an unfavorable mechanical situation is created with a long lever arm. Additionally, an unfortunate anatomical-mechanical arrangement occurs, with the stress-riser from the edge of the cup being across weak cancellous bone. Finally, femoral neck fracture can occur, because the bone is simply too weak in that particular patient.

Regardless of its cause, acute femoral neck fracture is probably the only theoretical indication for the use of a large-head, stemmed prosthesis, providing that the acetabulum is neither loose nor worn. These semicustom implants are available through any of the manufacturers who supply resurfacing prosthetic components. We do not, however, generally recommend the use of these implants because of the theoretical increase in wear and potential loosening associated with a large-diameter head.

Dislocation of resurfacing prosthetic components rarely occurs, because of the enhanced stability afforded by large-diameter interfaces. When dislocation does occur, it is usually due to malposition of the acetabular component: a technical error. The problem of a poorly placed acetabular component is accentuated by protrusion of the polyethylene beyond the acetabulum itself, so that it impinges against the femoral neck. Acetabular loosening may ensue, or the femoral head may be levered out of the acetabulum in the early post-operative period. The most common situation is for the acetabulum to be placed too vertically. Instability then occurs in adduction when the femoral neck inferiorly impinges on the protruding polyethylene and the head tends to superolaterally slide out. Malposition of the femoral component is a rare cause of dislocation. It may be related to a pre-existent deformity on the femoral side, such as the marked increase in anteversion seen with CDH. Hips having undergone a previous medial displacement osteotomy may also be prone to dislocation from the prominent lesser trochanter levering on the ischium. Repeat dislocation always requires revision if a specific technical error (of placement) can be identified.

The general principles of revision for an infected arthroplasty are detailed elsewhere in this book. In this context, an advantage of the resurfacing arthroplasty is the preservation of bone stock and the consequent enhanced stability of the hip which remains even after removal of all prosthetic components. Regardless of other considerations, removal of prosthetic components to leave an iliofemoral coaptation is the procedure we would recommend in the face of sepsis. In this procedure, both components and all polymethylmethacrylate are removed. Soft-tissue debridement is performed as indicated by the extent of sepsis, fibrosis, and ectopic ossification, but it is desirable to leave the soft tissues as intact as possible to enhance stability. Further technical considerations as dictated especially by sepsis are discussed elsewhere in this book.

Stability of the iliofemoral coaptation is influenced by the size of the femoral neck remnant, the state of the superolateral rim of the acetabulum, and the presence of soft-tissue contractures or stabilising structures. In any event, some shortening must occur. Because of these considerations, some have recommended routine transfer of the greater trochanter; in our limited experience, trochanteric transfer has not always been required.

Post-operative treatment ideally consists of 6 weeks in light skeletal traction

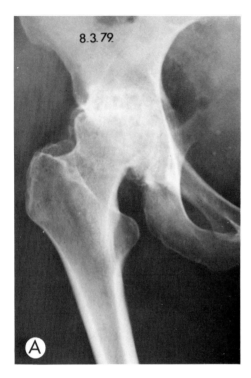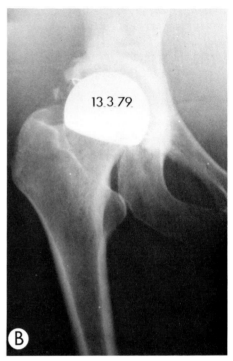

Fig. 9-2. Four x-rays of the right hip in a 45-year-old female with rheumatoid arthritis whose resurfaced hip failed 17 months post-operatively. **A.** Pre-operative. **B.** Early post-operative. Note uncovered P.E. lateral and medial cement mass. **C.** Failure by loosening and femoral neck erosion (*not* fractured; appearance of femoral neck is from bone loss and is fairly typical for a rheumatoid patient.) **D.** Revision to stemmed (straight, Müller) THA using acetabular reinforcement ring and mesh ('Mexican hat').

followed by 6 weeks non-weight-bearing. During the period of traction, an abducted position is maintained. It is extremely important to avoid a flexed, adducted, externally rotated position. After the first few days of traction, the patient is encouraged either to lie flat without a pillow under the affected limb, or to sit up with the opposite limb over the side of the bed. This increases abduction and avoids fixed flexion. As the patient will most likely be short on the affected side, even if abduction were to become fixed it would not be as unfavorable as fixed abduction or a relative loss of abduction. Limited passive flexion to the hip is instituted as soon as tolerated (usually within the first week). Active flexion is instituted when the traction is removed. The ideal compromise between motion and stability has not yet been determined, but it seems to us wise to err in the direction of stability, seeking eventually a stable, comfortable hip with 0°–60° of flexion, and no other motion.

Few of these procedures have been performed. The follow-up time is short so that information on the ultimate function of the hip is limited and anecdotal. Limited though they may be, reports are encouraging.[4,22] It is apparent that one of the real advantages to a hip resurfacing arthroplasty is that in the event of complete failure or sepsis, a reasonably functional result may still be obtained. There is

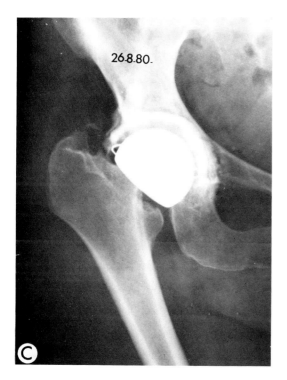

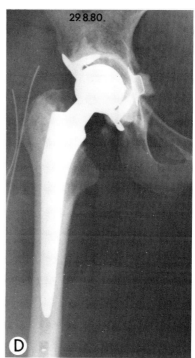

probably no indication to perform an excision arthroplasty similar to that described by Girdlestone, or to that performed when prosthetic components are removed from a stemmed hip arthroplasty.

A special note should be made about failure related to an underlying disease process. This may include the inflammatory arthropathies (Fig. 9-2), so-called rapidly progressive osteoarthrosis,[17] or any metabolic process affecting bone, including post-menopausal osteoporosis, renal osteodystrophy, etc. In the absence of trochanteric osteotomy, the mechanical mode of failure in these conditions is usually settling and loosening of the femoral prosthesis due to resorption and/or erosion of underlying bone. We now appreciate that patients falling into these diagnostic categories are not suitable candidates for resurfacing procedures. Therefore, no attempt should be made to exchange the implant for another resurfacing prosthesis. In the absence of sepsis, replacement with a stemmed prosthesis is the procedure of choice. During the revision operation, a remnant of femoral neck should be maintained until the acetabulum has been reconstructed and sepsis ruled out.

We recommend conversion to a stemmed prosthesis, regardless of the technical feasability of exchange for another surface replacement, in any patient over the age of 60 years. A conventional stemmed arthroplasty is known to provide a satisfactory, relatively long-term, functional joint in these patients, whereas the long-term results of even primary resurfacing procedures are as yet unknown. Secondly, rapidly progressive osteoarthrosis occurs only in this age group.[17]

Rapidly progressive osteoarthrosis has been little appreciated in North America, possibly because a conventional total hip arthroplasty effectively "cures" the

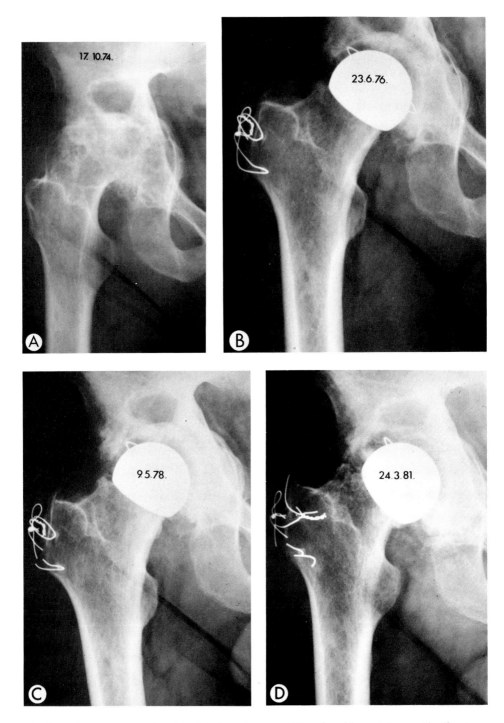

Fig. 9-3. Six x-rays of the right hip in a 41-year-old male with post-traumatic (fracture-dislocation) osteoarthrosis. **A.** Pre-operative. **B.** One year post-operative; a notch in the superior femoral neck can easily be seen. **C.** Three years post-operative. The notch has increased in size, but the hip remains asymptomatic and the patient is very active. **D.** Failure

disease process by removing all affected bony tissue. In Europe, where osteotomies have held a stronger following, this disease has been cited as an etiological explanation for failure of osteotomy in some patients.[17] A resurfacing procedure, like an osteotomy, preserves bone stock and is thus equally subject to failure if the preserved bone is diseased and thus is either too weak to support a prosthesis or continues to resorb.

The final patient group deserving special recognition is the physiologically (as well as chronologically) young patient with good bone stock and a long life expectancy. In this group an iliofemoral coaptation (Fig. 9-3) or removal arthroplasty is the recommended procedure, regardless of the mode of failure, since it is appealing to leave these patients with an implant-free hip. It must, however, again be emphasised that no long-term results are available following this procedure.

Another revision procedure, mentioned here almost solely for historical perspective, is that of arthrodesis. This method is another of the theoretical advantages of resurfacing over stemmed arthroplasty. Arthrodesis following a failed resurfacing hip replacement may be technically difficult, since some bone will inevitably have been lost, but it is feasible and has been successfully performed.[18] In the presence of sepsis, arthrodesis becomes increasingly difficult. Any of the para-articular or extra-articular augmentations, such as those described for fusion of a tuberculous hip, may have to be employed. In view of the theoretical difficulty of fusing a failed

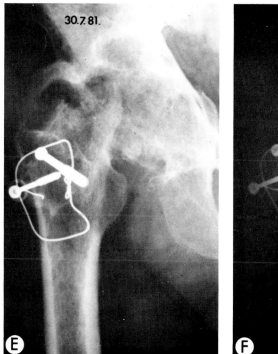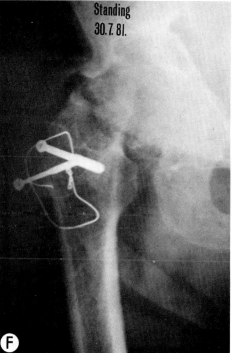

has occured by gross loosening 70 months following resurfacing. **E.** Revision, in spite of aseptic failure in this young, active patient, was to iliofemoral coaptation with transfer of greater trochanter. **F.** Weight-bearing roentgenogram 3 months following revision.

resurfaced hip and the relatively unfavorable long-term results of hip arthrodesis performed on adults, we do not, save in exceptional circumstances, recommend arthrodesis as a viable revision procedure for a failed hip surface replacement. We have not ourselves attempted this operation.[13,19,20] Formation of ectopic bone may be more of a problem in resurfacing than in conventional arthroplasties because of the narrow gap between the femoral neck and the pelvis, especially when compared to the wide space allowed by the relatively small metallic neck of a conventional prosthesis. Additionally, many of those patients for whom resurfacing is indicated (young adults, possibly with post-traumatic osteoarthrosis) are already at high risk for ectopic ossification. In spite of this, we have not found ectopic ossification to be a common problem in resurfaced hips; we have never revised a hip purely because of ectopic ossification. When ectopic ossification does occur, it usually presents as pain between 3 and 6 weeks post-operative. This pain is readily distinguished temporally and qualitatively from both the pre-operative pain and the usual post-operative, incisional-type of pain. Range of motion may not be appreciably affected at first; and, even when fully matured, ectopic ossification may not necessarily cause a functionally important interference with motion. Roentgenographic evidence may not be apparent for several months, but it is always visible at 6 months. The early pain usually resolves as the ectopic ossification matures on roentgenograms. Since ectopic bone usually reforms after removal, and since the functional result by the end of the first post-operative year is usually tolerable, we do not recommend revision surgery for this complication.

Fracture of prosthetic components as a mode of failure has not, to our knowledge, been observed as it has in conventional hip replacement, so that revision for this possible complication is never necessary in practice.

RESULTS OF REVISION SURGERY

One of the alleged advantages of a resurfacing procedure is that it can, with relative ease, be converted to a conventional, stemmed arthroplasty. It should be apparent from the above discussion that considerations, especially on the acetabular side, may render revision or reconstruction of a failed surface replacement arthroplasty almost as difficult as that for a stemmed arthroplasty. At present, little is actually known about the long-term results of hips having been revised from a surface replacement to a stemmed arthroplasty. It is therefore of interest to compare surface replacement hips which have been revised with conventional, cemented, metal-on-plastic hips which have also been revised. The failure rate for conventional hip revisions has been reported around 25 percent; but a rate of 66 percent has also been noted.[2,6,15,21] Our personal experience suggests that the outcome of revision for a failed surface replacement (in the short-term) falls somewhere between the generally expected outcome of a primary conventional hip arthroplasty and that of a revision procedure for a failed stem arthroplasty.

A formal review has not at this time been completed, but we have 41 patients in whom a surface replacement arthroplasty has failed and has been revised, and who have been followed for at least 6 months (Table 9-1). One hip has been revised and followed twice (see below). The maximum follow-up in this group is 8 years, with an average follow-up of 2 years and 5 months. The age range in this patient

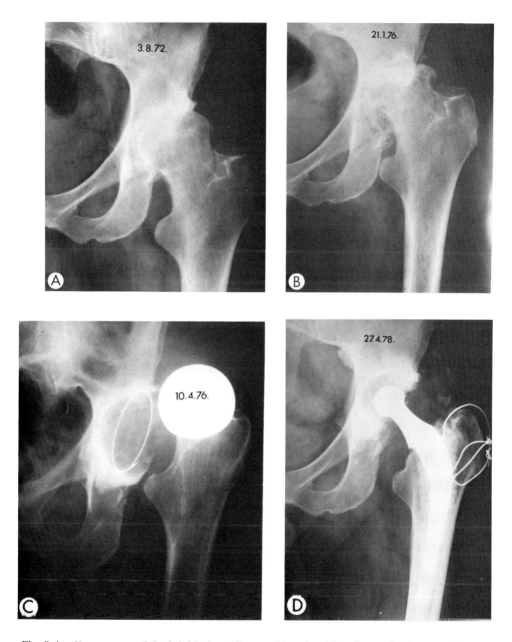

Fig. 9-4. Four x-rays of the left hip in a 62-year-old male with a diagnosis of osteoarthrosis.
A. Four years pre-operative. **B.** Two months pre-operative. Incidentally, although the time
is too long for accurate comparison with the previous roentgenograms, the marked shortening
and bone destruction as well as the patient's age suggest rapidly progressive osteoarthritis
(see text). **C.** Early post-operative roentgenogram showing the hip dislocated. The acetabulum
has been placed too vertical: there is little superior coverage and, worse, there is a large
protruding lip of polyethylene inferomedially. **D.** Following revision to a Charnley THA.

Table 9-1
Summary of our Follow-up Experience
with Revised Surface Replacement

Revised for infection: 2 (5%)
1. Resurfacing → resurfacing → stem (neck fracture)
2. Resurfacing → stem → Girdlestone (infection)

One additional hip became infected subsequent to revision. Therefore, infection rate at follow-up of revisions is 5%.

Revised to another resurfacing prosthesis: 5
Failed : 3 (60%)
1. Femoral neck fracture: 1
2. Loosening: 2

Revised to conventional stemmed prosthesis: 31
Failed : 3 (10%)
1. Sepsis: 2 (1 infected at time of revision)
2. Loosening: 1

---

group is 38 to 81 years of age, with an average of 61. Approximately equal numbers of males and females, as well as right and left hips, are represented. As might be expected, the majority of these failures have been converted to stemmed arthroplasties; 11 of the Charnley design (Fig. 9-4) and 20 of the Müller (Figs. 9-2 and 9-5) or straight stemmed Müller design. Five failed resurfacing prostheses were revised with another resurfacing prosthesis for either one or both components (Fig. 9-6). In three additional hips, the acetabulum was untouched, but the femoral side was replaced with a large-diameter head, stemmed prosthesis (Fig. 9-7). Three patients were converted to iliofemoral coaptation. One hip has been revised and followed twice, so that there are 42 revisions in this group. Of the total of 42 revised hips, 6 (14 percent) have subsequently failed.

Three of the five revisions to another resurfacing prosthesis have failed (60 percent). One of these had initially an acetabular defect (probably Brodie's abscess), which was debrided elsewhere prior to the first surface replacement. This exchange of one resurfacing to another resurfacing prosthesis failed 3 years following the revision; the hip was subsequently converted to a straight-stemmed Müller prosthesis. Another of the failed resurfacing revisions originally loosened secondary to sepsis and was revised with another resurfacing prosthesis using antibiotic-impregnated cement. The resurfacing revision subsequently loosened; histological evaluation revealed avascular necrosis but no signs of infection. Rerevision to a stemmed prosthesis was performed, and the hip functions satisfactorily 2 years following this second revision. The other resurfacing prosthesis which subsequently loosened did so at 2 years and has not as yet been revised.

Thirty-one hips were revised from a double-cup to a conventional stemmed prosthesis (22 mm or 32 mm head diameter). Three (10 percent) of those have subsequently failed. One was infected at the time of revision and eventually was converted to a Girdlestone excision arthroplasty; one became infected following revision surgery and now also has a Girdlestone (Fig. 9-8); the third has recently been revised to another stem for aseptic loosening of the femoral component.

Two hips were originally revised for infection. One was revised to another double-cup, which was in turn revised to a stemmed prosthesis following loosening, as mentioned above. This hip now functions well 2 years following the second revision. Another revision was to a stemmed prosthesis which was eventually converted to a Girdlestone when it, too, became infected (Fig.9-8). A third hip was revised to a stem for mechanical loosening, but the stem became infected and was converted to a Girdlestone. (All three of the infected hips have been discussed). It is important to realize that the incidence of infection generally increases with additional operations; all of these hips obviously had had one, and in some instances, more than one, previous operative procedure.

Follow-up data for those still-functioning revision arthroplasties is presented in Table 9-2. Briefly, the majority of these patients are pain-free or have only mild pain which does not interfere with activity. In none of these patients is their walking ability affected by the replaced, revised hip; the range of motion in most of these patients is within a "normal" physiologic range, considering their age. In summary, it can be stated that in those revision hips which are still functioning, function is comparable to a similar group of primary, conventional, stemmed hip arthroplasties.

MODIFICATIONS TO DIAGNOSIS AND TREATMENT

Some important design changes have been made in certain prostheses which considerably alter diagnostic and revision techniques. Wagner's change to a ceramic femoral component has been noted. For over 1 year we have been undertaking a

Table 9-2
Summary of Results in Successfully Revised Hips

Pain	
None	75%
Occasional, mild, associated with activity	20%
Continuous, but mild	5%
Severe, intermittent	0%
Severe, continuous	0%

Walking Ability	
Over 1 hr	47%
30–60 min	17%
0–30 mins.	29%
Indoors only	8%
Unable	0%

Range of motion

(*Total range.* Flexion − Extension + Abduction − Adduction + Rotation, minus any contracture. 140° is considered requisite for normal activity.)

Over 210°	16%
141–210°	56%
71–140°	28%*
0–70°	0%

*Includes 3 hips (or 9%) with significant radiological ectopic ossification.

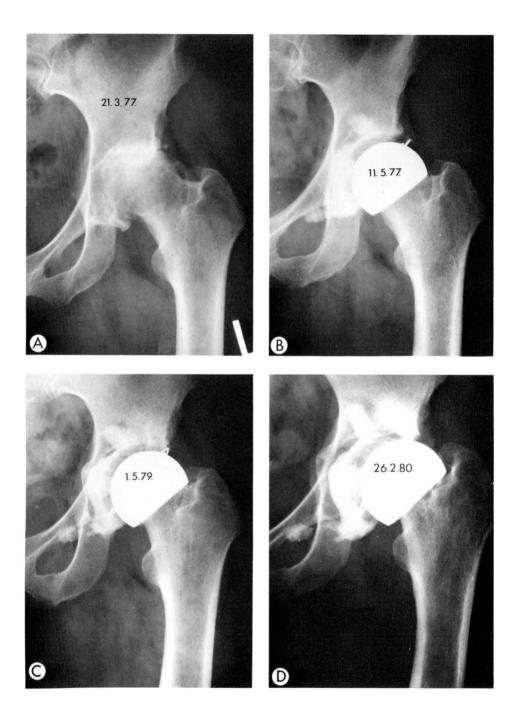

Fig. 9-5. Six x-rays of the left hip in a 52-year-old female with osteoarthrosis. The resurfaced hip failed 38 months post-operatively. **A.** Pre-operative. **B.** Early post-operative. Note laterally and medially overhanging polyethylene and large mass of medial cement. **C.** Two years later; acetabulum is apparently loose and has shifted vertically. Femoral component may have settled into more varus. **D.** Nine months later (35 months post-operatively); both components have obviously moved, but symptoms remain mild. **E.** Additional settling and

214

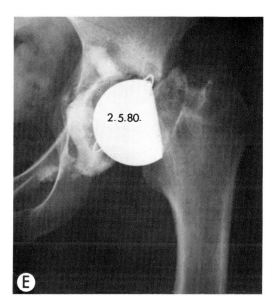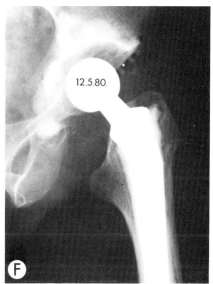

movement have occured; the femoral component has completely fallen off. **F.** Revised to straight-stem Müller THA using custom acetabulum with HMWPE centering pegs.

clinical trial on the use of another radiolucent non-metallic material for femoral resurfacing. This material allows roentgen evaluation of bone-cement and prosthesis-cement interfaces within the femoral component. Furthermore, bone scans performed through these components show virtually no shielding (Fig. 9-1).

Ceramic femoral components are extremely brittle and can, allegedly, be fractured by striking them with a hammer or mallet at revision surgery.[22] We have no personal experience with this technique. The material with which we are experimenting can be cut with a bone saw and then removed from the femur, causing minimal bone damage.

It is becoming apparent that, especially with the large-diameter femoral head required in a resurfacing prosthesis, the acetabulum need not approximate a hemisphere. Acetabulae with a subtended angle of 140° (as opposed to 180°, as in a hemisphere) have been functioning quite satisfactorily for well over a year. The Indiana conservative hip has an acetabulum with a subtended angle of 150°.

The ramifications of using a smaller angle acetabulum are several. Obviously, the total area of contact will be lessened. Theoretically, this has a favorable effect on the rate of production of wear debris. A smaller subtended angle incurs a proportionally smaller requisite outside diameter for a given sized internal radius of curvature. (Fig. 9-9). Thus a smaller cavity in the pelvis is required. It also means that prosthetic overhang outside the pelvis is eliminated; and, finally, conventional-thickness polyethylene can be used, by offsetting the articular surface.

Based on our assessment of the causes of loosening, smaller acetabular components should theoretically reduce the incidence of failure, and therefore of revisions. Since current techniques involve the removal of only minimal bone (no more than for a conventional 32 mm prosthesis), revision operations should be facilitated on the acetabular side and their results more predictable.

The other development of note, even though not in widespread use, is the use

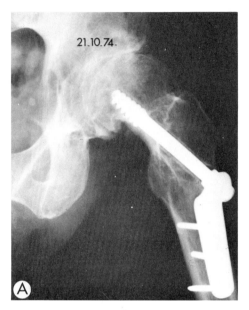
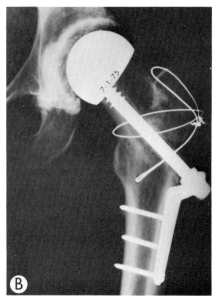

Fig. 9-6. Five x-rays of the left hip in a 40-year-old female with a "failed" osteotomy. Failure by loosening of both components occured 43 months post-operatively. **A.** Pre-operative, with "sliding nail" in place. **B.** Early post-operative. Note protruding acetabular component, especially medially. Femoral component is in more varus than is ideal. **C.** Failure by loosening of both components. **D.** Early post-operative x-ray following revision of both components. The hip screw has been removed to allow shortening of the femoral neck remnant for replacement of a prosthesis. **E.** Twenty-two months following revision to another resurfacing prosthesis; function is excellent but complete radiolucent line around the acetabulum is worrisome, as is relatively lateral position of the acetabular component.

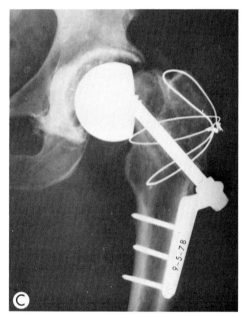

of a technique of fixation which does not require PMMA. Since less total material is implanted, revision surgery should be easier. Additionally, there is evidence that PMMA itself may contribute to bone loss through osteoclastic resorption as well as by direct mechanical erosion in a loose implant.[7] PMMA may also add to prosthesis three-body wear by the presence of acrylic debris.

The current thrust of development in resurfacing prostheses is toward smaller implants and the use of more chemically and mechanically biocompatible implants. These should facilitate the diagnosis and treatment of failed arthroplasties. Hope-

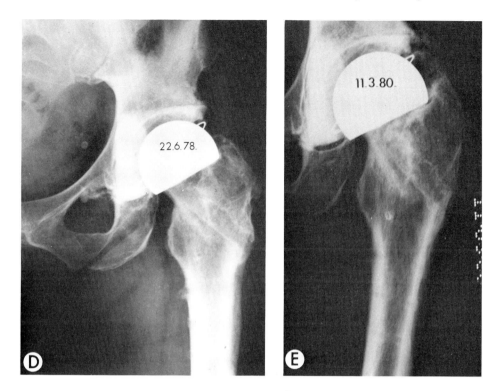

fully, they will substantially diminish the currently unacceptable failure rate in resurfacing hip arthroplasties.

CONCLUSIONS

Revision operations for a failed resurfacng procedure must, like revision for a failed conventional hip arthroplasty, be related to complications. Only certain complications will inevitably require revision; some complications never require revision. Specific to revision surgery for resurfacing prostheses, we consider the complications of sepsis, aseptic loosening, femoral neck fracture, and recurring dislocation as complications which always require revision (Fig. 9-10).

Ectopic bone formation, regardless of its relationship to hip surgery in conventional hip arthroplasties, is not a complication which necessarily requires revision in surface replacement of the hip. In our experience, the result in a hip with ectopic ossification is usually not totally unacceptable by 1 year following the replacement arthroplasty. Unexplained pain and trochanteric problems are two situations which sometimes require revision. Perhaps because of the subtlety of roentgenographic signs, the incidence of unexplained pain in resurfacing procedures may be higher than the incidence in conventional hip arthroplasty; usually, however, the underlying cause for the pain becomes clear if an expectant approach is adopted. The analysis and treatment of trochanteric problems are identical to those for conventional hip arthroplasties, and do not of necessity involve the prosthesis. In this summary, we will consider complications and the inherent diagnostic and

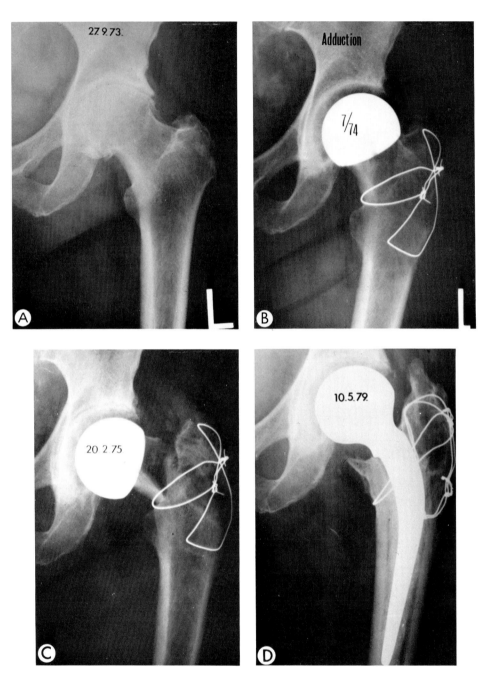

Fig. 9-7. Four x-rays of the left hip in a 63-year-old male with osteoarthrosis. **A.** Pre-operative. **B.** Four months post-operative x-ray in full adduction. Limitation may be partially attributed to medial protrusion of acetabular component. **C.** Failure by femoral neck fracture 11 months post-operatively. **D.** Revision with large-diameter head, stemmed THA. (we would now revise this to a standard, stemmed prosthesis.)

revision difficulties in resurfacing hip arthroplasty in comparison to similar difficulties in a conventional hip arthroplasty.

Considering first the diagnostic difficulties: aseptic loosening provides a different problem on the acetabular compared to the femoral side. Diagnosis of aseptic loosening on the acetabular side of a resurfacing hip arthroplasty is virtually the same as that for a conventional total hip arthroplasty. On the femoral side, however, diagnosis is much more difficult because the bone-prosthesis-PMMA interfaces are all invisible to x-ray. The usual signs of aseptic loosening, that is, changes in the interfaces, are therefore obscured; other signs, such as a change in position or angle of the prosthesis; settling of the prosthesis on the femoral neck; notching and/or progression of the size of a notch; if slight, can only be detected on serial, perfectly standardized roentgenograms.

The diagnosis of a fractured femoral neck in a resurfacing prosthesis is obvious on x-ray. (Stem fractures which may occur in a conventional hip replacement, are obviously impossible in a resurfaced hip.) Recurring dislocations, an early complication, are also obvious on x-ray.

The diagnosis of septic failure in a resurfaced hip compared to the diagnosis of sepsis as a cause of failure in a conventional hip replacement can also be considered on the acetabular vs the femoral side. Diagnosis on the acetabular side is, again, virtually identical to that of a conventional replacement. On the femoral side, the usual x-ray signs of shaft osteitis are absent. The hip looks more benign on x-ray, especially in the light of the relatively high incidence of otherwise benign radiolucent lines on the acetabular side seen after resurfacing arthroplasty. Progressive narrowing of the femoral neck is one sign highly suggestive of sepsis (Fig. 9-8).

Avascular necrosis of the resurfaced femoral head was an early concern in surface replacement. It is now known that this is not an inevitable finding in surface-replaced hips; but it remains possible that it occurs in some hips causing failure on the femoral side. It is our experience, however, that the pre-operative diagnosis of avascular necrosis is currently not possible in a femur resurfaced with

Table 9-3

Diagnosis of Failed Hip Arthroplasty:
Resurfaced Compared with Conventional

Faced with a complication requiring revision—is a resurfaced hip better, or worse, than a conventional hip arthroplasty?

Diagnostically?

Complication

Aseptic loosening:	Acetabulum—the same
	Femur—different, double-cup harder to diagnose.
Femoral neck fracture:	Different—does not occur in conventional hip replacement (but stem fracture does not occur in resurfaced arthroplasty).
Recurrent Dislocation:	The same
Sepsis:	Acetabulum—the same diagnostically as conventional hip.
	Femur—a different diagnosis than conventional hip, more difficult.

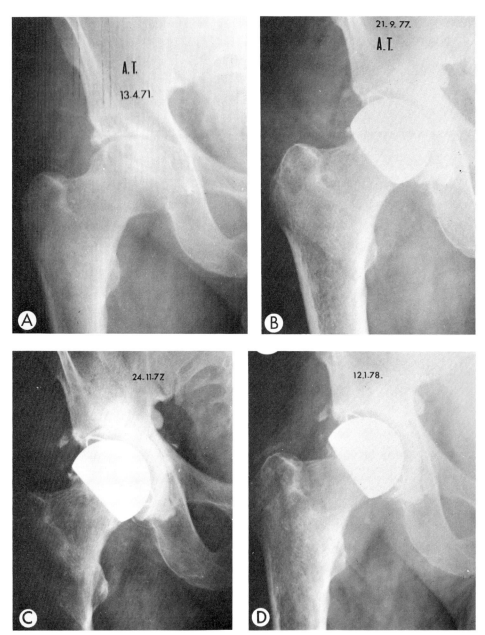

Fig. 9-8. Eight x-rays of the right hip in a 67-year-old male with osteoarthrosis. **A.** Six-and-a-half years pre-operative. **B.** Early post-operative. **C.** By 2 months post-operative, a complete periacetabular radiolucent line is apparent and there is a suggestion of femoral neck resorption. **D.** Two months later (4 months post-operative). Femoral neck narrowing is definite. **E.** By 11 months post-operative, neck narrowing is dramatic (see text for diagnosis of failure). **F.** Conversion of the septically failed hip was to a stemmed THA (using antibiotic-impregnated cement); but by 5 months following revision, the hip again appears suspicious. **G.** Eleven months following revision. Sepsis is indicated by osteolysis, periostitis, and widening radiolucent lines. **H.** Conversion to a Girdlestone has been performed. In retrospect, considering the bone changes, this hip would have been better served by simply removing the prosthetic components at the first revision.

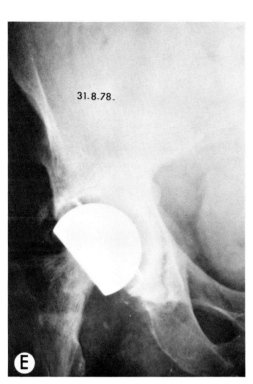

31.8.78.

E

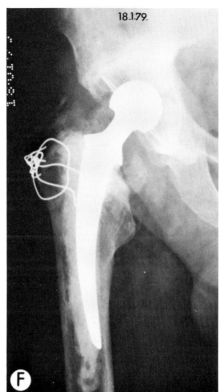

18.1.79.

F

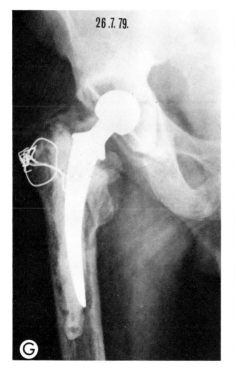

26.7.79.

G

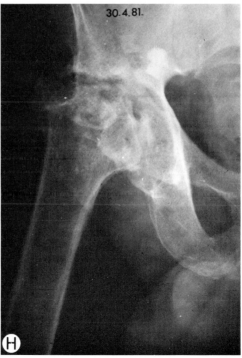

30.4.81.

H

a metal component since, as previously noted, bone scans are unreliable and x-rays are obviously impossible in these circumstances.

The surgical treatment of specific complications within a resurfaced hip can likewise be compared to the treatment of similar complications occurring in a conventional stemmed hip arthroplasty. In the instance of aseptic loosening in a double-cup, both components will usually be loose; this is not necessarily the case with a conventional hip replacement. The exposure requisite for the revision of a failed resurfacing hip is generally more difficult than that required for a conventional hip; more visibility is required and the fibrous reaction (possibly due to wear debris) may be more severe. Exposure for conversion to another double-cup is made even more difficult by the fact that a medially placed trochanteric osteotomy may severely compromise the result. For a revision to a conventional hip, trochanteric osteotomy will not compromise the result; it may be necessary for exposure. If the femoral component of a resurfaced hip is loose, the remnant of the femoral stump is usually insufficient for secure fixation of another double-cup; insertion of a stem, however, can be accomplished as easily as in a primary hip replacement, and is far easier than revision of a stemmed, conventional hip replacement.

On the acetabular side, bone loss with the early prostheses was often significant because of the insertion techniques and the hemispherical (or nearly hemispherical) components employed. This disadvantage of the earlier resurfacing prostheses is no longer present with the current insertion techniques and design of acetabular components.

If the femoral component of a double-cup is not loose it is extremely difficult to remove it without damaging underlying bone. In this instance, it is probably better either to leave the femoral component intact or to insert a stemmed prosthesis. Still, the primary rule of revision surgery for a failed resurfacing prosthesis is to maintain the integrity of the femoral canal until the possibility of sepsis has been eliminated.

Femoral neck fracture is of course unique to resurfaced hips. Revision to a conventional hip replacement represents no special problems (especially as compared with revision for stem fracture in a conventional total hip arthroplasty). We

Fig. 9-9. An example of how reducing the acetabular component to less than a hemisphere results in a smaller prosthesis having the same thickness of the polyethylene layer. In this hypothetical resurfacing acetabular component, the internal diameter is defined as being 45 mm and the concentric polyethylene is 6 mm thick. A hemispherical component will then have an outside diameter of 57 mm; a component reduced by 40° will have an outside diameter of only 50 mm.

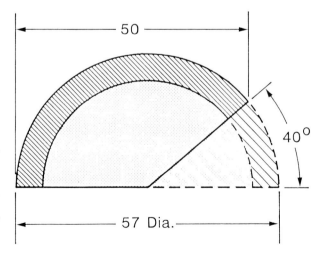

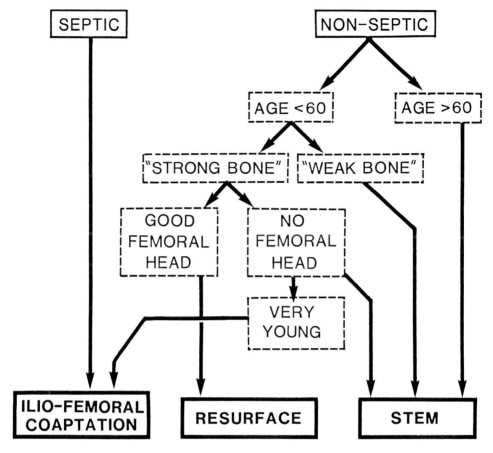

Fig. 9-10. Flow chart of usually recommended procedures for a failed resurfacing prosthesis.

do not advise the use of oversized diameter, semicustom femoral components in this instance because of the long-term problems theoretically related to a large weight-bearing surface. Our recommendation is conversion of both components to a conventional 22 mm or 32 mm head stemmed prosthesis.

Recurrent dislocation is almost always related to malplacement of the acetabular component in a vertical or anteverted position. Revision of a resurfacing prosthesis is comparable to revision for a conventional hip prosthesis. In addition to reorientating the acetabular component, it is also important to be certain that the margins of the prosthesis are entirely covered by bone.

In the case of sepsis, debridement and conversion of a double-cup is considerably easier than a similar procedure for a conventional, stemmed prosthesis with the canal partially filled with PMMA. Present concerns regarding insertion of a new prosthesis at the time of debridement are basically the same as for a conventional hip replacement, with the following additions:

1. There is probably no place for conversion of a septic double-cup to another double-cup, since the femoral stump inevitably will prove inadequate.
2. If a septic double-cup is converted to a conventional stemmed prosthesis

Table 9-4
Treatment of Failed Hip Arthroplasty:
Resurfaced Compared with Conventional

Complication	Treatment
Aseptic loosening	Acetabulum: worse in earlier double-cups; present generation is same. Femur: easier in surface replacement.
Femoral neck fracture	Different, but compared to revision for a stem fracture in a conventional hip replacement, double-cup is technically an easier procedure.
Recurrent dislocation	May be considerably different. Dislocation in a resurfaced hip is virtually always secondary to acetabular malposition, in which case revision is not very difficult. Recurring dislocation in conventional, stemmed replacement may be due to both or either; if due to malposition on the femoral side, revision surgery can be tedious at best.
Sepsis	Once exposure is obtained, surgical debridement is far easier in a surface replacement. Conversion of a surface replacement failed in the presence of sepsis to a stemmed arthroplasty is technically easier and theoretically safer than similar conversions for a stemmed prosthesis. Excision arthroplasty for a surface replacement is predictably a far better hip than a similar excision of all components in a septically failed conventional total hip arthroplasty. In a surface replacement hip there will not be any large dead space in the femoral canal.

which in turn becomes septic, the patient is much worse than he or she would have been prior to the first procedure. Therefore, we believe that (save in exceptional circumstances), nothing should be done other than removal of the double-cup prosthesis and debridement. This is especially true in view of the theoretically better functional results of this procedure compared with a similar Girdlestone procedure performed for a septic conventional hip replacement.[9]

3. Nonetheless, conversion of a septic double-cup to a conventional, stemmed arthroplasty is theoretically less hazardous than replacement of a stemmed hip with another stemmed hip, since the femoral shaft has not been previously violated in a resurfaced hip.

REFERENCES

1. Aubriot J, Insler HP: Unpublished data, 1980.
2. Buchholz HW, Elson RA, Engelbrecht E, et al: Management of deep infection of total hip replacement. *J Bone and Joint Surg* 63(B):342-353, 1981.
3. Buchholz HW: Personal communication, 1981.
4. Cameron HU: Personal communication, 1981.
5. Capello WJ, Wellman, HM: Unpublished data, 1978.
6. Carlsson AS, Josefsson G, Lindberg, L: Revision with gentamycin-impregnated cement for deep infections in total hip arthroplasties. *J. Bone and Joint Surg* 60(A):1059-1064, 1978.

7. Chambers TJ: The cellular basis of bone resorption. *Clin Orthop* 151:283-293, 1980.

8. Charnley J: *Low Friction Arthroplasty of the Hip.* New York, Springer-Verlag, 1979.

9. Clegg J: The results of pseudoarthrosis after removal of an infected total hip prosthesis. *J Bone and Joint Surg* 59(B):298-301, 1973.

10. Freeman MAR: Some anatomical and mechanical considerations relevant to surface replacement of the femoral head, *Clin Orthop* 134:19-24, 1978.

11. Freeman MAR: Unpublished data, 1981.

12. Furuya K, Tsuchiya M, Kawachi S: Socket cup arthroplasty, *Clin Orthop* 134:41-44, 1978.

13. Greiss ME, Thomas RJ, Freeman MAR: Sequelae of arthrodesis of the hip. *J of the Roy Soc Med* 73:497-500, 1980.

14. Head WC: Wagner surface replacement arthroplasty of the hip. *J Bone and Joint Surg* 63(A):420-427, 1981.

15. Hunter GA, Welsh RP, Cameron HU, et al: The results of revision of total hip arthroplasty. *J Bone and Joint Surg* 61(B):419-421, 1979.

16. Lange DR, Whiteside LA, Lesker PA: Femoral head circulation: Blood flow measurements in normal and arthritic canine femoral heads. *Trans 25th Annual ORS (vol. 4),* San Francisco, p 14, 1979.

17. LeQuesne M, DeSeze S, Arnouroux J: Coxarthrose destructive rapide; *révue de Rheumatisme* 37:721, 1970.

18. Müller ME: Personal communication, 1980.

19. Stewart MJ, Coker TP: Arthrodesis of the hip, *Clin Orthop* 62:136-150, 1969.

20. Stinchfield FE, Cavallero WU: Arthrodesis of the hip joint *J Bone and Joint Surg* 32(A):48-57, 1950.

21. Turner R: Revision arthroplasty in the USA. *Symposium: Revision arthroplasty,* Sheffield, England, 1979.

22. Wagner H: Double-cup resurfacing for the arthritic hip. *George Perkins Symposium.* London, 1981.

Peter P. Anas and
Arnold D. Scheller, Jr.

10

Femoral Hemiarthroplasty Revision Arthroplasty

The "arthroplasty era" of the hip was initiated through the pioneer efforts of Smith-Petersen with his introduction of the mold arthroplasty in 1939.[23] His work clearly established that arthroplasty could achieve significant relief for many who suffered from hip disease. A further advancement occurred with the development of the medullary-stem femoral prosthesis, which was introduced by the Judet brothers in 1948,[14] and subsequently improved and popularized by Austin Moore and Thompson.[18,24] Hemiarthroplasty allowed treatment of a diverse range of hip disorders for which the mold arthroplasty was not suited. Problems such as intracapsular hip fractures, nonunions, and avascular necrosis responded well, and continue to be prime indications for hemiarthroplasty.

There have been many series published in the orthopedic literature which demonstrate the success of hemiarthroplasty surgery. Apley, Hinchley, and Sarmiento report satisfactory results in 84-92 percent of patients.[2,12,21] One study by Salvati indicates that 90 percent of patients sustain their beneficial results for 5 years or more.[20] However, as with all arthroplasty procedures, there is a significant failure rate due to multiple causes. Reported failure rates for the hemiarthroplasty procedure range between 7 and 16 percent.[2,12,20] To examine this question of failure from another perspective, it is instructive to note that two extensive series of total hip replacements list failure of a hemiarthroplasty as the surgical indication in 15 percent of cases.[5,16]

Hemiarthroplasty surgery is a procedure of proven benefit for many painful conditions of the hip, and will predictably provide sustained therapeutic results for approximately 85 percent of patients. The main indication resides in the management of hip fractures, of which there are some 200,000/year in the United States. The procedure is of established benefit in other conditions which involve pathology of the femoral head with preservation of acetabular cartilage. These include avascular necrosis, nonunion, and neoplasm. Failure will occur in 10-15 percent of

227

Table 10-1
Etiology of Painful Hemiarthroplasty

Acetabular complications

Acetabular wear
Protrusio

Femoral complications

Aseptic loosening
Malposition
Subsidence—Shortening
Calcar resorption
Recurrent dislocation
Shaft fracture
Component fracture
Incorrect femoral head size

Infection

Septic loosening

Heterotopic bone

Periarticular complications

Soft-tissue contracture
Abductor weakness
Trochanteric bursitis
Limb-length inequality
Sciatic neuritis

Referred Pain

Lumbar spine disease
Genitourinary pain
Inguinal or obturator hernia

hemiarthroplasties, and management of selected cases may be achieved by revision to a total hip arthroplasty. This chapter will attempt to enumerate the potential causes of a painful hemiarthroplasty, develop a logical approach to evaluation of this condition, and consider management with special emphasis upon surgical conversion total hip replacement.

HEMIARTHROPLASTY FAILURE

Failure of a hemiarthroplasty will be defined as the occurence of severe pain, loss of motion, deformity, or instability which incapacitates a patient and necessitates surgical intervention. It is important to understand that a hemiarthroplasty will by no means render a diseased hip normal or absolutely asymptomatic. With few exceptions, patients who have undergone replacement of the femoral head will perceive some degree of discomfort in that hip. Sarmiento has reported similar observations in his review of hemiarthroplasty.[21] There is, however, a distinct subgroup of patients who experience severe and unremitting symptoms and need further treatment. These patients require a thorough diagnostic evaluation, and the surgeon requires an appreciation for the technical complexities and exigencies encountered in revision surgery.

Table 10-1 conveniently lists the potential mechanisms producing pain in a hemiarthroplasty; conditions are listed in order of significance. The problems of acetabular deterioration and femoral loosening are the most frequent causes of hemiarthroplasty failure. Infection and heterotopic bone are less frequent offenders and are covered in Chapters 7 and 15. The periarticular and referred sources of pain must be painstakingly diagnosed, since these are nonsurgical problems which are manageable by conservative measures. When approaching a patient problem or radiograph, it may be helpful to consider such a catalogue of potential problems to assure that a comprehensive evaluation has been made.

It is of significance that many of these complications are predictable sequelae of hemiarthroplasty surgery, and probably occur to some extent in the vast majority of patients. The introduction of a metallic prosthesis into a human joint is an anomalous, nonphysiologic situation. Upon completion of post-operative rehabilitation (6 to 12 months), the hemiarthroplasty is functioning maximally and will commence upon an inexorable course of deterioration. The extent and rate of deterioration vary with the individual patient, operation, and surgeon. It is for this reason that a surgeon must not anticipate or predict a "normal" hip, and must enlist the understanding and cooperation of his or her patient in the long-term care of a prosthetic joint. Discomforts which the patient experiences are manifestations of deterioration and wear. Most patients will coexist with this situation and the prosthesis will function within acceptable limits. In others, the rate of deterioration will exceed patient tolerance, and symptoms will dictate the necessity for evaluation and treatment.

Acetabular Wear

Acetabular deterioration occurs because of the articulation between hyaline cartilage and metal. The normal synovial joint provides for congruent articulation between two hyaline cartilage surfaces, which are supported by a composite of subchondral and trabecular bone, allowing a physiological transmission of static and dynamic forces through the weight-bearing surfaces to the cortical shaft of the femur. These hyaline surfaces function within a physiological milieu of nutritive and lubricating synovial fluid. A metallic femoral head destroys this physiologic balance. The hyaline cartilage of the acetabulum must articulate with an incongruent and unyielding metallic surface which exhibits an increased coefficient of friction. Acetabular cartilage must inevitably deteriorate in a fashion analogous to pure degenerative joint disease (Fig. 10-1).

Acetabular deterioration proceeds as a function of several variables, the most significant of which probably is the condition of the acetabular surface at the time of prosthetic implantation. A healthy articular surface will survive for a longer duration, which explains the observation that a hemiarthroplasty undertaken for femoral disease, such as a fracture, will provide better results than one performed for a process such as osteoarthritis, where both femoral and acetabular articular

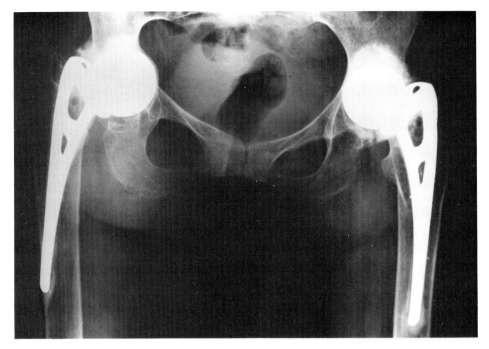

Fig. 10-1. Acetabular wear and protrusion are demonstrated in this 65-year-old female with rheumatoid arthritis, 6 years following bilateral hemiarthroplasties. Also note varus malposition of stem on left.

surfaces are diseased. Hemiarthroplasty patients who possess a radiographic joint space of significant thickness may anticipate superior function over those who have lost joint space. Size of the prosthetic femoral head will influence this variable, since an improper size will fail to homogenously transmit joint forces. Incongruence produces areas of excessive stress transmission and consequent damage to the acetabular surface.

The status of the subchondral and trabecular bone which supports the acetabular surface also plays a role in determining the durability of a hemiarthroplasty. Patients with ostoepenia, inflammatory arthroses, and Paget's disease exhibit weakened mechanical support of the chondral surface. A metallic femoral head may initiate subchondral microfracture and accelerated articular wear. This process may extend beyond articular degeneration and produce protrusio acetabulae as the entire osseous support structure yields.

Femoral Complications

Hemiarthroplasty components demonstrate an inherent potential for deterioration and failure on the femoral side of the joint (Fig. 10-3). Femoral complications most often manifest as inadequacy of intramedullary fixation. Anchorage within the medullary canal of the femur is based upon an interference fit between metal and bone, collar-calcar contact, and bone growth into stem fenestrations.[9] Absolute fixation of an intramedullary component is rarely, if ever, achieved. This observation is shared by many authors, and is expressed in the works of Coventry, Evarts, and

Sarmiento.[6,9,21] The basis for femoral loosening resides in the inadequacy of interference fit and bone ingrowth. Factors which exacerbate the loosening problem are high physical demand on the hemiarthroplasty, improper stem-canal ratio, and osteopenia. A loose prosthesis will move within the medullary canal and produce pain. Motion may remain continuous or the prosthesis may resettle into an improper position. Malposition will most frequently occur in a retroverted or varus orientation; either attitude may cause pain or awkward gait (Fig. 10-2).

Calcar resorption and associated subsidence of the femoral component are additional failure modes which cause malfunction and pain. Subsidence of a prosthesis leads to shortening of the limb which in turn causes functional abductor weakness, impingement of the greater trochanter on the iliac wing, reduced range of motion, and short limb gait. The etiology of calcar resorption is unknown, but theoretical causes include poor local blood supply after surgery or trauma, excessive compressive forces produced by the collar on the calcar, and the phenomenon of stress-shielding. Osteopenia and lack of firm fixation of the medullary stem may exacerbate calcar resorption, since even greater forces will be transmitted to the calcar.

Innovations have recently been introduced in an effort to alleviate the problems

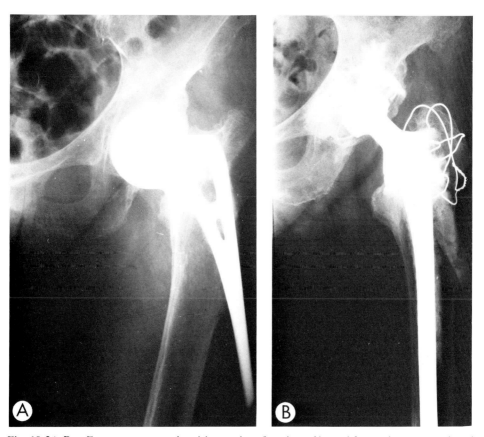

Fig. 10-2A,B.   Extreme varus malposition and perforation of lateral femoral cortex produced pain and necessitated revision to total hip replacement.

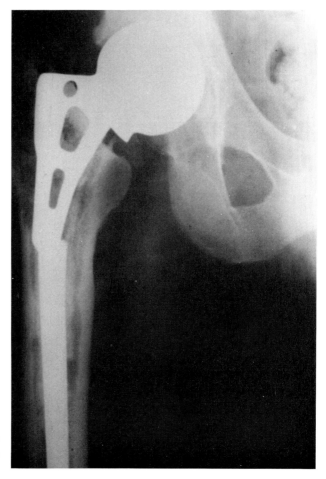

Fig. 10-3. Fracture of hemiarthroplasty stem prior to revision.

of acetabular wear and femoral loosening. The development of the bipolar hemiarthroplasty implants, such as the Bicentric (Howmedica), Bateman (3M Company), and Giliberty (Zimmer) types, was an attempt to limit acetabular wear through a reduction in motion between the prosthesis and acetabulum. While these ingenious devices have intriguing theoretical advantages, their efficacy has yet to be demonstrated.[7] The use of acrylic cement to enhance intramedullary fixation of the hemiarthroplasty has been advocated,[9] but remains a controversial matter and has not entirely overcome the problem of femoral loosening. The approach to diagnosis and management of a painful bipolar prosthesis is the same as any other hemiarthroplasty, whereas the management of a cemented hemiarthroplasty is analogous to the revision of a cemented femoral component of a total hip prosthesis (Fig. 10-4).

Infection

Infection must always remain a consideration in the evaluation of a painful hemiarthroplasty. This is perhaps the most serious complication in the field of joint replacement and may present in the early post operative period, or at any subsequent point in the patient's life. All previously mentioned modes of acetabular and femoral failure may be precipitated or exaggerted by the presence of infection. Infection may manifest in an acute, fulminating manner, or as an indolent process that is clinically indistinguishable from nonseptic failure. Infection must be ruled out pre-operatively in all cases of failed hemiarthroplasty, since its presence has direct implications in management.

DIAGNOSTIC APPROACH

The standard diagnostic approach of history, physical, and radiologic examination should be applied in the evaluation of a paiful hemiarthroplasty. Many helpful clues may be derived from each phase of evaluation; departure from this comprehensive approach may court error. Information concerning duration, location, progression, and character of a patient's discomfort may suggest the underlying cause of pain. The temporal relationship of pain to the original surgery is often of import, as are the original diagnosis for which the hemiarthroplasty was performed,

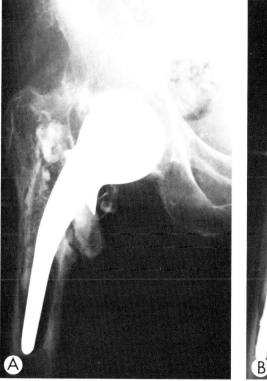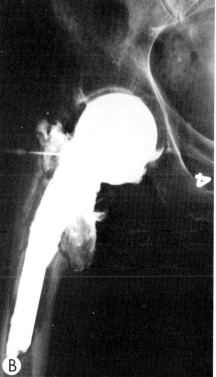

Fig. 10-4A,B. Failure of cemented hemiarthroplasty 6 months after surgery. Aspiration and arthrogram demonstrated loosening and no infection. Patient was converted to total hip replacement.

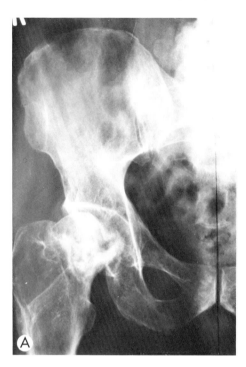
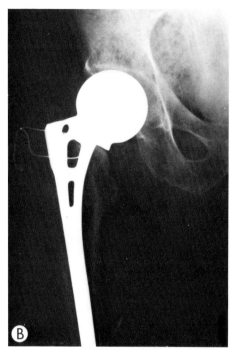

Fig. 10-5A–D. Serial films of patient who underwent hemiarthroplasty for avascullar necrosis complicating a subcapital fracture. Note loss of joint space indicating acetabular wear and subsidence of prosthesis into femoral canal. Revision to total hip replacement provided complete pain relief.

a history of previous surgery of the involved hip, and any history of local or systemic infection.

Pain which localizes to the groin and is exacerbated by weight-bearing is indicative of acetabular wear, whereas pain associated with femoral loosening is commonly referred to the thigh, knee, or occasionally the entire lower extremity. The onset of pain in the immediate post-operative period suggests early post-operative infection, improper prosthetic size, or malposition. Pain which has a later onset and has been slowly progressive over time typifies the inexorable process of acetabular wear or femoral loosening. A history of progressive limb shortening, loss of motion, or abnormal position of the foot during gait are all typical of femoral loosening with subsidence and toggle. Any evidence of infection, wound drainage, erythema, or prolonged swelling is important to elicit. Likewise, one should assess underlying medical problems, such as diabetes, rheumatoid arthritis, corticosteroid therapy, or any general debility which may predispose to infection. Inquiry should also be directed at obtaining information about the lumbrosacral spine, gastrointestinal, and genitourinary tracts which may cause referred pain to the hip area.

Physical examination should include the standard orthopaedic parameters of stance, gait, range of motion, and strength, together with assessment of previous surgical scars, movement of soft-tissue planes, and inguinal adenopathy. The gait must be observed for an antalgic component, functional length, and excessive in-

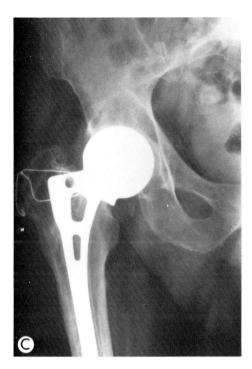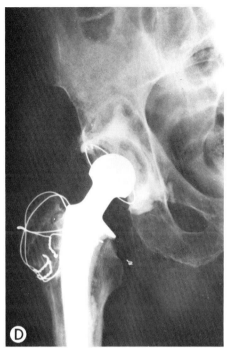

toeing or out-toeing. A study of hip motion may demonstrate instability, malposition, or impingement. Weakness of the abductor musculature may significantly contribute to pain about the hip, instability, and poor gait mechanics. Tell-tale signs of infection such as erythema, fluctuance, and inguinal adenopathy should be sought. Neurovascular examination will assist in the exclusion of referred sources of pain. (Chapter 1 expands upon the clinical evaluation of painful arthroplasties.)

Radiographic Assessment

The radiologic studies of assistance in the evaluation of a painful hemiarthroplasty are the plain films, arthrogram, and bone scan. Plain films are indispensible; a routine series should include the anteroposterior (AP) projection of the pelvis and both hips, together with a frog-lateral and true-lateral of the involved side. This permits evaluation from several viewing angles. If surgical revision is planned, then an anteroposterior and lateral film of the entire femur should be evaluated, since a longer-stem prosthesis commonly is required. The optimal radiographic assessment is provided by study of serial films from initial surgery to the present. Subtle pathologic alterations may then be observed over time (Fig. 10-5).

An orderly assessment of the radiograph begins with an evaluation of overall bone density and trabecular pattern for evidence of osteopenia, which can contribute to various modes of failure or complicate surgical revision. The joint space is then observed for acetabular wear and narrowing, best examined through comparison of serial films. The uncommon finding of an enlarging joint space over a short time course is an indication of sepsis, as granulation tissue or purulence expand the joint space. An additional sign of infection on the acetabular side is the loss or absence

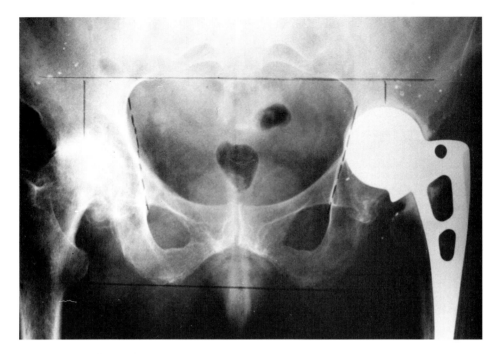

Fig. 10-6. Radiographic assessment demonstrates osteopenia, acetabular wear, protrusio, superior migration of acetabulum, calcar resoption, and sclerotic bone reaction at prosthetic interface and tip.

of a sclerotic reaction "eye brow sign" in the subchondral acetabular roof. Loss of the sclerotic eye brow sign is consistent with infection. Attention should next be drawn to the acetabulum for evidence of protrusio, defined as inward migration of the femoral head beyond the ilioischial line (Fig. 10-6).

The femoral side of the joint should be scrutinized next for the size relationship of the prosthetic head and acetabulum, quality of calcar bone stock, the bone-prosthetic interface of the intramedullary stem, and the alignment of the stem within the medullary canal. A wide or widening interface about the prosthetic stem is an indication of sepsis, as is a progressive dissolution of bone stock. Much has been written of the sclerotic bone resection about the prosthetic tip as both an indicator of firm fixation and loosening. Most authors report that it is a]sign of loosening,[1,21] whereas we have observed it with equal frequency in painless and painful arthroplasties. It has not been a helpful sign in our experience.

A change in the position of the intramedullary stem indicates loosening and will generally manifest as a varus tilt. Stem orientation in both AP and lateral planes should be studied in regards to future reaming of the medullary canal, since following a tract which is not centered within the canal may result in shaft perforation. The relative length of the proximal femur may be judged by comparison of the lesser trochanters to a tangential line connecting the two ischial tuberosities. A long or short neck should be compensated for during revision. The degree of prosthetic anteversion or retroversion may be determined by a method similar to that used in assessing femoral anteversion in children, but this technique offers little benefit over the clinical examination of internal and external rotation.

Radionucleotide studies may be of some value in the assessment of a painful hemiarthroplasty. Painful arthroplasties will demonstrate increased uptake of technesium pyrophosphate as a nonspecific indicator of increased regional blood flow, and may result from mechanical loosening or infection. A negative bone scan would preclude loosening or infection, but a positive scan will not distinguish between the two. A gallium or tagged white cell scan will distinguish infection.[19] These are, however, expensive and time-consuming endeavors to demonstrate infection, whereas hip aspiration and the arthrogram are direct and valuable techniques which we consider mandatory to complete the pre-operative evaluation.

THERAPY AND REVISION SURGERY

Nearly all painful arthroplasties should undergo a trial of conservative therapy. The principle modes of conservative treatment include weight reduction, ambulatory aids, reduced activity, and physical therapy. Physical therapy is directed at improving range of motion, abductor strength, and gait abnormalities. These conservative modalities combined with judicious use of anti-inflamatory and analgesic medications will relieve many patients. Others will prefer the permanent use of an ambulatory aid and limited activity rather than revision surgery. Some will experience inadequate pain relief from conservative measures or will have a clear indication for revision surgery. Severe pain, protrusio acetabulae, gross femoral loosening, and infection constitute absolute indications for surgery, with pain relief being the principal indication.

The surgical procedures which may be of use in the management of a painful hemiarthroplasty include: (1) conversion to a total hip replacement; (2) exchange of the hemiarthroplasty component; (3) debridement of heterotopic bone; and (4) removal of the hemiarthroplasty, joint debridement, and conversion to a resection arthroplasty. Exchange of a hemiarthroplasty component may be considered in the rare situation of an over-sized or undersized prosthesis in the early post-operative period. Heterotopic bone may be a cause of pain and limited motion, and if the hemiarthroplasty itself is functioning well, a procedure limited to the debridement of heterotopic bone may be undertaken (Chapter 15). The Girdlestone procedure is indicated in cases of infection and severe loss of bone stock in the acetabulum or proximal femur.

CONVERSION OF HEMIARTHROPLASTY TO TOTAL HIP REPLACEMENT

The following discussion will consider, in detail, the conversion of a hemiarthroplasty to a total hip replacement, as performed at the New England Baptist Hospital. It will be followed by a section addressing the problems and complications unique to hemiarthroplasty revision. Table 10-2 outlines the pre-operative program followed by our patients in preparation for surgery.

The surgical principles of hemiarthroplasty revision include a wide transtrochanteric approach with extensive soft-tissue release to facilitate exposure of the failed endoprosthesis and femoral canal. Exposure is followed by prosthetic

Table 10-2
Pre-operative Program

Day 1

Admission and Orthopaedic Examination

Laboratory studies
  CBC, ESR, chemistry profile
  Electrolytes, urinalysis and culture
  PT/PTT, platelet count, bleeding time
  EKG, impedance plethysmography
  Crossmatching of blood (4-6 units)

Radiology
  CXR
  AP pelvis, frog and true lateral of prothesis
  AP and lateral of femur
  Hip aspiration and arthrogram

Nightly iodine or hexachlorophene scrubs

Day 2

Medical evaluation

Anesthesiology evaluation

Physical therapy evaluation and training

Pre-operative surgical planning

Day 3

Surgery

---

extraction; preparation of the medullary canal; acetabular reconstruction; component selection and fixation; and trochanteric reattachment. It is paramount that a broad selection of acetabular and femoral components are available to insure that intraoperative contingencies may be met. Careful planning from the pre-operative films will provide an indication of appropriate component size; templates are useful for this purpose. However, final judgement of component size must be reserved until intraoperative assessment of skeletal anatomy, trial prosthetic reduction, range of motion, and soft tissue tension. Table 10-3 lists the component sizes used in a review of 100 hemiarthroplasty revisions, and offers an indication of the broad selection of component sizes which should be available at surgery.

Proper management of the femoral canal is critical to the maintenance of sound acrylic fixation of the femoral component. Furthermore, the proper length of the femoral stem is that which bypasses the previous component. It is our thesis that the proximal femoral canal of a failed hemiarthroplasty is ill-suited for sound acrylic fixation, due to the proliferation of a fibrous membrane and a sclerotic bone reaction at the failed prosthetic interface. In addition to the problem of cement fixation, there is also a problem of stress transmission. The proximal femoral cortex is generally thinned and weakened because of the previous hemiarthroplasty and the necessary preparation for a revision arthroplasty (color plate V). The transition area from the "abnormal" cortex to the normal distal cortex acts as a stress-raiser and a potential point of failure.

Table 10-3

Components Used in 100 Hemiarthroplasty Revisions*

Femoral Components		Acetabular Components	
Stem length	Neck length	Outside diameter	
8 inch (2%)	30 mm	45 mm	(58%)
9 inch (10%)	36 mm	51 mm	(27%)
10 inch (17%)	42 mm	56 mm	(11%)
12 inch (81%)	45 mm	66 mm	(4%)
	52 mm		
	62 mm		

*Figures in parenthesis indicate percentage of use.

In order to overcome the problems of fixation and stress transmission it becomes necessary to bypass the end of the failed prosthesis with a longer femoral component. The optimal length of a revision stem is not known, but certain factors guide the decision. Engineering analysis has shown that for a cylinder, which most closely approximates the femur, one must bypass a stress-raiser by a distance twice the diameter of the cylinder in order to reach an area of normal stress distribution. We therefore conclude that optimal bone-cement fixation and pattern of femoral stress transmission require a stem length which bypasses the previous prosthesis by a minimal distance of twice the femoral shaft diameter.

The standard femoral component design for revision surgery of the hip has been the Aufranc-Turner 12-inch revision stem. This component has proven both suitable and reliable. In a review of 173 cases (Hamati and Turner, 1979, unpublished ms.) of revision hip procedures followed for 5 years, there has been only a single case of nonseptic loosening. Although bone-cement fixation is increased with the long stem, there are theoretical reservations concerning the routine use of a 12-inch femoral stem. Reservations include the problem of stress-shielding and disuse atrophy of the proximal femur, together with the extraordinary complexity required to revise a failed 12-inch stem. To this end, we have proposed and follow a set of guidelines to aid in selection of proper stem length when revising a failed hemiarthroplasty (Table 10-4).

On the day of surgery, the patient is brought to the operating room where general anesthesia is administered. Patients are monitored with central venous

Table 10-4

Guidelines for Selecting Length of Revision Stem

Revision Stem Length Must:

Pass pathologic cortical tube created by removal of failed prosthesis,

Penetrate distal cancellous mantle for improved bone-cement interface, and

Reach a point beyond pathologic cortical tube where stress pattern becomes normal (for a cylinder, this distance is twice the diameter).

Recommended Minimum Revision Stem Length:

Failed stem	Revision stem
5 inch (125 mm) stem	150 mm stem
7 inch (175 mm) stem	250 mm stem

catheters, arterial lines, and indwelling Foley catheter. During the procedure we strive for milliliter-for-milliliter blood replacement to avoid a hypotensive response to acrylic monomer. The patient is placed in the lateral position upon a translucent operating table that will accommodate a flouroscopic C-arm. The extremity is scrubbed for 10 minutes with iodine scrub solution from the costal margin to the mid-calf, and then painted with tincture of iodine. Routine draping is carried out with a double layer of cloth sheets, a disposable lap sheet which is impervious to water, and a sterile cloth bag opposite the surgeon to eventually accommodate the anteriorly dislocated extremity which will overhang the edge of the operating table. Proper draping should expose the iliac crest, should a bone graft be required, and the lateral thigh to the supracondylar area, in case distal femoral perforation necessitates exposure of the femur.

The standard incision is centered over the tip of the greater trochanter and is extended in the proximal direction to a point which marks the intersection of a tranverse line at the level of the anterior superior iliac spine and a longitudinal line at the posterior border of the greater trochanter. The incision is then extended along the midline of the femoral shaft approximately 8 inches. It may be extended in either direction should conditions warrant. We attempt to utilize previous skin incisions if possible. The standard incision may deviate approximately 1 inch anterior or posterior to the greater trochanter and femoral shaft if previous incisions so dictate. Otherwise, a new, parallel incision is made. Transversing a previous incision which is at least 1 year old has not caused wound problems in our experience. Previous scars may be excised for cosmetic reasons, but it is best deferred until the time of closure when final assessment of tissue-tension is made.

Dissection is then carried through the subcutaneous tissues and fascia lata in line with skin incision, while palpating the lateral femoral shaft to assure a position posterior to tensor fascia lata and anterior to the tendon of gluteus maximus. Proximal to the greater trochanter, the fibers of gluteus maximus are split bluntly, taking care to observe for occasional bleeders. The bursa of the greater trochanter is then opened and, if possible, preserved for subsequent closure. The anterior and posterior borders of the abductor musculature are then identified. Great care is taken to preserve the integrity of the abductors, since they have often been unwittingly damaged during prior surgery and are crucial to the stability and fuction of a total hip replacement. With the leg in flexion and external rotation, it is possible to superiorly retract the anterior borders of the gluteus minimus and medius, and identify a border of demarcation between the insertion of these tendons onto the greater trochanter and the origin of vastus intermedius. This border indicates the anterior boundary of the trochanteric osteotomy. While in this region, it is also helpful to identify the anterior and inferior hip capsule, which may be cleared with a periosteal elevator and incised. The hip is then brought into extension and internal rotation. The posterior border of the osteotomy is established by releasing remnants of the short external rotators and exposing the posterior capsule. The origin of the vastus lateralis is then released from the vastus tubercle with the coagulation knife; the trochanter is osteotomized at this level.

The depth of the trochanteric osteotomy should be sufficient to include the entire insertion of the abductor musculature, and not so deep as to entirely destroy a cancellous bed for subsequent reattachment. An osteotomy based at the vastus tubercle and directed parallel to the lateral cortex of the femur will generally fulfill these requirements. The trochanter must be osteotomized for proper exposure and preparation of the medullary canal; it will also simplify removal of the hemiarthroplasty implant by allowing greater access to fenestrations. Trochanteric osteotomy is a potential cause of post-operative complications due to avulsion, nonunion, and bursitis. Attention to detail in the osteotomy, preservation of cancellous bed, and secure reattachment will alleviate many of the potential difficulties.

The trochanter is then superiorly retracted onto the lateral wing of the ilium, taking care to preserve the abductor tendon and separating it from superior capsule. The entire capsule may now be exposed and capsulectomy undertaken. Cultures of synovial fluid and capsular tissue are obtained at this point. With a bone hook about the neck and distal traction, the hip is gently dislocated anteriorly by flexion, adduction, and external rotation. The leg is placed in the sterile cloth bag. Dislocation is potentially hazardous because of the large lever arm of the femoral shaft and the potential for producing a shaft fracture. If dislocation is not readily achieved, the obstruction must be isolated and corrected. A common cause is osteophyte formation about the acetabular rim, producing a bottle-neck effect. This must be osteotomized before dislocation. Another frequent obstruction to dislocation is incomplete capsulotomy of the inferior capsule.

Once dislocation has been achieved, the prosthesis must be removed from the femoral shaft. Femoral shaft fracture is a hazard during this maneuver. Prosthetic removal should commence by dissection of all soft tissue and bony overgrowth at the junction of femur and prosthetic neck. The femoral component may then be dislodged with a slap-hammer extractor inserted into the fenestrated collar, or the prosthesis may be drive out with a bone set and mallet, striking the collar of the implant upwards and driving the component out. Should these maneuvers fail to provide the desired result, a flexible osteotome may be driven alongside the prosthesis to release soft-tissue or osseous adhesions within fenestrations. A thin-blade reciprocating saw may be used in a similar fashion. Note that trochanteric osteotomy allows greater access to the fenestrations. Patience, care, and perservance will prevail; the component will yield. Should all else fail, the femoral cortex may be anteriorly windowed, to release the fenestrations and drive the component upwards.

Once the femoral head is dislocated and extracted from the femoral canal, there will be clear access to the acetabulum. A complete circumferential capsulectomy is performed in order to gain full exposure of the acetabulum, relieve soft-tissue contractures, allow proper adjustment of neck length, and facilitate delivery of the femur from the wound for subsequent preparation of the medullary canal. It rarely becomes necessary to release the psoas tendon to gain sufficient exposure. The acetabulum is then reamed with standard Mira reamers or the Midas Rex pneumatic tool, according to surgeon's preference. Reaming should extend partway through subchondral bone to achieve a cancellous interface suitable for cement fixation. The medial wall may be thinned due to medial migration of the previous hemiarthroplasty, and extra care must be taken to avoid penetration. Anchorage holes are then made in the ilium, ischium, and pubis. The proper acetabular component is that which is covered superiorly to at least 75 percent of its extent when placed in 35°–40° abduction from the horizontal, while allowing for a 2–4 mm circumferential cement mantle. The acetabulum is cemented in this position with 15°–20° of forward flexion.

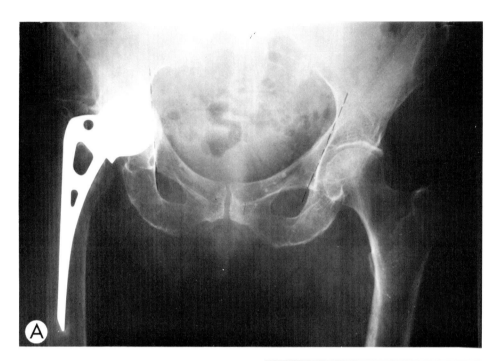

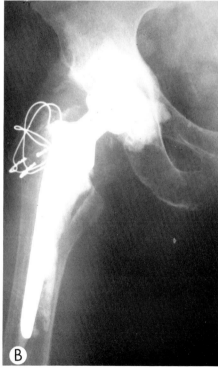

Fig. 10-7A, B. Revision of hemiarthroplasty to total hip replacement. Note poor bone-cement interface due to faulty preparation of proximal canal and short stem. Femoral component at risk for loosening.

Attention is now directed to the femoral canal, which is delivered from the wound, and the flouroscope is draped and brought into position. The surgeon may be seated so as to look directly into the medullary canal. A fiberoptic headlight is of much assistance. All reactive membrane from the previous bone-metal interface must be debrided, and the distal medullary canal is entered. Membrane and sclerotic bone may be removed with curetttes and rasps (Fig. 10-7A, B) The optimal tool, however, is the Midas Rex pneumatic instrument. We also prefer to open the distal canal with this instrument, under direct vision with the flouroscope. It may also be possible to enter the distal femoral canal with a set of flexible Kuntchner reamers, which are also used to expand the distal canal once it is opened. At this juncture, the trial femoral component is introduced into the femur and examined under direct flouroscopic visualization to insure position within the canal and abssence of femoral perforation. Once the stem has been found to fit, the proper neck length is determined on the basis of ease of reduction into the acetabulum, range of motion, stability, and knowledge of pre-operative limb lengths.

Prior to final preparation of the canal, three wires for trochanteric fixation are introduced through the drill holes in the proximal femur. With the leg held in abduction, the trochanter is brought down to the trochanteric bed of the femur and its position is adjusted to place it under slight tension. Two #18 stainless steel wires are then longitudinally inserted through the lateral cortex; a third is transversely inserted. Final preparation for cementing is completed by thorough lavage, femoral brushing, suction, and packing. Three to four packages of acrylic cement are then introduced into the canal in a retrograde fashion, using a cement gun. A low-viscosity technique is preferable. The prosthesis is then introduced at 10° anteversion, and further pressurization of the cement is achieved by delivering the stem into the canal. Excess cement is debrided and the remainder is allowed to dry. A final flouroscopic examination of the entire shaft is performed in two planes to observe for shaft perforations and cement extrusion.

The hip is then reduced and a final inspection and irrigation of the wound is made. The leg is supported in abduction and the greater trochanter is secured with three wires. A meticulous tenodesis of the vastus lateralis over the greater trochanter is performed. This reinforces trochanteric fixation and aids in preventing avulsion. External rotators are reattached when present, and the wound is closed over suction drains. Sterile dressings and compressive bandage spica are applied, and the patient is transferred from the operating table to his or her bed. The patient is then placed in balanced suspension with Buck's traction. X-rays of the femur and pelvis are obtained in recovery room to insure against dislocation during transfer from the operating table.

OPERATIVE PROBLEMS AND COMPLICATIONS

Protrusio Acetabulae

Protrusio acetabulae is not an uncommon sequel to hemiarthroplasty and is prevalent in osteoporosis and inflammatory arthropathy. It is defined as medial migration of the femoral head beyond the ilioischial line, and may be graded as mild, moderate, or severe. Three basic approaches to management attempt to achieve lateralization of the femoral head beneath the weight-bearing dome of the acetabulum. Mild-to-moderate degrees of protrusio may be lateralized by utilizing a thicker medial mantle of cement or, preferably, an oversized acetabular component. Cases of severe protrusion or medial wall deficiency may be managed by bone grafting the medial wall and inserting a protrusio shell about the acetabular rim. Minimal or no reaming of the medial wall is preferred, but the remainder of the acetabulum is prepared as usual. Fresh frozen allograft or autograft is then fashioned to cover the medial defect and lateralize the cup. A thin layer of gelfoam overlies the graft; acrylic cement, protrusio shell, additional cement, and the acetabular component are introduced in that sequence. (Chapter 5 provides a detailed discussion of protrusio and other problems of acetabular deficiency.)

Femoral Shaft Fracture About a Hemiarthroplasty

This situation may be managed by revision to a long-stem total hip replacement. Extensive surgery is required and must be weighed against prolonged traction or casting. If the hemiarthroplasty did not provide satisfactory function prior to femoral fracture, this may be a further indication for revision arthroplasty. The technique requies exposure of the shaft fracture by extending the standard incision along the lateral thigh and elevating the vastus lateralis. The hip joint is routinely managed in preparation of the acetabulum and proximal femur. Prior to cementing the femoral component, the fracture must be anatomically reduced and held in place with a Lohman clamp or temporary cerclage wires. Cement and femoral component are then introduced. Bone grafting of the fracture site is optional, but we prefer to use it routinely. (Fig. 10-8). (See chapter 6 for further details.)

Femoral Shaft Perforation

This complication may result from reaming of the femoral canal with hand or power tools. It may be identified at the time of occurrence or following cementing of the stem. In either situation, the defect must be exposed by splitting or elevating the quadriceps muscle. Digital pressure applied during introduction of cement and prosthesis will obstruct extrusion of cement into soft tissues; hardened cement may be chipped and removed with an osteotome. Flouroscopic examination during reaming and following cementing will reveal this problem and allow correction. Extruded cement should not be allowed to remain in soft tissue since it may produce painful irritation and permits a permanent stress-raiser to exist. All perforations should be bone grafted.

Problems of Trochanteric Reattachment

Osteotomy of the trochanter is required for appropriate exposure in revision arthroplasty, but may induce difficulty in obtaining and maintaining secure trochanteric fixation. The trochanter may be thin, porotic, or fracture during surgery. Inadequacy of the femoral trochanteric bed may delay union, and difficulty may be encountered in drawing the trochanter down to the femoral bed if significant length has been restored to the femoral neck. Several maneuvers may be employed to overcome these problems: Relative length may be gained by elevation of the

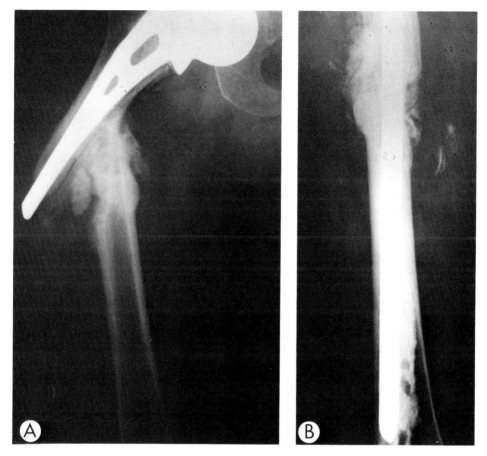

Fig. 10-8A, B.　Inability to maintain alignment and delayed union of femoral shaft fracture were managed by conversion to total hip replacement.

abductors from the lateral ilium, taking care to preserve the superior gluteal artery and nerve as they exit from the sciatic notch. The trochanter may also be attached with the hip in wide abduction, subsequently adducting the limb over 2 to 3 weeks. A porotic or fractured trochanter may be reinforced with trochanteric mesh. An inadequate bed may be supplemented with bone graft or fixation may be achieved with the Voltz Bolt (Howmedica). This device has provoked trochanteric bursitis in numerous instances and should be resorted to only in desperation. If there is absolute inadequacy of the trochanter, the abductor tendons may be tenodesed to the vastus lateralis or fascia lata. Chapter 11 is dedicated to a comprehensive review of trochanteric problems.

Infected Hemiarthroplasty and Girdlestone Procedure

Deep infection of a hemiarthroplasty is a perplexing situation, requiring a high index of suspicion for diagnosis and combined medical and surgical expertise in management. Deep infection may be broadly categorized into low-grade indolent sepsis, produced by low-virulence sensitive organisms; high grade aggressive sepsis produces exuberant granulation, purulence, sinus tract formation, and frank osteomyelitis. Indolent sepsis may be diagnosed by pre-operative aspiration, or retrospectively recognized as the result of positive intra-operative cultures. Indolent sepsis produced by sensitive organisms may be managed by extensive soft-tissue debridement, antibiotic-impregnated cement, and prolonged post-operative antibiotic treatment. This approach has led to an 80 percent long-term success rate (see Chapter 13).

Aggressive sepsis produced by Gram-negative organisms or highly resistant Gram-positive strains is an indication for the Girdlestone procedure. The presence of osteomyelitis, unhealthy or inflamed soft tissues, and sinus tracts frankly contraindict revision surgery. The Girdlestone procedure is also indicated in situations of extensive proximal femoral bone stock loss or an unstable pelvis. (An unstable pelvis is defined as acetabular deficiency or fracture, to the extent that independent motion of the ilioischial, iliopubic, or ischopubic portion(s) of the acetabulum exists.) The Girdlestone procedure is performed through the standard approach, with complete debridement of unhealthy tissues, prosthetic removal, and trochanteric reattachment with a single wire. Constant skeletal traction through the proximal tibia is maintained for a period of 3 weeks, utilizing 15–20 pounds of weight. The patient is then ambulated on crutches during the fourth week, with skeletal traction applied at night. This has proved a suitable salvage procedure allowing a painless pseudoarthrosis and ambulation with either crutches or cane.

POST-OPERATIVE CARE

Post-operative care emcompasses prophylaxis against infection, thromboembolism, and respiratory disease, together with a program of physical rehabilitation. Our general approach is outlined in Table 10-5 and discussed in chapter 16. Aspirin is currently our drug of choice for prophylaxis against thromboembolism; it is combined with elastic stockings and post-operative monitoring by impedance plethysmography. In cases of a positive pre-operative history for thromboembolic disease, we prefer to prescribe coumadin to the patient, starting the evening of surgery. Post-operative abnormalities on impedance plethysmography are further evaluated by venogram; therapy is initiated according to the latter. Prophylactic antibiotics are maintained for 48–72 hours pending the final results of intra-operative cultures and tissue pathology. A physical therapy treatment plan is detailed in chapter 16.

SUMMARY

Proximal femoral hemiarthroplasty remains a sound therapeutic modality for treatment of subcapital fractures and pathologic lesions about the femoral head and neck. Although the surgical implant renders considerable benefit, it is not free of complications and failure. This chapter discusses the clinical manifestations of failure and a logical therapeutic plan for failed hemiarthroplasties.

The scope of therapy ranges from modifying a patient's hip demands and expectations to revision hip arthroplasty. When conservative measures fail and the

Table 10-5
Post-operative Care

Prophylaxis against infection

—Antibiotic (cephalosporin) at time of incision

—Post-operative antibiotic 48-72 hours pending return of intraoperative cultures

—Antibiotic-impregnated cement

Prophylaxis against thromboembolism

—Acetylsalicylic acid (aspirin), 10 gr twice daily

—Coumadin, if patient has a positive history of thrombophlebitis

—Elastic stockings, elevation, and early motion

—Impedance plethysmography, every 3 days

Respiratory therapy

Incentive respirometry, hourly at bedside

Physical Therapy (daily visit by therapist)

Day 0 to 21: Balanced suspension, bedrest
  Day 1: Gluteal, quadriceps, calf-muscle setting exercises hourly
  Day 3: Active assisted range of motion to hip, four times daily

Day 21, or earlier if trochanteric fixation is adequate
  Dangle leg at bedside
  Walk with three-point, touch-down, crutch gait
  Prone lying at least 30 minutes twice daily
  Discharge to home when ambulating comfortably with three-point gait.

—4 months
Transfer from two crutches to one crutch, if patient is comfortable and trochanter is united

—Six months
Transfer to one cane for use outside the home

---

acetabulum is involved, we advocate revision to a total hip replacement. A method of pre operative analysis and the surgical technique with emphasis on problems germane to revision hemiarthroplasty is presented.

REFERENCES

1. Amstutz HC, Smith RK: Total hip replacement following failed hemiarthroplasty. *J Bone and Joint Surg* 61(A):1161–1166, 1979.
2. Apley AG, Millner WF, Porter DS: Follow-up study of Moore's prosthesis in treatment of osteoarthritis of the hip. *J Bone and Joint Surg* 52(B):638–647, 1969.
3. Aufranc OE: Constructive hip surgery with the vitallium mold. A report of 1000 cases of arthroplasty of the hip over a fifteen-year period. *J Bone and Joint Surg* 39(A):237–248, 1957.
4. Barr JS, Donovan JF, Florence DW: Arthroplasty of the hip. *J Bone and Joint Surg* 46(A):249–266, 1964.

5. Beckenbaugh RD, Ilstrup DM: Total hip arthroplasty. *J Bone and Joint Surg* 60(A):306–313, 1978.

6. Coventry MB: Salvage of the painful hip prothesis. *J Bone and Joint Surg* 46(A):200–212, 1964.

7. Drinker H, Murray WR: The universal proximal femoral endoprosthesis. *J Bone and Joint Surg* 61(A):1167–1174, 1979.

8. Dupont JA, Charnley J: Low-friction arthroplasty of the hip for failure of previous operations. *J Bone and Joint Surg* 54(B):77–87, 1972.

9. Evarts CM, Gingras MB: Cemented versus non-cemented endoprostheses, in Murray WR (Ed): *The Hip.* Proceedings of the Fifth Open Surgery Meeting of the Hip Society. St. Louis, CV Mosby, 1977, pp. 75–85.

10. Gringas MB, Clark JC, Evarts CM: Prosthetic replacement in femoral neck fractures. C.O.R.R. 152:147–157, 1980.

11. Heywood-Waddington MB: Use of the Austin Moore prosthesis for advanced osteoarthritis of the hips. *J Bone and Joint Surg* 48(b):236–244, 1966.

12. Hinchley JJ, Day PL: Primary prosthetic replacement in fresh femoral neck fractures. *J Bone and Joint Surg* 46(a):223–240, 1964.

13. Hunter GA: Should we abandon primary prosthetic replacement for fresh displaced fractures of femoral neck. C.O.R.R. 152:158–161, 1980.

14. Judet J, Judet R: The use of an artificial femoral head for arthroplasty of the hip. *J Bone and Joint Surg* 32(B):166–173, 1950.

15. Lunceford EM: Use of the Moore self-locking vitallium prosthesis in acute fractures of femoral neck. *J Bone and Joint Surg* 47(A):832–841, 1965.

16. McBeath AA, Foltz RN: Femoral component loosening after total hip replacement. C.O.R.R. 152:147–157, 1980.

17. Müller ME: Total hip replacement: planning, technique, and complications, in Cruess RL, Mitchess NS (Eds): *Surgical Management of Arthritis of Lower Limb.* Philadelphia, Lea & Febiger, 1975.

18. Moore AT: A metal hip joint. A new self-locking vitallium prosthesis. *South Med J* 45:1015–1918, 1952.

19. Reing MC, Richin PF, Kenmore PI: Differential bone scanning in evaluation of painful total joint replacement. *J Bone and Joint Surg* 61(A):933–938, 1978.

20. Salvati E, Wilson PD: Long-term results of femoral head replacement. *J Bone and Joint Surg* 55(A):516–524, 1973.

21. Sarmiento A: Austin Moore prosthesis in the arthritic hip. C.O.R.R. 82:14–23, 1972.

22. Sarmiento A, Gerard FM: Total hip arthroplasty for failed endoprosthesis. C.O.R.R. 137: 112–117, 1978.

23. Smith-Petersen MN: Evolution of mold arthroplasty of the hip joint. *J Bone and Joint Surg* 30(B):59–75, 1948.

24. Thompson FR: Two-and-a-half years' experience with a vitallium intramedullary hip prothesis. *J Bone and Joint Surg* 36(A): 489–502, 1954.

Walter G. Krengel, Jr. and
Roderick H. Turner

11

Trochanteric Revision

Inadequate union of the greater trochanter is but one of the unsolved problems confronting the hip surgeon. The rate of the inadequate union varies from 5 percent[2] to 17.5 percent.[20] The competent greater trochanter is very important for proper functioning of the hip. The leverage attained by an intact long lever arm greatly aids the functioning of the abductor muscles and lessens the load on the hip joint (demonstrated by Pauwels,[19] discussed in further detail later in this chapter). When the hip joint load is lessened, this should result in prolonged life of the prosthesis-cement composite by decreasing both wear rate and potential loosening.

Correcting trochanteric problems and establishing a competent, secure trochanter are desirable goals for the hip joint surgeon. In revision surgery, this is even more important because the trochanter is usually osteotomized and there may be significant problems with the trochanter related to repeated operations and/or demineralization secondary to disuse. Trochanteric reattachment is an extremely important part of revision surgery; it must be addressed with the same precision and intensity as any other phase of this complex surgical exercise.

This chapter stresses the mechanical importance of the greater trochanter, identifies common clinical maladies, and discusses surgical techniques for insuring enduring trochanteric fixation.

BIOMECHANICAL CONSIDERATIONS

A long-intact abductor lever arm decreases the load on the hip joint.[19] Pauwels' studies clearly demonstrate that lateral transfer of the greater trochanter reduces hip joint forces and moments.[19] His work does not indicate that simple distal transplantation of the trochanter adds much to the abductor moment arm. An

249

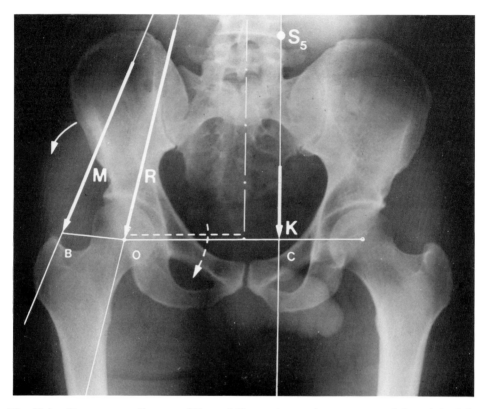

Fig. 11-1. Force vector diagram of Pauwels[19] superimposed on an x-ray of the pelvis. OC is the lever arm of the body weight K. OB is the lever arm of the abductor muscular force M.

analysis of the force vector diagram superimposed on an x-ray of the pelvis summarizes and mechanically demonstrates Pauwels' contributions to our understanding of the abductor lever arm (Fig. 11-1). The lever arm (**OC**) of the body weight (**K**) is approximately three times greater than the lever arm (**OB**) of the abductor muscular force (**M**). Forces must be three times greater than body weight in order to maintain body balance. Therefore, it is most appropriate to move the trochanter laterally and increase the abductor lever arm (**OB**) as much as possible, in turn decreasing the abductor work load.

Trochanteric integrity following hip replacement allows physiologic action of the hip abductors in order to balance the body during stance phase of gait, and to decrease the forces transmitted across the implanted hip. An intact greater trochanter establishes a dynamic lateral support buttress for the hip arthroplasty composite.

In the case of abnormal anatomy, such as a loss of femoral neck length, two important events occur: First, the abductor lever arm (**OB**) is shortened. Second, the contractile force of the hip abductors is further decreased, as the individual muscle-fiber units must initiate contraction from a position shorter than their normal resting length. Dowben[9] has quoted the classic works of Gordon and Huxley[8] and Zierler et al[24] in his discussion of the tension generated in muscle fibers during isometric muscular contraction. The authors establish that maximum tension is generated in a muscle fiber, and hence in a muscle unit, when the unit contracts from a position as close as possible to its normal resting length.

Consequently, distal transplantation of the greater trochanter is only recommended when the abductor muscle length has been shortened by factors such as migration of the prosthetic components on either side of the joint, dislocation, component breakage, bone resection, or other factors. Trochanteric transplantation beyond that distance required to re-establish normal abductor length risks stretching the muscle beyond its physiologic limits and creates undue tension on the trochanteric repair. (The reader is referred to Chapter 3 for further discussion of biomechanical and engineering principles.)

INDICATIONS FOR TROCHANTERIC OSTEOTOMY

In one of the few randomized simultaneous clinical studies, Mallory reported better abductor strength in 25 patients who had trochanteric osteotomy when compared to 25 patients whose surgery was done without trochanteric osteotomy.[15] Thompson et al reported fewer post-operative complications in patients whose sugery was done without trochanteric osteotomy when compared to those patients who had an osteotomy.[20] Note that Thompson's most difficult cases often required trochanteric osteotomy, so his is not a truly comparable series.

Parker et al found that trochanteric osteotomy was associated with a one-unit increase in the intra-operative blood transfusion requirements.[18] This short-term follow-up study further showed that the early post-operative complications were more common, and that the operative time was longer, when the trochanter was transplated. A longer follow-up study of 12 patients treated by the same surgeons as those studied by Parker et al[17] was done by Wiesman et al.[23] Studies by force-plate gait analysis of this group of patients indicated that the patients whose surgery was performed without trochanteric transplantation had more normal hip function than those whose trochanter had been transplanted.

The clinical results in regard to relief of pain, functional rating, and range of motion were not significantly different in the two groups studied by Wiesman et al.[23]

The authors of this volume agree in the following recommendations about trochanteric osteotomy and transplantation:

1. Most primary hip operations can be adequately performed by a careful surgical approach without trochanteric osteotomy. We prefer the postero-lateral approach; those well schooled in the anterior-lateral approach may prefer it.
2. Complex hip problems with distorted anatomy, contractual deformity, or severe loss of motion are best approached with trochanteric osteotomy, even for primary hip surgery. (Examples: CDH, ankylosed hips, severe protrusio acetabulae, etc.)
3. Trochanteric osteotomy facilitates exposure in the morbidly obsese patient.
4. Trochanteric osteotomy is preferred in most revision total hip arthroplasties.

5. Whenever the trochanter is transplanted, the surgeon should have a careful preoperative plan for reattachment; he or she should be certain that fixation is secure prior to wound closure.

TROCHANTERIC BURSITIS

Some trochanteric problems are major and require re-operation; others are minor in nature and can be treated non-operatively. It is important to differentiate between symptomatic and asymptomatic trochanteric problems, and to isolate those cases that have significant trochanteric pathology. This latter group may range from simple bursitis to painful displaced and non-united trochanters. Patients with simple bursitits may be relieved by systemic non-steroidal anti-inflammatory agents.

If the etiology of trochanteric pain is in doubt, a diagnostic injection of 10 to 20 cc of a local anesthetic agent may clarify the issue. If the pain is not relieved within 10 to 20 minutes, the surgeon can be suspicious that the etiology of the pain is not trochanteric bursitis.

If the local anesthetic relieves trochanteric pain, then an injection of the bursal sac with steroids with relatively insoluble chemical bonds, such as acetate salts, may give prolonged or even permanent relief.

If trochanteric fixation devices such as wires or bolts prominently protrude, they may cause a chronic bursitis that only temporarily responds to injections. Repeated trochanteric injections are not advised because of the remote, but serious, risk of infection.

Surgical removal of any offending devices is indicated if symptoms are not relieved after a few injections. At surgery, only the prominent offending portion of the device should be removed. Wires that are solidly embedded should be cut flush where they exit the bone. Heavier devices, such as bolts, can be cut with metal cutting instruments, such as the diamond wheel attachment available with the Midas Rex drill. Attempts to forcefully extract metal embedded in cement risks unnecessary immediate cement fracture or creates cement defects which can lead to future fatigue fracture of the cement.

Trochanteric surgery should be treated with the same care and respect given any major hip operation. At the time of wire removal, any inflamed or redundant trochanteric bursa should be removed. Careful bacteriologic studies of the fluid and tissue should be obtained, inlcuding aerobic, anaerobic, and fungal cultures. When the enlarged bursa is removed, closed suction drainage and a compression dressing will help to obliterate the dead space.

Post-operatively, the patient should remain on crutches for 2 weeks and then on a cane until he or she demonstrates a negative Trendelenburg gait.

DELAYED UNION AND NON-UNION

Delayed union of the greater trochanter is present when there is x-ray evidence of trochanteric separation 3 months following surgey. Patients with proven delayed union should be kept on crutches and should have a half-inch lift added to their contralateral heel. If union is not achieved by 6 months, then non-union of the trochanter is present and further crutch protection is based solely on the presence or absence of symptoms. Some patients with non-union develop sufficient strength to sustain a negative Trendelenburg gait. Others may have a Trendelenburg gait, yet be perfectly comfortable with the full-time use of a cane.

The most important aspect in the history of the patient with suspected trochanteric pathology is pain. One must analyze the pain in relationship to its character, duration, and precipitating causes. Only a small number of patients with trochanteric non-union have sufficient pain to warrant a repeated attempt at trochanteric fixation.

Serial standard radiographs are the most helpful guidelines in elucidating bony trochanteric problems. They can delineate migration of the trochanter, delayed union, and fractured fixation devices. Not only can the internal devices break, but they can also migrate, which is particularly common with broken wires. Broken wires can travel a considerable distance; small broken pieces of wire can even migrate between the femoral head and the acetabulum (Fig. 11-2). Such interposition creates a high friction system between the femoral head and the acetabulum. As a result, loss of fixation of one or both of the components is likely within a few years.

Patients with an established trochanteric non-union and wide separation of the trochanteric fragment will usually require a cane for support, although some

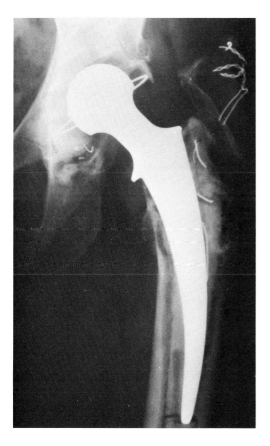

Fig. 11-2. Broken wire interposed between the femoral head and the acetabulum.

patients manage without any external support (Fig. 11-3). Other patients experience severe abductor weakness which may be perceived as a sensation of instability and which can progress to subluxation and/or recurrent dislocation. Severe instability and the presence of pain are two indications for re-attachment of the greater trochanter as an isolated procedure (Fig. 11-4A,B). In still other patients, the trochanteric problem is only part of the overall failed total hip, and one that requires attention at the time of the total hip revision (Fig. 11-5A,B). In a final group of patients, a delayed union of the trochanter may be wrongly incriminated as a source of pain. Subsequent trochanteric union will not relieve the hip pain in this latter group (Fig. 11-6A,B).

FURTHER DIAGNOSTIC STUDIES

The surgeon must sometimes resort to techniques more sophisticated than standard x-rays, including serial x-rays, tomography, arthrography, and radio-nuclide bone scanning. Hip arthrography with color subtraction techniques can often be helpful, and can delineate subtle x-ray changes. Arthrography and other sophisticated diagnostic studies, such as tectnetium and gallium scans, are discussed in detail in Chapter 2.

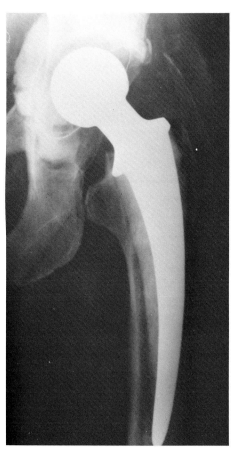

Fig. 11-3. Sixty-eight-year-old female with asymptomatic left hip, with excellent range of motion and negative Trendelenburg.

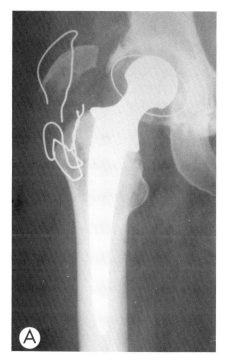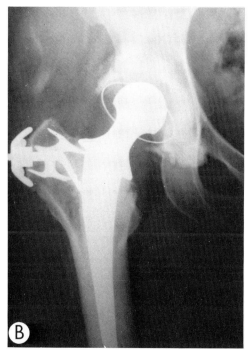

Fig. 11-4A. Fifty-six-year-old female with a painful displaced trochanter with positive Trendelenburg and an excellent range of motion.
Fig. 11-4B. Volz bolt fixation of a healthy greater trochanter.

TROCHANTERIC FIXATION

Techniques

Many techniques have been devised for securing the trochanter, which leads to the realization that no single method is perfect. Most hip surgeons have adjusted their techniques as improved materials and techniques have replaced older ones. Among the securing devices used are bolts, screws, tension wires, circlage wires, figure-eight wires, and synthetic sutures and tapes In the United States, the most popular method uses wire (both stainless steel and cobalt-chrome alloys). A strong caliber of wire should be used, specifically 16- to 18-gauge. Some techniques imbed the wire in cement; in others, the wire or wires are wrapped around the proximal femur and/or the femoral component. Clarke et al presented evidence that the usual cause of wire breakage is fatigue failure rather than tension failure.[5] This breakage is primarily seen when a wire is damaged, kinked, or is subjected to a stress-raiser where it exits the cement.

Careful preparation of the trochanter and adjacent femoral bed for re-attachment is critical to successful trochanteric repair. Meticulous and tedious soft-tissue debridement of both the trochanter and femoral bed is important. Obtaining a flat bone-to-bone contact surface is ideal, but is often impossible. The use of cancellous bone graft is often necessary to fill gaps in the contact of bony surfaces. When

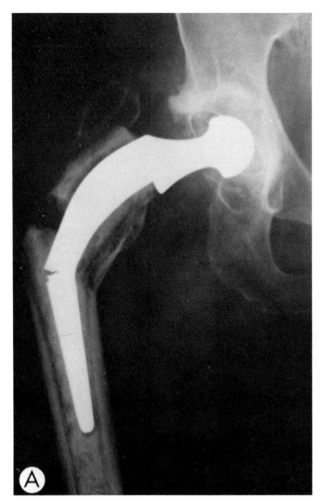
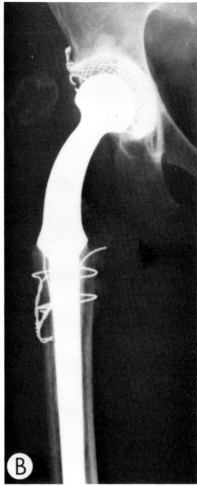

Fig. 11-5A. Nonunion of greater trochanter with broken prosthetic stem and fractured femoral shaft.
Fig. 11-5B. Postoperative x-ray showing proximal femoral replacement. Lateral soft tissues were repaired.

performing revision surgery, the surgeon should always harvest and save any available bone in case it is needed at the time of wound closure for trochanteric grafting.

Charnley has written that surgeons who are skilful in securing the trochanter have fewer trochanteric problems than less-skilled surgeons.[2] Independent of Charnley's study, Amstutz reported that technical errors at the time of surgery and osteopenia of the trochanter and femur are the most common causes for separation of the trochanter.[1]

Regardless of the skill and experience of the surgeon, certain patients represent substantially increased risk for trochanteric problems. These include patients with marked osteopenia, patients with multiple joint involvement, revision patients, as well as patients who are overweight or untrustworthy. Patients with extensive upper extremity disease, such as arthritis, paralysis, or contractures, may find it impossible to protect their transplanted trochanter even with optimum use of their crutches.

If good bone substance is present in the greater trochanteric fragment, consideration can be given to the use of the Volz trochanteric bolt.[22] This bolt provides the strongest compressive force at the osteotomy site of any available fixation device, but it does create some central weakness in the trochanteric fragment. Volz has experimental data indicating that any devices penetrating the trochanter create significant stress-raisers, which may result in trochanteric fracture.[21] This supports the use of braided wires which are secured by a crimping clip rather than knotted or twisted. Volz has further devised a two-pronged fixation clip to be used in conjunction with braided wire to further secure the trochanter[21] The fixation clip wraps around the top of the greater trochanter and prevents proximal migration, thus relieving the braided wires of tension stresses. If these laboratory experiments are borne out by clinical studies, this promises to be an excellent trochanteric fixation system.

When the revision does not require changing the previously cemented femoral component, the Mayo technique (as popularized by Coventry[6] is recommended for securing the trochanter. The single-tension wire passes through drill-holes lateral to the prosthesis. The transverse wire is added in patients whose trochanter is "slight" or "porotic" (Fig. 11-7).

A similar technique utilizing two transverse wires has been reported by Harris and Crothers and is recommended where trochanteric bone is good.[11] Harris and Jones have advocated the use of wire mesh as a reinforcement for trochanteric fixation when dealing with osteoporotic trochanters and with trochanteric non-union.[12] All surgeons undertaking revision total hip surgery should be familiar with the mesh technique because it allows fixation of greater trochanters with poor-

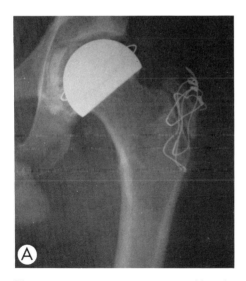
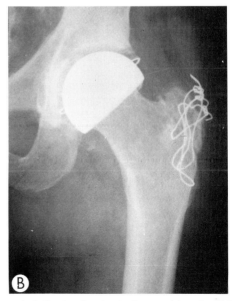

Fig. 11-6A, B. Forty-seven-year-old male, three months postoperative Tharies resurfacing, who had hip pain attributed to trochanteric delayed union. Serial x-rays revealed the trochanter to have achieved solid union, but the patient was still symptomatic.

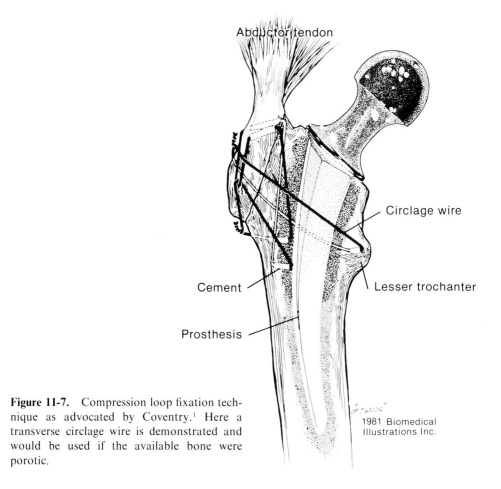

Abductor tendon

Circlage wire

Cement

Lesser trochanter

Prosthesis

1981 Biomedical
Illustrations Inc.

Figure 11-7. Compression loop fixation technique as advocated by Coventry.[1] Here a transverse circlage wire is demonstrated and would be used if the available bone were porotic.

quality bone; simpler methods are likely to fail (Figs. 11-8 and 11-9). Harris has reported 500 successful trochanteric unions out of 503 osteotomies.[10]

Often the trochanteric fragment is atrophic and porotic. Because of the porosity of the bone, the wires easily pull through the weak bone. The two vertical wires should therefore be placed through the abductor tendon directly over the trochanteric fragment, rather than through the bone. With this technique, of course, one or two circumferential wires are utilized, but no wires go through the weak trochanteric fragment (Fig. 11-10). This technique is a slight modification of that described by Harris and Crothers.[11]

SEVERE TROCHANTERIC PROBLEMS

Multiple methods are available to encourage approximation of the chronic proximally migrated trochanter to the femur. One is usually able to approximate the trochanter to the femur by removing all the superior capsule and scar tissue down to the muscle and tendon of the gluteus minimus. The origins of the minimus and medius can be stripped from the lateral face of the ilium by dissecting them off the ilium with an elevator, beginning at the lateral lip of the acetabulum. In rare instances, the surgeon must utilize a secondary incision along the crest of the ilium and strip the gluteus medius, minimus, and tensor fascia off the ilium and let these muscles slide. Even less frequently, one may need to "Z-lengthen" the gluteus medius–minimus muscle-tendon unit. This is fraught with the possibility of leaving a very small strip of the abductor tendon attached to the small devascularized trochanteric fragment, making it a procedure of last resort. The surgeon occasionally is confronted with absence of the trochanter; the patient has a proximal lateral deficiency of bone. One may then attempt to graft a piece of the iliac crest to the adjacent bone to construct some trochanteric bone mass (Fig. 11-11A,B,C).

When special proximal femoral replacement prostheses are utilized and there is no possibility of approximating the bone surfaces, then woven polyester fiber tape can be utilized to approximate the abductor and vastus lateralis fascia.

POST-OPERATIVE MANAGEMENT

The post-operative management for revision trochanteric surgery should be carefully outlined to the patient; it will be discussed in Chapter 17. If trochanteric fixation is at all tenuous, the patient is kept in balanced suspension for 21 days.[12]

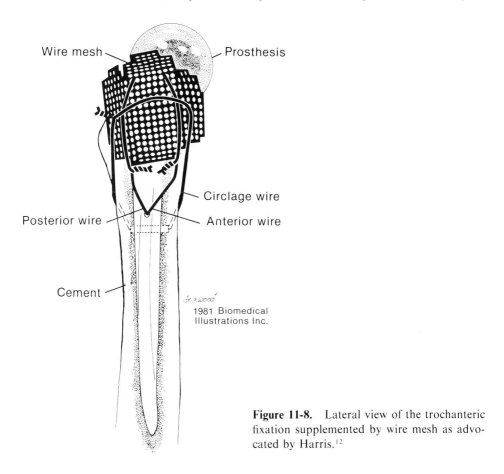

Wire mesh

Prosthesis

Circlage wire

Posterior wire

Anterior wire

Cement

1981 Biomedical
Illustrations Inc.

Figure 11-8. Lateral view of the trochanteric fixation supplemented by wire mesh as advocated by Harris.[12]

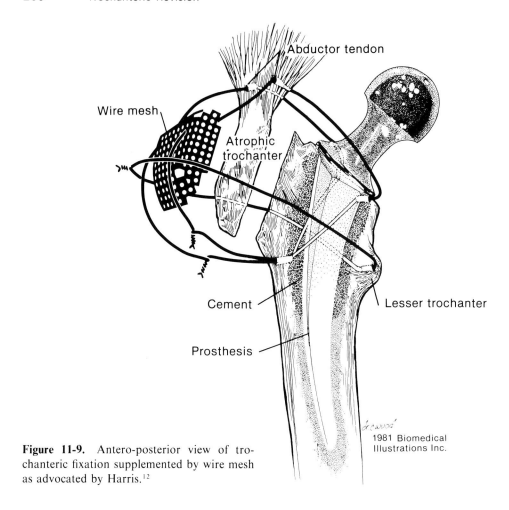

Figure 11-9. Antero-posterior view of trochanteric fixation supplemented by wire mesh as advocated by Harris.[12]

This allows the physical therapist to utilize passive abduction during the early soft-tissue healing phase. The patient is then encouraged, after 21 days, to actively contract the abductors. In extremely unstable situations, one can resort to a 1½ leg spica or to abduction splints which are more readily acceptable to patients than a solid spica cast. The abduction splint should be applied from the thigh down to the area proximal to the medial malleolus. The use of fixed abduction boot casts is not advised as the knee has a tendency to fall into internal rotation when the patient is abducted, and can place a great deal of torque on the transferred trochanter as well as precipitate posterior dislocations. Boot casts have the additional disadvantage of being very uncomfortable to the patient.

Following removal from balanced suspension, the patient is carefully started on crutch walking, with limited weight bearing. Crutch walking is advised for 4 to 6 months following all revision total hip arthroplasties. If trochanteric fixation is tenuous, protection should be continued until there is radiographic evidence of solid healing or the patient progresses to a negative Trendelenburg gait.

SUMMARY

Trochanteric fixation is uniquely important in revision total hip arthroplasty because of the need for a transtrochanteric approach and because of the usually encountered condition of osteopenic bone. The rationale for trochanteric transplantation has been presented, as have several techniques for achieving fixation even in the face of adverse conditions, such as non-union, shortening, and osteopenia.

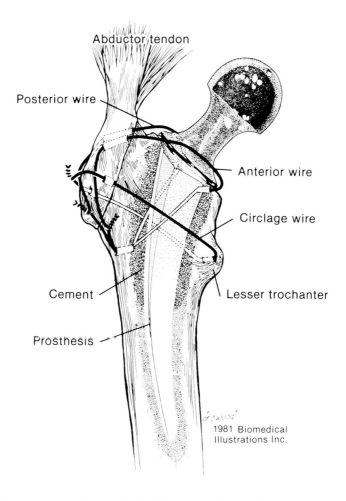

1981 Biomedical
Illustrations Inc.

Fig. 11-10. Three-wire technique useful for the fixation of atrophic greater trochanter. Note that the anterior and posterior wires pass around the medial aspect of the prosthesis and through the abductor tendon. No wires pass through the atropic trochanteric bone.

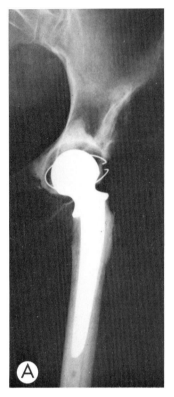 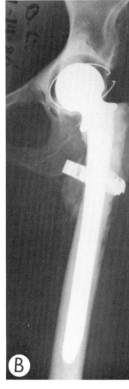 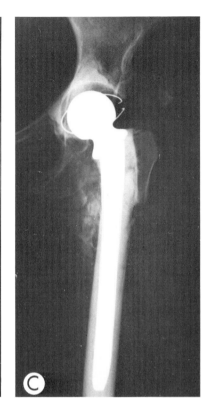

Fig. 11-11A. Thirty-seven-year-old patient with congenital dysplasia of the left hip. Multiple previous operations left the patient with dissolution of lateral femoral bone stock.

Fig. 11-11B. Bone grafts to the proximal femur and trochanteric area are held in place by circumferential fixation.

Fig. 11-11C. Bone grafts have consolidated and fixation has been removed. Abductor function was improved.

BIBLIOGRAPHY

1. Amstutz HC, Maki S: Complications of trochanteric osteotomy in total hip replacements. *J Bone and Joint Surg* 60(A): 214–216, 1978.
2. Boardman KP, Bocco F, Charnley J: An evaluation of a method of trochanteric fixation, using three wires in the Charnley low friction arthroplasty. *Clin Orthop* 132:31–38, 1978.
3. Charnley J: Transplantation of the greater trochanter in arthroplasty of the hip. *J Bone and Joint Surg* 46(B): 191–197, 1964.
4. Charnley J, Ferreira ASD: Transplantation of the greater trochanter in arthroplasty of the hip. *J Bone and Joint Surg* 46(B):191–197, 1964.
5. Clarke RP, Shea WD, Bierbaum BE: Trochanteric osteotomy. *Clin Orthop* 141:102–110, 1979.
6. Coventry, MD: The surgical technique of total hip arthroplasty, modified from Charnley, as done at the Mayo Clinic. *Orthop Clin N Amer* 4:473–482, 1973.
7. Dowben RW: Contractility with special reference to skeletal muscle, in Mountcastle VB (ed): *Medical Physiology.* New York, CV Mosby Co, 1980, pp. 82–119.

8. Gordon AM, Huxley AS, Julian FJ: The variation in isometric tension with sarcomere length in vertebrate muscle fibers. *J Physiol* 184:170–192, 1966.

9. Greenwald AS, Nelson CL: Biomechanics of the reconstructed hip. *Orthop Clin N Amer* 4:435–447, 1973.

10. Harris WH: Four wire technique. Scientific exhibit, presented at the American Academy of Orthopedic Surgeons Annual Meeting, Las Vegas, February, 1981.

11. Harris WH, Crothers OD: Reattachment of the greater trochanter in total hip replacement arthroplasty—a new technique. *J Bone and Joint Surg* 60(A): 211–213, 1978.

12. Harris WH, Jones WN: The use of wire mesh in total hip replacement surgery. *Clin Orthop* 106:117–121, 1975.

13. Izadpanah M: Ergebnisse der Trochanter Major-Fixation, bei 181 Hüftgelenks-Total-endoprothesen unter dem speziellen Hinweiss auf die Zuggurtungsteosynthese. *Z Ortho* 117:938–941, 1979.

14. Johnston RC, Brand RA, Crowninshield RD: Reconstruction of the hip. *J Bone and Joint Surg* 61(A):639–652, 1979.

15. Mallory TH: Total hip replacement with and without trochanteric osteotomy. *Clin Orthop* 103:133–142, 1974.

16. Markoff KL, Hirschowitz DL, Amstutz HC: Mechanical stability of the greater trochanter following osteotomy and reattachment by wiring. *Clin Orthop* 141:111–121, 1979.

17. Parker HG, Wiesman HG, Ewald FC, et al: Comparison of immediate and late results of total hip replacement with and without trochanteric osteotomy. *J Bone and Joint Surg* 56A:1537, 1974.

18. Parker HG, Wiesman HG, Ewald FC, et al: Comparison of pre-operative, intra-operative and early post-operative total hip replacement with and without trochanteric osteotomy. *Clin Orthop* 121:44–49, 1976.

19. Pauwels, F: Die Bedeutung der Biomechanik für die Orthopädie. IX Congr Internat Chir Orthop et de Traumatol, II. Vienna, 1963. Wien, Verlag der Wiener Med Akademie, 1965, pp 1–32.

20. Thompson RC, Culver JE: Role of trochanteric osteotomy in total hip replacement. *Clin Orthop* 106:102–106, 1975.

21. Volz RG: Personal communication, January, 1981.

22. Volz RG, Brown FW: Painful migrated ununited greater trochanter in total hip replacements. *J Bone and Joint Surg* 59(A):1091–1093, 1977.

23. Wiesman HJ, Simon SR, Ewald FC, et al: Total hip replacement with and without osteotomy of the greater trochanter. *J Bone and Joint Surg* 60(A):203, 1978.

24. Zierler KL Maseri A, Klassen G, et al: Muscle metabolism during exercise in man. *Trans Assoc Am Physicians* 81:266–273, 1968.

Kim R. Sellergren,
Arnold D. Scheller, Jr., and
John McA. Harris, III

12

Total Hip Instability and Revision Arthroplasty

Instability in the total hip arthroplasty (subluxation or dislocation of the femoral component from the acetabular component) is one of the more frequent complications. In the 1975 Mayo Clinic series analyzing 3,204 total hip replacements, dislocation was the second most common cause for re-operation.[12] However, in their 1974 evaluation of 2,012 arthroplasties,[4] when all complications were taken into account, dislocation was the most frequent complication. In Fackler and Poss' series of 1,433 arthroplasties, dislocation was again the most common complication.[9] Reported incidences range from 0.5[5,7] to 5 percent.[2,8] Most of the larger and more recent series published have dislocation rates of 3 percent or less.[4,5,7,9-13] The magnitude of the problem is not to be underestimated, because anywhere from 20[7] to 75 percent[5] of the dislocations require at least another general anesthetic for reduction, many require re-operation.

The repeat surgery is not without morbidity.[11] Patients with multiple dislocations have a slower rehabilitation, as measured by gait velocity and single limb support time, and their cost of care is increased by longer hospitalizations and more surgery.[2] A small but finite number eventually require resection arthroplasty.[10,14]

This chapter evaluates a variety of etiologies for instability, the possible methods of avoiding instability, and the various procedures for dealing with it should it occur. Most studies unfortunately were retrospective, and precise methods of measurement were not always used. Statistical analysis was seldom done in the published series. Much of the available information therefore remains anecdotal. There does, however, appear to be enough general agreement amongst experienced reconstructive surgeons that the practitioner can find some guidance.

265

ETIOLOGY OF INSTABILITY

Prior Hip Surgery

There is a definite association between previous hip surgery and a higher incidence of dislocation. In Lewinnek's series, six of nine dislocating total hips had previously had surgery.[11] In Fackler and Poss' series, only 1.8 percent of hips not previously operated on dislocated. In contrast, 5.5 percent of hips previously operated on dislocated. Of those hips which had had a previous total hip arthroplasty, 20.8 percent dislocated.[9] Seventy-five percent of the dislocations in Eftekhar's series, 32 percent of the dislocations in Khan's series, and 80 percent of the dislocations in Evanski's series had been previously operated on.[5,8,10] (No figures are given for how many of their non-dislocating hips had had previous surgery.) This dislocation may be related to damage to the hip abductor muscles. The tension of these muscles is necessary for stability of the total hip replacement; each successive operation may weaken them more (Fig. 12-1).

Overall Medical Condition

Neither age, sex, nor the primary pathologic joint process necessitating hip replacement affected the incidence of dislocation.[4,5,9,12-14] However, some authors felt that the overall physical condition of the patient might have a bearing on the rate of dislocation. Fackler and Poss noted that the incidence of severe medical or neurologic problems (including alcoholism, uremic psychosis, senile dementia, cerebral palsy, and muscular dystrophy) was 14 percent in their control group, 22 percent in those patients who experienced a single dislocation, and 75 percent in those with recurrent dislocations.[9] Khan noted that of his 142 dislocations, 9 patients were confused, 7 had neurologic disorders, and 33 had disorders of other joints in the same limb.[10] No similar analysis was made of those patients in his series whose hips did not dislocate.

Surgical Experience

A lower dislocation rate has been noted with the more experienced surgeon. Fackler and Poss noted that the most experienced surgeon in their series had a lower dislocation rate,[9] as did Lewinnek (0.5 percent for the most experienced surgeon, as opposed to 3 percent overall).[11]

Time of Dislocation

All series showed that the bulk of dislocations occur less than 6 weeks post-operatively. Ninety percent of dislocations in the Mayo Clinic experience occurred at less than 3 months.[4] Sixty-seven percent of dislocations in Lewinnek's series,[11] 68 percent in Fackler's series,[9] 71 percent in Pellicci's series,[13] and 65 percent in Khan's series[10] occurred during the 6-week period following initial hip arthroplasty. These early dislocations can often be attributed to poor positioning of the patient in the early post-operative period, and a lack of patient understanding or cooperation in avoiding positions that risk dislocation. In Khan's series of 142 dislocations, 7 were

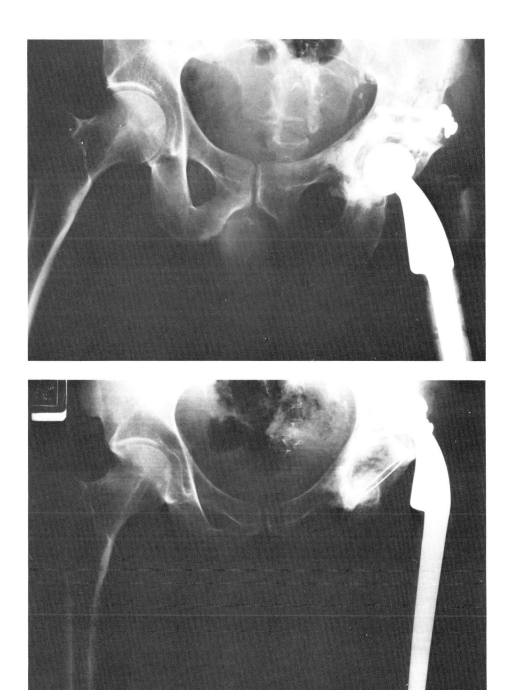

Fig. 12-1. Abductor weakness from multiple previous surgeries, leading to dislocation.

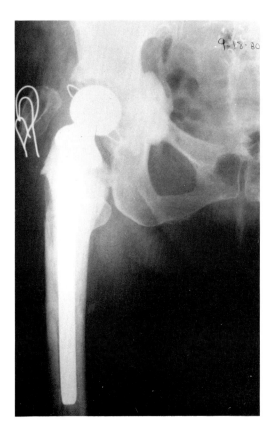

Fig. 12-2. Trochanteric nonunion associated with dislocation.

felt to be dislocated as they left the operating room. Another 31 dislocated in hyperflexion; 38 dislocated by rotating the hip, some in flexion and some in extension.[10] Twelve of the 14 dislocations in Pellicci and Salvati's series occurred in hyperflexion (8 while the patient was getting out of a chair).[13]

Of those patients with late dislocations, (greater than 6 weeks post-operatively) trauma was more likely to be a factor. In Khan's series, of the 10 dislocations due to trauma, 9 occurred late.[10] Two of the three dislocations in Lewinnek's series which occurred more than 30 days post-operatively were due to falls.[11]

Surgical Approach

Surgical approach to the hip was not felt to be a significant factor in dislocation, except possibly as it related to trochanteric osteotomy. Ritter found that there was an increased incidence of trochanteric non-union in dislocating and subluxing hips, but it was not statistically significant.[14] Ten percent of dislocations in the 1974 Mayo Clinic series were associated with trochanteric non-unions, but no figures are given for the overall percentage of trochanteric non-unions.[4] Etienne's series showed that trochanteric non-unions were associated with 29 percent of dislocations (Fig. 12-2), although again no figures are given as to their overall trochanteric non-union rate.[7]

Component Malposition

A commonly cited reason for dislocation is component malposition. Not all authors accurately measured the positions of the components, either in the dislocated or the non-dislocated hips; among those who did attempt to measure position, an ideal component position was not strictly agreed upon. Most authors indicated, however, that when the components were placed outside of the range of positions which they felt to be correct, the rate of dislocation increased. We believe the correct position of the acetabulum should be less than 50° of abduction (the angle formed with the horizontal plane), and from 5° to 15° of anteversion. Acetabular and femoral retroversion are to be strictly avoided. The femoral component should be placed in a neutral varus-valgus position with 5°–10° of anteversion.

In Lewinnek's series, all three of the anterior dislocations were associated with anteversion of the acetabulum of greater than 25° (Fig. 12-3).[11] None of the posterior dislocations were associated with malposition of components. However, there were no acetabula which were more than 4° retroverted in the series. Additionally, the acetabula of dislocating hips did not have a significantly different angle of tilt (angle from the horizontal) from that of the non-dislocating hips.[11] Ritter's series revealed that of seven dislocating hips, three had component malposition.[14] One acetabular cup and two femoral components were too anteverted (Fig. 12-4). Ritter did not define what he regarded as "too anteverted," but his surgical goal was 0°–10° of anteversion for all femoral components, and 30° of anteversion for the McKee-Farrar acetabulum which dislocated.[14] Eftekhar's series

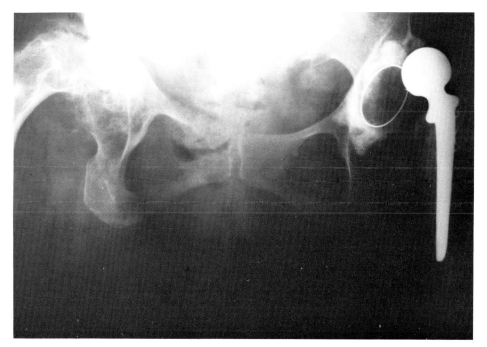

Fig. 12-3. Acetabular component with extreme anteversion and abduction. Femoral component dislocated.

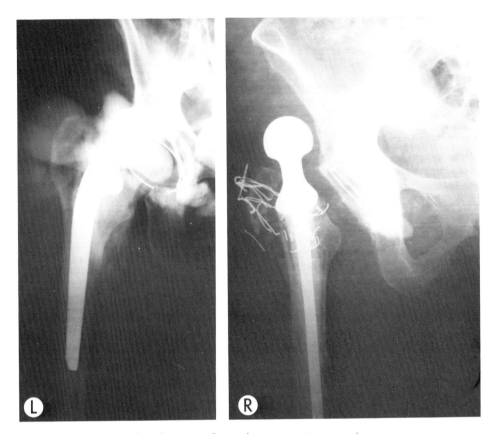

Fig. 12-4.   Two examples of extreme femoral component anteversion.

of eight dislocations included two which he believed were due to poor placement of the components, but he does not tell us how they were malpositioned.[5] He does make a point of saying that the Charnley femoral component should not be anteverted more than 5° and the acetabulum should have an angle of 45° from the horizontal. He also stresses that the acetabulum should not be placed too cephalad, nor should the femoral neck be shortened too much (Figs. 12-5, 12-6).[5] In Khan's series of 142 dislocations, it was felt that an acetabulum was malpositioned if it was anteverted more than 15°; if it was too vertical (made an angle of greater than 50° with the horizontal); or if it was more than 1 cm superior to the opposite side (Fig. 12-7).[10] The femoral component was considered malpositioned if it was anteverted more than 15°. He found that the most common errors of the acetabulum were that it was too anteverted (33 cases), too vertical (35 cases) (Fig. 12-8), too superior (17 cases), or retroverted (13 cases). The most common femoral component errors were too much anteversion (22 cases), or too much retroversion (11 cases).[10] Pellicci and Salvati found that of their 14 dislocations, 7 had acetabular malposition.[13] One was too anteverted (37°) and resulted in an anterior dislocation; the others were unspecified. Fackler and Poss defined component malposition as being anteversion of the femoral component of more than 25° or retroversion of either component. They found that 6 percent of their controls had component malposition, and 44 percent of their dislocations had malposition. Femoral retroversion was the most common error they encountered (Fig. 12-9). They noted that the position of the reattached trochanter following trochanteric osteotomy was critical: those patients who had trochanteric osteotomies and subsequently dislocated had a mean trochanter-to-head distance of 5 mm less than their pre-operative values, compared to a 2 mm increase in the control group.[9] They concluded that if a trochanteric osteotomy is done, it must be reattached in both a lateral and distal position so as to re-establish the trochanter-to-head distance.[9] They also found that not performing a trochanteric osteotomy was associated with almost a two-and-a-half times greater dislocation rate. Too much valgus of the femoral component, in their experience, resulted in a decreased trochanter-to-head distance, and an increased chance of levering of the component against the acetabulum (Fig. 12-10), thus increasing the chance of dislocation in two ways.[9] Etienne, Cupic, and Charnley did not speak specifically to the issue of malposition of the components.[7] They did, however, believe that two changes had been important in reducing their incidence of dislocation from 1.4 percent in 1966 to 0.2 percent in 1974. These were the more distal placement of the acetabulum, accomplished by reaming at right angles to the long axis of the body (Fig. 12-11), and the development of the long posterior wall (LPW) socket (Fig. 12-12), which made posterior dislocations less likely.[7] The Mayo Clinic series found that of their 46 dislocations, at least 30 were posterior; of these,

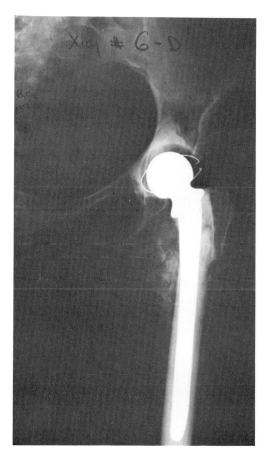

Fig. 12-5. Short neck femoral component associated with dislocation (relocated here).

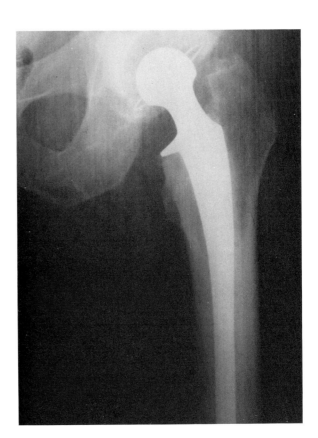

Fig. 12-6. A relatively shortened femoral neck. A regular neck femoral component was used, but the neck was cut quite distally, which allows early trochanteric impingement with abduction. Note the decreased head to trochanter distance.

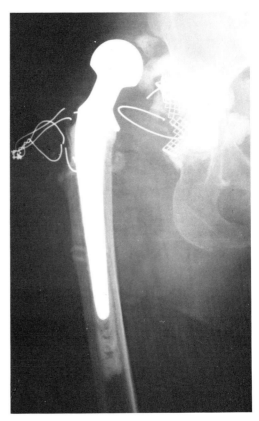

Fig. 12-7. Overly cephalad placement of acetabular component, femoral component dislocated.

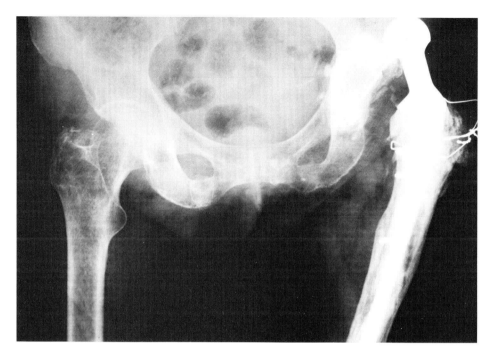

Fig. 12-8. Overly vertical acetabulum associated with dislocation.

at least 23 had acetabular retroversion (Fig. 12-13). At least 11 dislocations were anterior; of these, 10 were felt to be due to acetabular anteversion. Few were operated upon, however, and radiographs were not accurate enough to make specific measurements.[12]

Prosthetic Design

The type of prosthesis seems to have little to do with the dislocation rate. Many surgeons have the impression that the 22 mm head prosthesis is inherently more unstable, but Ritter, who did a statistical analysis of his results, failed to show that the type of prosthesis made any difference.[14] Charnley, exclusively using a 22 mm prosthesis, has one of the lowest dislocation rates.[7] Eftekhar had a 0.5 percent dislocation rate using the 22 mm prosthesis.[5] It has been shown, however, in laboratory studies by Amstutz and Markolf,[1] that different prostheses have differing ranges of motion before impingement of the neck on the rim of the acetabulum occurs. This is influenced by the head-to-neck diameter ratio (Fig. 12-14). The higher the ratio, the greater the possible range of motion without impingement. Obviously, a larger head diameter permits a larger head-to-neck diameter ratio without unduly reducing the size of the neck. A larger head also means that if the socket is equal in depth to the radius of the head, the head must be pulled farther out of the socket before it begins to ride up over the rim and possibly dislocate (Fig. 12-15).[1] This is another reason why those who favor the use of the 22 mm head prosthesis stress the importance of (1) keeping the acetabulum placed at least as caudal as the original acetabulum; (2) not shortening the neck of the femur too much; and (3) both distally and laterally transferring the trochanter.

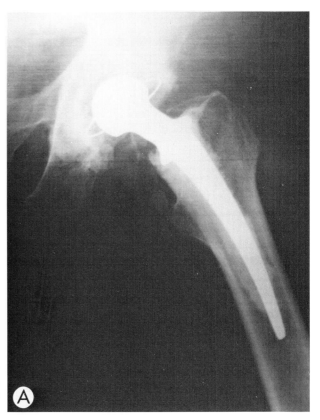

Fig. 12-9. Excessive retroversion of femoral component. Note that retroversion is more apparent in lateral view.

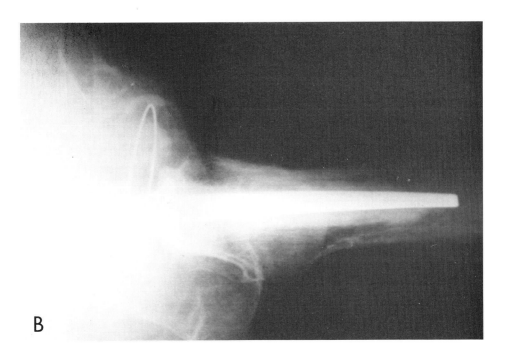

B

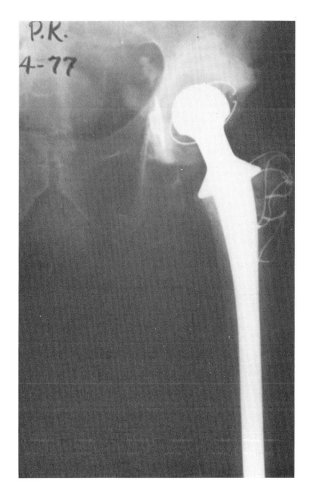

Fig. 12-10. Excessive femoral component valgus, associated with dislocation.

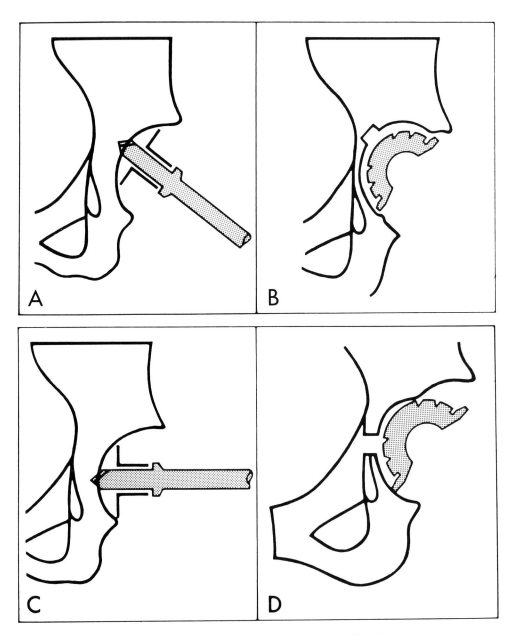

Fig. 12-11. Importance of reaming at right angle to long axis of body to keep acetabulum in anatomical position. (A, B) Reamer directed too cephalad and cup placed too cephalad. (C,D) Correct direction of reamer and placement of cup. (From Charnley J: *Low-Friction Arthroplasty of the Hip.* New York, Springer-Verlag, 1979.)

276

These maneuvers are designed to keep the necessary tension on the soft tissues to prevent the small head from riding out of the socket (Fig. 12-16). Eftekhar also stresses not resecting the inferior capsule unless it is necessary for exposure since this capsule also contributes to stability.[6]

Impingement: Extra-articular vs Intra-articular

Other factors mentioned by various authors as being related to dislocation include remnants of methacrylate or osteophytes around the rim of the acetabulum which allow the femoral neck to lever out (Fig. 12-17).[4,5,12,13] Other causes may be the presence of foreign bodies (fragments of methacrylate, wire, or bone) in the acetabulum (Fig. 12-18),[11] and an over-deepening of the acetabulum, such that the femoral neck can lever on the rim.[5] The presence of too much fluid in the capsule was cited by Ritter as one reason why the artificial hip would dislocate in the sitting position (Fig. 12-19).[15] He feels that the fluid, when pressed upon by the soft tissues when the patient is in a sitting position (i.e., when the two components are no longer being pressed together by the patient's body weight), acts to force the two components apart and dislocate the hip.

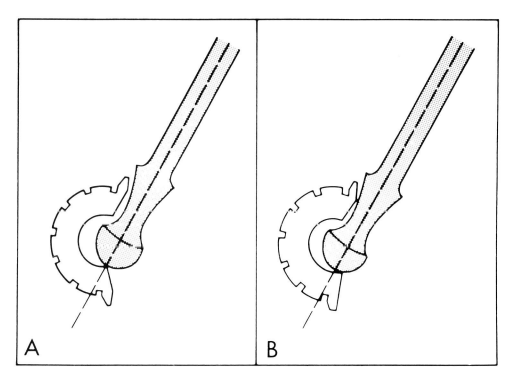

Fig. 12-12. (A) Standard socket. (B) Long posterior wall (LPW) socket, allowing greater motion without dislocation. (From Charnley J: *Low-Friction Arthroplasty of the Hip.* New York, Springer-Verlag, 1979.)

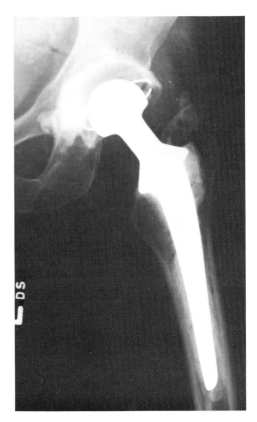

Fig. 12-13. Acetabular retroversion. Note that the anteroposterior view alone may be misleading. The true lateral view better reveals the acetabular retroversion.

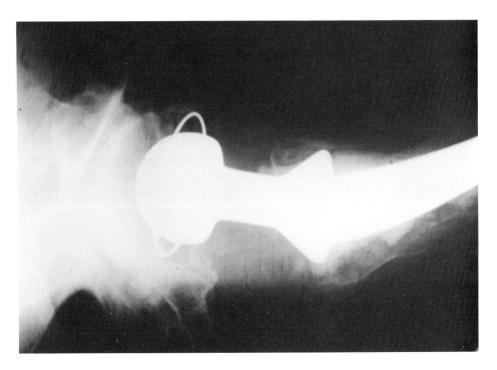

Prosthesis	Head diameter (mm)	Head-neck diameter ratio	Flexion*	Internal rotation in flexion	Abduction in extension	External rotation in extension
Charnley	22 0	1.74	80	0†	42	42
Bechtol	25 4	2.00	93	2	45	52
Harris	26 0	2.03	93	3	57	66
Trapezoidal-28	28 0	Long axis of neck 1.72–2.01 Short axis of neck 2.97–3.24	114	36	60	74
Aufranc-Turner	32 0	Long axis of neck 2.00 Short axis of neck 2.32	101	14	56	69
Müller	32 0	1.98	96	6	57	68

*The flexion reported here is measured at 0° abduction and 0° external rotation; increases in either abduction or external rotation will increase the given angles.

†At 90° of flexion and 0° of abduction the femur was in external rotation.

Fig. 12-14. Increased head-to-neck diameter ratio leads to a greater in vitro range of motion before impingement occurs. (From Amstutz HC, Markolf KL: Design features in total hip replacements, in *The Hip*, Proceedings of the Second Open Scientific Meeting of the Hip Society, 1974. New York, CV Mosby Co, 1974, pp 111-124.)

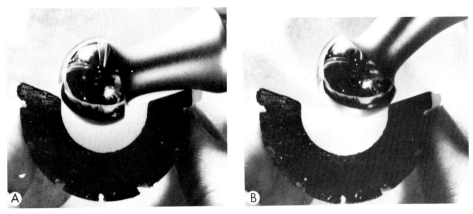

Fig. 12-15. Dislocation may occur (A) due to the neck levering on the rim or (B) due to the head pulling directly out of the acetabulum. A larger head must be pulled farther out before it will slip over the rim. (From Amstutz HC, Markolf KL: Design features in total hip replacements, in *The Hip,* Proceedings of the Second Open Scientific Meeting of the Hip Society, 1974. New York, CV Mosby Co, 1974, pp 111–124.)

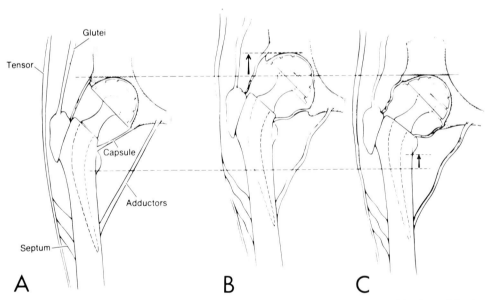

Fig. 12-16. (A) Correct soft tissue tension is maintained by accurate positioning of both components. (B) The acetabulum has been placed too cephaled; "effective neck length" is reduced and soft tissue laxity results. (C) Excessive shortening of the femur results in similar laxity; a short neck component or a component placed in excessive varus or valgus may do the same thing. (From Eftekhar NS: *Principles of Total Hip Arthroplasty.* New York, C.V. Mosby Co., 1978.)

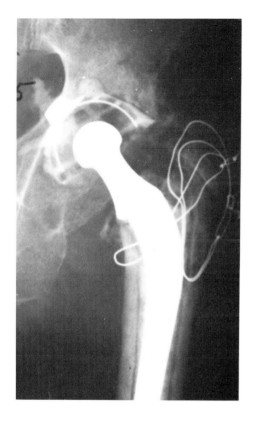

Fig. 12-17. Osteophyte impingement associated with dislocation.

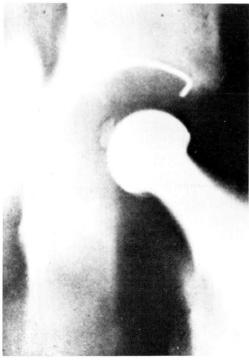

Fig. 12-18. Tomogram showing foreign body (methacrylate) in acetabulum. (From Eftekhar NS: *Principles of Total Hip Arthroplasty.* New York, C.V. Mosby Co., 1978.)

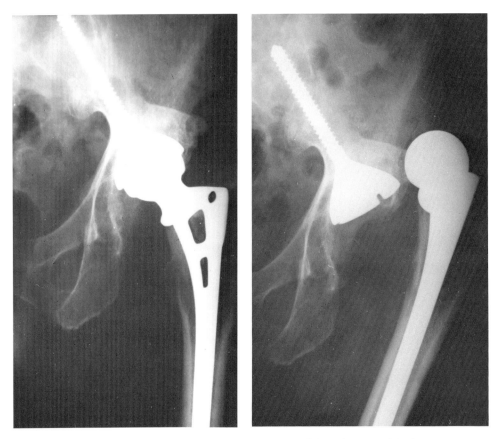

Fig. 12-19. An infected Ring arthroplasty that led to dislocation, possibly from increased fluid pressure.

ORTHOPAEDIC MANAGEMENT

The overall prognosis of the dislocated total hip arthroplasty is relatively good. A high percentage can be reduced without operative intervention. In the 1974 Mayo Clinic series, 76 percent of the dislocations were successfully reduced closed.[4] In the series by Fackler and Poss, 71 percent of the dislocations were reduced closed using intravenous diazepam.[9] Another seven patients (21 percent) had their hips reduced under spinal or general anesthesia; one was reduced without anesthetic; only two patients required primary open reduction. Six of those dislocations initially treated closed eventually required further surgery (18 percent). One avulsed greater trochanter was reattached, one distal femoral osteotomy was done to correct excessive femoral anteversion, and four patients had revision arthroplasty.[9] In the 1974 Mayo Clinic series, only 16 of 60 dislocations (27 percent) were not successfully treated closed.[4] Three of these 16 were successfully reduced open; eight were eventually revised; one was left dislocated due to the patient's overall medical condition. In Charnley's study, only 22 percent of the dislocations since 1971 have recurred; only one has required re-operation.[7]

Most authors do not speak extensively about their treatment regimens for the dislocated total hip. Ritter, in his 1976 series, treated five of seven patients in plaster pants. Two patients later subluxated, but none apparently redislocated.[14] In his 1980 article, Ritter stressed the importance of relocating the hip under general anesthetic, examining it for range of motion and for positions of dislocation, and aspirating the hip. Aspiration is performed both to remove excess fluid which might be the cause of the subluxation or dislocation, and to obtain material for culture, because Ritter believes that infection can be a cause of dislocation.[15] If the cultures are negative and surgical intervention is not indicated, the patient should avoid extremes of motion for 6 weeks. Any malposition of components or of trochanter or any bony or methacrylate impingement must be surgically corrected if it continues to produce dislocation. Fackler and Poss found that traction or suspension following dislocation did not reduce the rate of further dislocation; they recommend the use of guided ambulation as soon as possible after reduction, with instruction to avoid extremes of position.[9] They did, however, find that two patients with recurrent dislocations were successfully treated with traction and plaster immobilization, for 6 weeks in one case and 12 weeks in the other, both without further dislocation.[9]

It is difficult to propose any hard-and-fast rules concerning the etiology of and therapy for dislocating arthroplasties. The experiences of different surgeons have not been the same; results have not always been reported in such a way as to permit the use of statistical analysis; and accurate radiographic measurements cannot always be made. Some general conclusions can be drawn, however, and should be remembered in primary hip arthroplasty in order to prevent instability and dislocation.

The age, sex, and hip pathology of the patient seem to have little bearing on the outcome. Patients with a history of previous hip surgery, and those with multiple medical problems (particularly neurologic problems which make post-operative cooperation difficult), are at higher risk for post-operative dislocation.

The more experienced surgeon will probably have a lower dislocation rate. The choice of surgical approach is not critical, but if the trochanter is detached, care must be taken to reattach it in a distal and lateral position so as to maximize the distance between the trochanter and the femoral head, and to re-establish proper soft-tissue tension so as to hold the hip in place.

The choice of prosthesis is also not critical. Under laboratory conditions, some prostheses, particularly those with larger heads and larger head-to-neck diameter ratios, have more inherent stability (evidenced by larger ranges of motion without impingement). In clinical situations, though, good results can be obtained with large or small head sizes, depending on one's training and experience. One must be aware, however, of the requirements of whichever prosthesis one is using. Particularly with the 22 mm head prosthesis, proper component positioning and proper maintenance of soft-tissue tension is very important. The acetabulum must not be too superiorly placed; this can be partially avoided by reaming at right angles to the long axis of the body rather than aiming the reamer somewhat cephalad in line with the natural angle of the acetabulum.

The femoral neck should not be over-shortened, as this will result in abnormally low soft-tissue tension. The patient should be held firmly in place on the operating room table by a reliable holding device, so that the surgeon will not be misled by changes in position during the surgery. This will allow accurate positioning of the components.

Neither component should be placed in retroversion with respect to the coronal plane. The femoral component should not be anteverted by more than 10°, and the acetabulum should not be anteverted by more than approximately 15°. Correct placement of the femoral component may be aided by flexing the patient's knee 90°. The neck of the femoral prosthesis can then be oriented so that it is at a right angle to the lower leg, and it will be at an approximately neutral position, neither anteverted nor retroverted. The proper anteversion can then be added.

Except in cases where the natural acetabulum is badly distorted by congenital dysplasia or osteophyte formation, the surgeon may find that it is the best guide for placement of the prosthetic acetabulum. Reaming as well as cementing in the acetabular component may be done at the same angle of anteversion as the natural socket. This is usually the most reliable way to restore the natural anatomy and range of motion of the hip. The acetabulum should not be too vertical; in other words, it should not make an angle of more than 50° with the horizontal plane.

The femoral component must not be placed in too much valgus, since this reduces the trochanter-to-head distance, leading to relative abductor laxity, and increases the possibility of levering against the acetabular rim. All osteophytes and excess cement must be removed from around the rim. The acetabulum must not be seated too deeply, to avoid neck impingement. Care must be taken not to leave any methacrylate, bone, or other foreign bodies within the acetabulum. The trochanter must be reattached both distally and laterally to reestablish soft tissue tension.

Range of motion testing should be done on the operating room table; if impingement or dislocation occurs, the etiology must be sought and the problem eliminated, even if this involves component revision. Post-operatively, the patient should be x-rayed to ascertain that the hip is properly located. Medical personnel must be careful in positioning the patient; the patient should be carefully instructed to avoid positions which risk dislocation, such as hip flexion with adduction and internal rotation. Failures in patient and staff cooperation may be responsible for the majority of the early post-operative dislocations.

Those patients who do dislocate can usually be treated by closed reduction. This is sometimes done with intravenous anesthesia, but may require general or spinal anesthesia. After the hip has been relocated, range of motion should be tested to determine the position of dislocation, relative stability and the causative factor. X-rays should be checked for malposition of components, foreign bodies in the acetabulum, osteophytes or methacrylate excrescences allowing levering out, and malposition of the trochanter, if it was detached. An aspiration should be done of the hip joint both to remove excess fluid and to rule out infection. Occasionally an open reduction will be necessary, but this does not necessarily require a revision of the components.

After relocation, the patient should be immobilized in traction or at bedrest in abduction for 3 weeks. The patient must be educated to avoid positions of dislocation. If the hip dislocates again, it can sometimes be successfully treated by 6 to 12 weeks of immobilization in traction or in plaster pants. If dislocation persists, surgical intervention may be necessary to correct the problem. This may involve revision of malpositioned components, removal of foreign bodies, reattachment of the trochanter, or plicating loose soft-tissue, depending on the etiology of the instability. If repeated revisions fail to achieve stability, a Girdlestone pseudar-throsis may be the eventual result, but this, in most series, is a rare occurrence. The following flow chart represents one approach to the dislocated total hip (Fig. 12-20).

Notice that it is possible to reach the bottom line of this flow chart (at which point the surgeon decides that the hip is (1) stable; (2) unstable, but nothing more can or should be done; (3) needs surgical correction; or (4) unstable, components should be removed) in one of three ways. This last row of alternatives can be reached (1) without ever doing an open surgical procedure, (2) during the initial open reduction, or (3) after the initial open reduction while the patient is recuper-ating. The treatment of a septic total hip has been dealt with in another chapter. Further surgical correction of a non-septic hip may involve advancing the trochanter distally to re-establish soft-tissue tension, plicating the capsule, or revising one or both components to correct malposition. If the decision is made not to revise the arthroplasty but it remains unstable with certain motions, bracing may be a good alternative.

Bracing

The brace that is used for stabilization of a chronically dislocating hip following total arthroplasty must be designed to specifically prevent motion and positions which lead to dislocation. Any brace intended to control the hip must include a pelvic belt, a connection that puts the potential for motion at the level of the anatomic hip joint, and an attachment to the lower extremity that is sufficiently secure to prevent the motion that must be blocked. The blocking of flexion or extension, as well as abduction and adduction, can be accomplished by a hip hinge with a single axis and appropriate stops. Immobilization to the point of only a few degrees of movement can be achieved by adding a drop lock to such a hinge. For such braces, it is probably adequate to hold the thigh by a lacer or strapping arrangement (Fig. 12-21). If dislocation occurs with rotation, the attachment to the leg almost invariably must go below the knee in order to achieve rotary control. If the only unstable position is one of internal or external rotation (i.e., control of flexion and extension is not a problem), a twister table (attached to the shoe and held to the thigh by a light cuff which only serves to prevent the cable from having excessive relative motion), will be adequate to prevent rotation (Fig. 12-22). If a combination of flexion or extension, abduction or adduction, and rotational control is needed, a long leg brace is almost certainly necessary. In order to save weight, the newer, molded thermoplastic braces probably represent the only feasible approach to a total long leg brace with hip hinge and pelvic belt.

Whatever brace is chosen must be functionally acceptable to both patient and physician. The brace will only be useful if it is sufficiently cosmetically acceptable, so that the patient will wear it, and it is sufficiently easy to don, so that the patient, or those involved in his or her care, can place it on the patient without tremendous effort. In addition, the brace must not make demands upon an already weakened muscle and bone structure. A very heavy or cumbersome brace may greatly inhibit the patient's ability to ambulate independently. A brace which so restricts motion as to hold the leg in a non-functional position may either increase the energy demands of ambulation to the point that the patient cannot tolerate them or hold

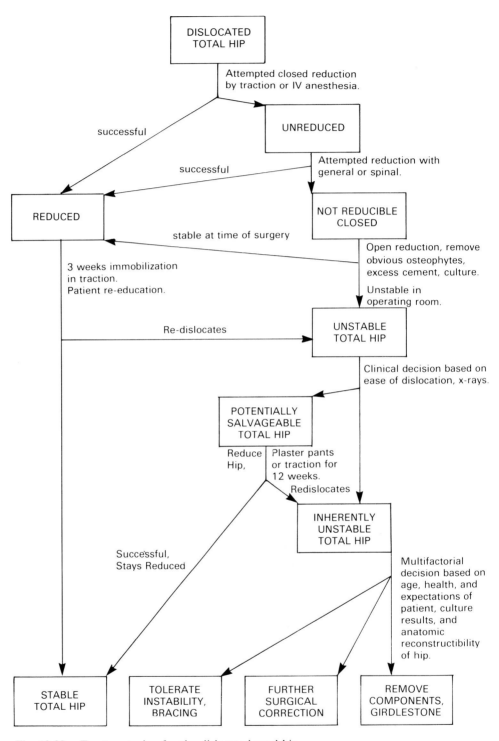

Fig. 12-20. Treatment plan for the dislocated total hip.

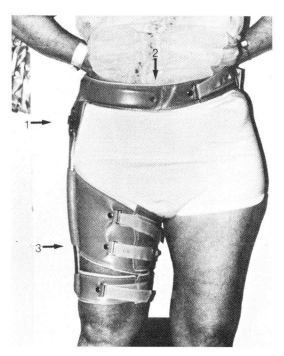

Fig. 12-21. Pelvic band with hip hinge and thigh cuff to control abduction, adduction, flexion, and extension. (From Eftekhar NS: *Principles of Total Hip Arthroplasty*. New York, C.V. Mosby Co., 1978.)

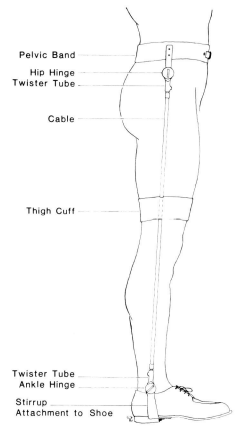

Pelvic Band

Hip Hinge

Twister Tube

Cable

Thigh Cuff

Twister Tube

Ankle Hinge

Stirrup

Attachment to Shoe

Fig. 12-22. Pelvic belt with twister cable that attaches to shoe to control rotation of hip.

287

the limb in such a position that the patient cannot sit or undertake even limited activities of daily living. Patently, such a brace is not an effective functional solution.

Finally, it must be remembered that hips with poor motors are subject to distortion forces secondary to the mass of the extremity below them. If this is a significant problem and further weight is added to the limb, particularly distally, in the form of heavy braces, the pendulum effects may impart motion to the hip which the hip motors cannot dampen or control. This may result in a limb which is uncomfortable and non-functional on the basis of that lack of control. More importantly, such pendulum motions may move the limb into a position where dislocation or other painful problems can occur. Bracing must give the necessary control to prevent dislocation without creating further stresses on the hip.

SUMMARY

Dislocation is the most common complication of total hip arthroplasty, occurring in 0.5 to 5 percent of cases. Age, sex, and hip pathology are not related to the incidence of dislocation. Multiple medical problems and previous hip surgery are associated with increased risk. Most dislocations occur less than 6 weeks postoperatively; most can be avoided by careful positioning of components, accurate maintenance of soft-tissue tension, and removal of all excess osteophytes and methacrylate. Medical personnel and the patients themselves must be educated in avoiding leg positions which may risk dislocation. When dislocation does occur, it may usually be treated without further surgery. When malposition of components or lack of patient cooperation renders the hip chronically unstable, revision, removal of the components, or bracing, may be necessary.

REFERENCES

1. Amstutz HC, Markolf KL: Design features in total hip replacements, in *The Hip*, Proceedings of the second open scientific meeting of The Hip Society, 1974. New York, CV Mosby Co, 1974, pp 111–124.
2. Chandler RW, Dorr LD, Perry T: Dislocation following total hip arthroplasty: Function and cost analysis. Accepted for publication, *J Bone and Joint Surg*.
3. Charnley J: *Low-Friction Arthroplasty of the Hip*. New York, Springer-Verlag, 1979.
4. Coventry MB, Beckenbaugh RD, Nolan DR, et al: 2,012 total hip arthroplasties. A study of postoperative course and early complications. *J Bone and Joint Surg* 56(A):273–284, 1974.
5. Eftekhar NS: Dislocation and instability complicating low-friction arthroplasty of the hip joint. *Clin Orthop* 121:120–125, 1976.
6. Eftekhar NS: *Principles of Total Hip Arthroplasty*. New York, CV Mosby Co, 1978.
7. Etienne A, Cupic Z, Charnley J: Postoperative dislocation after Charnley low-friction arthroplasty. *Clin Orthop* 132:19–23, 1978.
8. Evanski PM, Waugh TR, Orofino CF: Total hip replacement with the Charnley prosthesis. *Clin Orthop* 95:69–72, 1973.
9. Fackler CD, Poss R: Dislocation in total hip arthroplasties. *Clin Orthop* 151:169–178, 1980.

10. Khan MAA, Bruckenbury PH, Reynolds ISR: Dislocation following total hip replacement. *J Bone and Joint Surg* 63(B):214–218, 1981.

11. Lewinnek GE, Lewis JL, Tarr R, et al: Dislocations after total hip replacement arthroplasties. *J Bone and Joint Surg* 60(A):217–220, 1978.

12. Nolan DR, Fitzgerald RH, Beckenbaugh RD: Complications of total hip arthroplasty treated by re-operation. *J Bone and Joint Surg* 57(A):977–981, 1975.

13. Pellicci PM, Salvati EA, Robinson AJ: Mechanical failures in total hip replacement requiring re-operation. *J Bone and Joint Surg* 61(A):28–36, 1979.

14. Ritter MA: Dislocation and subluxation of the total hip replacement. *Clin Orthop* 121:92–94, 1976.

15. Ritter MA: A treatment plan for the dislocated total hip arthroplasty. *Clin Orthop* 153:153–155, 1980.

Roderick H. Turner,
Gerald B. Miley, and
Paul Fremont-Smith

13

Septic Total Hip Replacement and Revision Arthroplasty

More than 75,000 total hip replacements will be performed in the United States in 1982. A deep wound infection rate of 1 to 2 percent is acknowledged by most experienced reconstructive orthopedic surgeons, even with the use of laminar-flow clean air rooms and prophylactic antibiotics.[5,6] The emotion and economic impact of sepsis in a prosthetic hip could range from a bare minimum of $25,000 in hospitalization expenses for removal of the prosthesis and associated medical therapy, to a lifetime of total disability. Although local drainage and systemic antibiotic therapy may be successful in treating a select group of patients with acute sepsis and no evident loosening, definite therapy for established sepsis usually mandates total removal of the prostheses and massive debridement. Following removal and debridement, the decision must be made whether to leave the patient with a resection arthroplasty or to convert the patient back to a total hip replacement by revising both components.

HISTORICAL REVIEW

The surgical approach to hip disease in general was pioneered by Dr. Lewis A. Sayre in 1876.[67] Dr. Sayre, speaking in his lectures on orthopedic surgery and disease of the joints at Bellevue Hospital, described resection of the hip for the relief of hip joint disease. Girdlestone is generally credited with popularizing the resection surgical approach to tuberculosis and pyogenic hip sepsis.[25,26] In his classic monograph on constructive surgery of the hip, Aufranc first described the use of a cup arthroplasty associated with extensive debridement as treatment for hip sepsis.[2] Harris and Aufranc collaborated on a successful series of nine patients treated with cup arthroplasty in the face of known sepsis.[29]

291

REVISION TOTAL HIP ARTHROPLASTY
ISBN 0-8089-1466-9

Since the introduction of cement and total hip component systems, further opportunities have been provided for unusual and extensive forms of sepsis to be established. Fortunately, significant advances have taken place in antimicrobial therapy and in the surgical approach to revision arthroplasty in the face of sepsis.

Charnley has consistently advised against one-stage revision arthroplasty in the face of sepsis.[13] Hunter and Dandy have reported a disappointing 33 percent success rate when revision total hip arthroplasty was performed in the face of active sepsis.[33]

Wilson et al,[79-81] Salvati,[66] Turner,[72] and others have reported favorable results with revision total hip replacements in the face of sepsis largely without the benefit of antibiotic-impregnated cement.

Jupiter et al have described successful total hip revision in 14 of 18 patients with active infection, pointing out the uniquely unfavorable consequences of gram-negative infection and the *unusual* prolongation of hospital stay required for extensive antibiotic therapy.[34]

Fremont-Smith described 41 patients of which 39 were successfully treated utilizing one-stage revision and triple intravenous antibiotic therapy, followed by prolonged oral antibiotic suppression.[33] In this series, follow-up was short; only 25 percent of the patients had been followed over 2 years. Early results were very encouraging.

ANTIBIOTIC RATIONALE AND CLINICAL EXPERIENCE

Since 1970, an effective program of combined medical and surgical treatment of endoprosthetic sepsis has been undertaken at the New England Baptist Hospital. We continue to follow the intensive antibiotic program advocated by Fremont-Smith,[33] both in one-stage revisions and in Girdlestone excisional revisions. This program is derived from experience with the natural history of recurrent osteomyelitis. Analysis of treatment failures in various deep infections has led to an understanding of the phenomenon of "microbial persistence," so brilliantly elucidated by McDermott.[40,41]

McDermott showed that in experimental and clinical infections, certain bacteria may achieve a metabolic state in which they are "indifferent" to usually effective antibiotic therapy as chosen on the basis of *in vitro* antibiotic sensitivity testing. Bacteria in this state are called "persisters," and may be thought of as "hibernating." Although in a given clinical infection only a small percentage of the infecting organisms may enter into this phase, it is this group of cells which may, even years later, "reawaken," and cause recurrent invasive infection. Further work by Park[57] and Gordon[27] has confirmed the validity of McDermott's models in clinical osteomyelitis. Norden showed the effectiveness of double and triple antibiotic therapy treating *Staphylococcus aureus* osteomyelitis in a rabbit model.[55,56]

Infecting organisms may assume unusual bacteriologic characteristics when in the "persisting" phase, showing changes in morphology, staining properties, and cultural requirements.[19]

The antibiotic program, later discussed in more detail, has two important objectives: (1) To deliver high concentrations of three different classes of antibiotics to the tissues. Each chosen antibiotic is designed to kill the infecting bacteria by a different mode of action so that maximum bactericidal activity against the large majority of the bacterial population will be achieved. (2) To deliver prolonged oral therapy to suppress the small number of viable "persisting" organisms remaining unaffected by the intense antibiotic program.

We have done a detailed clinical follow-up study of 100 patients comprising 101 septic hip problems treated over 12 years and followed for a minimum period of 32 months, with a mean follow-up period of 48.5 months. All of these patients were treated with one-stage revision; the success rate has been 86 percent. During the same 10 years that these infected hips were undergoing one-stage revision surgery, 41 patients were treated by debridement and Girdlestone resection because of septic hip problems thought to be too severe for one-stage revision.

Although it is our current practice to use antibiotic-impregnated cement in all revision total hip arthroplasties, only 11 of the 100 patients reviewed were so treated. Consequently, the addition of antibiotics to acrylic cement will be separately treated later in this chapter.

PRE-OPERATIVE EVALUATION

The hallmark of success in treating endoprosthetic sepsis is close cooperation among the orthopedic surgeon, infectious disease consultant, anesthesiologist, physical therapist, nursing team, microbacteriology laboratory, and the orthopedic radiologist. Using a team approach, we have developed a systematic program for evaluating the painful and possibly septic hip.

Careful general medical evaluation of the patient must be undertaken prior to treatment of a septic hip. Little benefit will be derived from successfully reimplanting a prosthesis and eradicating sepsis if a stag-horn calculus remains as a continuing nidus for repeated gram-negative urinary tract infections which may seed a healthy hip. Early consultation for treatable sources of potential metastatic infection is essential prior to any reconstructive procedure. Stinchfield,[71] Downes,[15] D'Ambrosia,[17] Rubin,[65] and others have reported metastatic seeding via the hematogenous route. In the 100 patients discussed in this chapter, we have documented 10 cases of hip sepsis specifically seeded from foci of infection elsewhere in the body. Extraction of carious teeth, optimal treatment of psoriatic skin, healing of venous stasis ulcers, and eradication of any other foci of infection should be accomplished before making a final decision to proceed with any hip surgery.

The most dangerous potential sources of sepsis are those which involve gram-negative organisms. Dr. Camer will report in Chapter 17 on the high incidence and serious consequences of post-operative cholecystitis with the potential for abdominal anaerobic and/or gram-negative sepsis seeding of the hip. Urethral strictures, urolithiasis, and chronic bacturias need careful pre-operative evaluation and control. If urogenital surgery, cholecystectomy, or other procedures are indicated, they must always be done prior to elective hip surgery.

It is essential when reviewing the history that all old records, including nursing notes, be obtained and carefully reviewed. Many clues to the possible origins of sepsis have been found deep within a chart, yet absent from the final discharge summary.

Table 13-1.

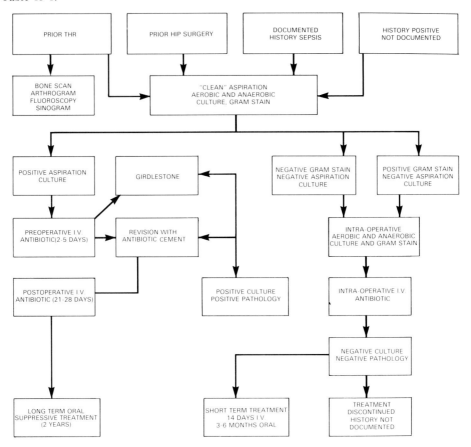

Table 13-1 outlines our pre-operative diagnostic work-up in schematic detail. Any patient with a painful hip and prior prosthetic surgery must be considered potentially infected until proven otherwise. A documented history (even remote) of sepsis and/or prior surgery also places any patient with a painful hip at increasing risk for infection. Radionuclide bone scanning is performed especially if the prior surgery was performed more than 12 months previous to the current problem. Septic loosening can usually be distinguished from mechanical loosening by selective radionuclide scanning. A negative or "cold" Gallium scan is useful in ruling out sepsis (see Chapter 2). Following the bone scan, aspiration and arthrogram are routinely performed. Any fluid recovered from the hip is sent for immediate Gram's stain and culture for aerobic and anaerobic organisms. Careful subculturing must be performed to detect indolent organisms. Draining sinuses may be evaluated by sinogram to demonstrate or rule out communication with the hip. If such communication between sinus and hip is not demonstrated by sinogram, the hip should be aspirated through a clean portal. Only after a complete and thorough investigation has been done can a decision regarding revision be made. Usually the final decision as to whether to do a one-stage revision or a resection has to be made at the time of surgery; this will be discussed later.

ANTIBIOTIC PROGRAM

Antibiotic management of the infected hip patient is the same, regardless of whether the surgeon elects a one-stage revision or a resection arthroplasty. The antibiotic program is chosen on the basis of (1) sensitivity testing to the organism by Bauer-Kirby* disc or by Auto-Bac 1† testing; (2) proven bone-penetrating qualities of the antibiotic; and (3) mode of action of the antibiotic.

Table 13-2 depicts the three major groups of antibiotics and their cellular area of action. Pre-operative intravenous (IV) antibiotic treatment referred to in Table 13-1, begins with institution of Group 1 and Group 2 (Table 13-2) antibiotics 2 to 5 days pre-operatively, if accurate bacteriologic data is available from aspirate cultures.

Massive cellulitis, edema, and drainage are indications for longer periods (7 to 14 days) of pre-operative antimicrobial treatment, in an effort to quiet down the host tissues. Those patients with drainage and unhealthy soft tissues will almost invariably be surgically managed by Girdlestone resection rather than by conversion to a new total hip replacement. (The flow of treatment decisions can be further followed on the right side of Table 13-1.) In the presence of a negative pre-operative aspiration culture, all antibiotics are withheld until definitive intra-operative cultures can be obtained. An empiric intravenous antimicrobial program is then selected and begun intra-operatively only after joint, soft tissue, and bone cultures are harvested. Adjustments in the drug selection are then made depending upon the results of intra-operative cultures.

Group 3 antibiotics (Table 13-2) are always started intra-operatively, in an effort to maximize the period of treatment after definitive debridement and surgery. An exception to the intra-operative institution of Group 3 (aminoglycoside) drugs is the patient in whom we planned to use aminoglycoside-impregnated cement.

Table 13-2
Three Groups of Drugs Used in Triple Antibiotic Protocol

	Antimicrobial agent	Site of action	Average dose (70 kg adult)	Duration of therapy
Group 1	Cefamandole Oxacillin Cephalothin	Interferes with cell wall "linkage"	2 gm IV every 4–6 hrs	21–28 days
Group 2	Clindamycin	Interferes at 50 S ribosomal subunit	600 mg IV every 6 hrs	21–28 days orally; 2 years, if appropriate
Group 3	Gentamicin Tobramycin Amikacin	Interferes at 30 S ribosomal subunit	80 mg IV every 8 hrs; 300 mg IV every 8 hrs (for amikacin)	10–14 days for Gram-positive organism(s); 21–28 days for Gram-negative organism(s)

*Bauer AW, Kirby WMM, Shreis JS, Turck M: Antibiotic susceptibility testing by a standardized single-disk method. Am J Clin Pathol 53:149–158, 1966.

†Autobac 1™ Instrumentation and Reagents. Distributed by Pfizer Inc. Patent 3,832,532.

Under these circumstances we recommend withholding systemic Group 3 antibiotics during the first 24 hours post-operatively. This is because high hematoma aminoglycoside levels are present by antibiotic leaching for 24 hours; possible toxicity is avoided by postponing systemic therapy for that period.

As indicated in Table 13-2, the duration of IV therapy post-operatively for Group 1 and Group 2 drugs is 3 to 4 weeks. Group 3 drugs are stopped after 14 days in gram-negative infections. The duration of therapy was initially mandated by patient tolerance and, in pre-aminoglycoside-monitoring years, by fear of renal complications. Our poor results with controlling sepsis in the presence of Gram-negative infections leads us to accept the additional risk of administering 4 weeks of aminoglycoside therapy in these difficult cases. Continuation of Group 3 drugs for the 4-week treatment period is usually possible if the patients are carefully monitored for ototoxicity, nephrotoxicity, and other complications.

Routine monitoring of all patients on triple therapy should include a complete blood count and differential count, as well as SGOT, creatinine, and urinalysis every 3 days. Audiovestibular monitoring is performed weekly. To achieve optimal therapeutic levels, aminoglycoside levels are measured 30 minutes before and 30 minutes after drug administration, once every 5 days or as clinically indicated. Patients on aminoglycoside therapy for more than 14 days and patients with *any* history of renal disease should have serum creatinine levels done every day, 7 days a week. It is critical to do a daily bedside examination of the patient, with attention to skin rashes, phlebitis, diarrhea, and monilial infection.

Upon completion of the triple parenteral therapy, oral suppressive antibiotic therapy is instituted. We strive for a 2-year oral treatment period. This has proved to be an elusive goal, due to poor patient compliance. Detailed review of patient cooperation shows that the average time patients continued regular oral medication was 13.2 months. Twenty-four patients took antibiotics for less than 12 months; of those 24, only 18 were considered successful by the criteria outlined below. Consequently, the precise duration of therapy remains an open question. Recurrence of infection with cessation of therapy in high-risk, eg, steroid-treated and/or immunosuppressed patients, has convinced us to continue oral treatment for a minimum of 2 years in this group. Patients who are on prolonged therapy with immunosuppressive drugs, cytotoxic agents, or steroids should be covered with oral antibiotics for life, or at least until these dangerous systemic drugs can be discontinued. For otherwise healthy patients, we strive for a 1-year minimum period of oral antibiotic treatment. Generally, we select a non-cell wall directed drug in Group 2, as seen in Table 13-2.

Table 13-3

Indications for a One-Stage Revision Arthroplasty

1. Organisms that are sensitive to at least three, and preferably six, antibiotics.
2. Gram-positive organisms.
3. Absence of superinfection and multiple organisms.
4. Healthy, well-vascularized tissues.
5. Absence of draining sinuses.
6. X-ray evidence of healthy femoral cortical bone.
7. Reasonably good bone, to support cement fixation, both in the acetabulum and in the femur.

Clindamycin is a proven drug for the treatment of osteomyelitis, and has a good antistaphylococcal spectrum, so it is usually chosen for long-term suppression when sensitivity testing permits. Cephalexin and ampicillin are other antibiotics often used for long-term oral suppressive therapy, depending upon the sensitivity pattern of the last organism(s) recovered.

The lack of good long-term oral suppressive antibiotics for the treatment of Gram-negative infections is undoubtedly part of the reason for the limited success in controlling this virulent type of infection by one-stage revision.

SURGICAL DECISION

The surgeon operating in the face of known sepsis should be prepared to do either a one-stage revision or a Girdlestone resection arthroplasty. Factors that favor one-stage revision are listed in Table 13-3. Of paramount importance is soft-tissue and bone quality. No amount of extensive surgery and intensive antibiotic treatment will offset the presence of disasterously unhealthy tissues. A representative

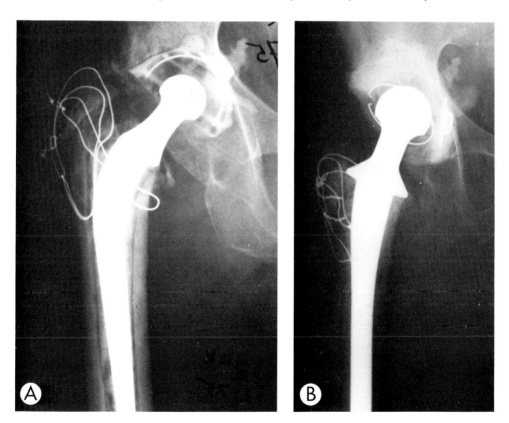

Fig. 13-1A. Pre-operative x-ray of an infected Bechtol total hip replacement. Note radiolucent lines at the bone-cement interface.

Fig. 13-1B. Post-operative x-ray shows a long-stem femoral component secured with radiolucent cement on the femoral side and radiopaque cement on the acetabular side of the joint.

case of a one-stage revision is seen in Figure 13-1A and 13-1B. Figure 13-1A shows an infected, loose, Bechtol-type prosthesis with a radiolucent shadow obvious at the bone-cement interface. The tissues were healthy and the offending organism was *Staphylococcus aureus* coagulase negative, so one-stage revision was performed to a long-stem Aufranc/Turner prosthesis, as seen in Figure 13-1B. Seven years post-operative, the patient is dry, healthy, and free of pain.

Factors favoring a Girdlestone resection are listed in Table 13-4. Although most of these indications are absolute, judgment must be used, especially when evaluating factors 2 and 3 of Table 13-4. We would not feel absolutely committed to resection arthroplasty in the presence of a low-virulence gram-negative organism that was sensitive to multiple antibiotics. The final decision is made at the time of surgery after weighing all factors.

An infected total hip replacement is seen in Figure 13-2A, with radiolucent lines around the bone-cement interface on both sides of the joint. Cultures from hip aspiration showed *Pseudomonas aeruginosa* infection; the soft tissues were edematous. Girdlestone resection was done; the post-operative x-ray is seen in Figure 13-2B.

SURGICAL APPROACH

Technique for One-Stage Revision

Revision arthroplasty in the face of sepsis should be approached as a very radical surgical debridement designed to remove all foreign materials and all tissues that are either devitalized or sequestered from the circulation sufficiently so that they might harbor micro-organisms. The lateral approach is recommended with trochanteric transplantation, as discussed in Chapters 4 and 11.

When the trochanter is osteotomized, it should be kept as small as possible, but it must be large enough to receive the insertion of the gluteus medius and minimus. Transplanting a large trochanteric fragment could risk having a trochanter too large to be nourished by the blood vessels coming through the scarred gluteus muscle complex. After trochanteric transplant, complete capsulectomy and extensive debridement are done to remove the dense scar and adhesions that invariably characterize infected hips. The femoral prosthesis, cement, and all granulomatous tissue are removed from the femur by the techniques described in Chapter 4. If one-stage revision is to be performed, it is absolutely essential to remove all of the

Table 13-4
Indications for a Girdlestone Resection

1. Virulent, resistant organisms.
2. Gram-negative organisms.
3. Two or more concominant strains of organisms.
4. Unhealthy and edematous soft tissues.
5. Draining sinus(es).
6. X-ray evidence of well-established osteomyelitis with bone erosion.
7. Severe loss of bone substance.

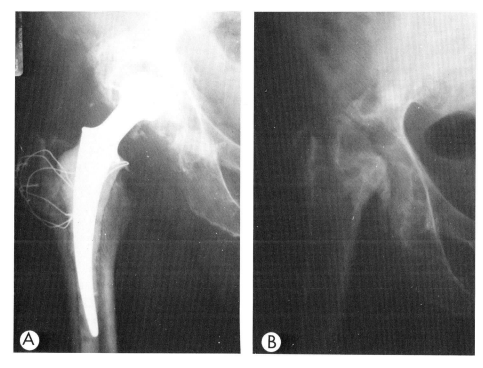

Fig. 13-2A.   Total hip replacement with *Pseudomonas aeruginosa* infection.

Fig. 13-2B.   Girdlestone resection following removal of all prosthetic components and cement.

previous cement. Failure to remove all cement commits the surgeon to a Girdlestone resection procedure.

The acetabular component will almost invariably be loose. It is removed by the techniques described in Chapter 5. It is important to remove the acetabulum from the inside of the acetabular cavity and not to try to pry the cement out of the softened pelvic bone, for fear of creating pelvic fracture(s). All of the acetabular cement is removed and the granulomatous membrane at the bone-cement interface is likewise carefully and thoroughly removed. Intrapelvic protrusions of cement should be removed in infected cases unless the surgeon feels that such removal would risk damage to intra-abdominal organs and/or vessels. If such damage is a possibility, then serious consideration should be given to a transabdominal removal of intrapelvic cement protrusions, to be discussed in Chapter 17.

After the removal of cement and granulomatous tissue, both the acetabulum and the femur are reamed back to healthy, bleeding bone if the bone is of sufficient strength to withstand power reaming. Careful attention should be given to remove no more bone stock than is necessary to create a clean healthy bed on both sides of the joint.

Once the decision has been made to implant a new total hip, the components are implanted with antibiotic-impregnated cement, with careful effort being given to optimum pressurization of the cement (discussed in Chapters 4 and 8).

Antibiotic wound irrigation with the pulsating jet should be voluminous and repetitive. Wound suction drainage is established with four separate suction tubes connected to portable wound suction units. Combined antibiotic inflow and suction drainage should not be necessary; the intravenous antibiotic can be delivered directly to the tissues if the debridement has been sufficiently extensive.

Wound closure is done simultaneously with completion of the debridement, as unhealthy and devitalized tissues are repeatedly debrided during careful layer-by-layer repair of the wound.

Rehabilitation and physical therpay activities following one-stage revision arthroplasty are the same as for other non-septic cases. The reader is referred to Chapter 18 for the details of these activities.

RESULTS OF ONE-STAGE REVISION ARTHROPLASTY

One hundred patients involving 101 infected hips with histologic evidence of acute and/or chronic inflammation associated with positive intra-operative cultures and/or positive pre-operative aspiration cultures of hip fluid were treated by one-stage revision surgery. Diagnoses in these 101 infected hips are seen in Table 13-5. All patients in this study were followed for a minimum of 32 months, or until death. The mean period of follow-up was 48.5 months.

Table 13-6 displays the 110 organisms recovered from the 97 patients with positive cultures. Twelve hips had mixed bacteriological cultures. Four patients had negative operative cultures, but were included because of the combination of a definite history of positive Gram's stain and confirmed histiologic evidence of sepsis. In these four patients, the wound cultures were modified by pre-operative antibiotic therapy.

All patients presented with pain; 77 percent reported pain at rest. Rest pain should be regarded as presumptive evidence of sepsis, as patients with non-septic mechanical loosening usually report that their pain is relieved specifically by rest.

Patients were graded as to functional outcome (Table 13-7).

Eighty-six percent of the patients were dry, free of pain, and ambulated with the support of a single crutch or less (Table 13-8).

Minor complications related to antibiotic therapy were seen in 42 of 101 hip cases and are listed in Table 13-9.

Although fully half of the patients treated reported loose stools at some time, only 14 patients reported five or more bowel movements per day. These 14 patients required minor modifications in the antibiotic program. Other minor complications such as rash, focal upper extremity phlebitis, moniliasis, etc, also responded to adjustments in specific antibiotics.

Table 13-5
Diagnoses: 101 One-Stage Revisions

Total hip replacements	47
Femoral endoprostheses	15
Fracture femoral neck	12
Cup arthroplasty	11
Girdlestone resection	10
Miscellaneous	6

Table 13-6
Culture Results (110 Positive Cultures)

Gram-Positive Isolates

Organism	Aspiration and/or Operative Culture	
Staphylococcus epidermidis	38	
S. aureus	23	
Micrococcus sp	1	
Streptococcus sp		
Enterococci	8	
Alpha-streptococci	3	
Beta-streptococci	4	
Group D streptococci	2	
Non-hemolytic streptococci	1	
Streptococci viridans	1	
Gram-positive cocci	2	
Diphtheroids	1	
TOTAL	84	(76%)

Gram-Negative Isolates

Organism	Aspiration and/or Operative Culture	
Escherichia coli	10	
Proteus mirabilis	4	
Pseudomonas aeruginosa	4	
Klebsiella pneumoniae	3	
Acinetobacter calcoaceticus	1	
Serratia marcescens	1	
Moraxella lacunata	1	
Gram-negative bacilli	2	
TOTAL	26	(24%)

Complications were deemed "major" when it was necessary to significantly decrease either the time or the triple-drug intensity of the therapeutic program. These major complications are seen in Table 13-10. The most severe complications were renal failure in two patients, one of whom required dialysis. There have been no cases of renal failure since aminoglycoside levels have been routinely monitored. In the two patients with enterocolitis, it was necessary to discontinue clindamycin therapy before completion of the protocol.

The mean duration of hospital stay for these 101 hip cases was 37 days, acceptable in the light of the magnitude of these septic problems.

GIRDLESTONE ARTHROPLASTY

Surgical Techniques

The principles and techniques discussed for one-stage revision arthroplasty are all applicable to Girdlestone resection. Any draining sinuses should be delineated

Table 13-7
Grades of Results

Grade I

Dry hip
Pain-free
Normal life-style

Grade II

Dry hip
Pain-free
Cane or crutch for stability or distant ambulation

Grade III

Dry
Painful; Medication needed
Limited mobility; Constant use of crutch or cane

Grade IV

Drainage
Constant pain
Further surgery suggested or performed

---

prior to the skin incision by injecting methylene blue dye into the sinus tract. The surgeon then attempts to excise everything that is stained by the dye as he or she dissects down to the depths of the wound. Debridement, capsulectomy, cement removal, granuloma removal, irrigation, and meticulous wound closure are as important in the resection patient as in the revision patient.

When there is considerable thinning of the femoral cortex, complete cement removal may be impractical and/or dangerous. When the surgeon believes that complete cement removal runs a high likelihood of fracturing the femoral shaft, he or she may be forced to leave some intramedullary femoral cement untouched.

On the acetabular side of the joint, complete cement removal rarely is a major problem. The decision to remove inaccessible intrapelvic cement through a separate anterior approach relates to realized or potential damage to adjacent vital organs, as will be discussed in Chapter 14.

Primary wound closure is possible in 90 percent of Girdlestone resections, and is performed in conjunction with a final debridement of the wound.

If certain extreme conditions prevail, it may be necessary to do open packing of the wound followed by delayed secondary closure. Such extreme conditions follow: (1) multiple draining sinuses with severe edema of the wound; (2) multiple virulent organisms recovered which are resistant to most or all antibiotics; and (3) gross pus found to be loculated in multiple separate pockets not well perfused by the systemic circulation.

If these extreme conditions prevail, open packing of the wound and dressing changes are done, under anesthesia if necessary, every 48 hours until the issues appear healthy enough to permit delayed secondary closure (usually 10 to 14 days). On rare occasions unhealthy wounds will have to be left to granulate in from the depths of the wound to the outer layers. This granulation process take months and sometimes even years, taxing the patience of both the surgeon and patient.

Table 13-8
Post-Operative Results of One-Stage Revision

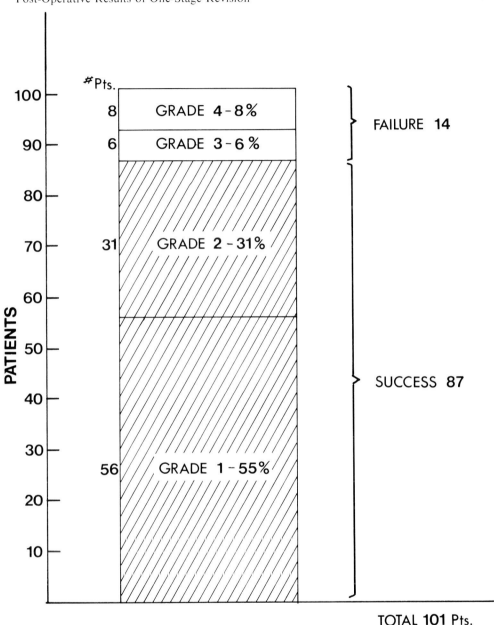

Physical Therapy Program

As Chapter 18 covers therapy programs for revision patients where the hip has been replaced, only those features unique to therapy for the resection arthroplasty patient need to be mentioned here. The principles of this post-operative program are very similar to those originally set forth by Girdlestone.[25,26]

Table 13-9
Minor Complications of Triple Antibiotic Therapy

Diarrhea	14
Rash	9
Phlebitis	9
Moniliasis	4
Drug fever	4
Pruritus	2
TOTAL	42

Post-operative therapy involves a prolonged period of skeletal traction for 24 hours/day in the first three weeks, 22 hours/day in the fourth week, and approximately 20 hours/day in the fifth week. In the fourth and fifth weeks, the 2-to-4 hours a day out of skeletal traction is used to start the patient on a program of sitting, stretching, and early ambulation. Ambulation is first assisted with a walker; the patient is then graduated to two crutches. The patient is never allowed to stay out of skeletal traction for more than 1 hour at a time until the completion of the fifth post-operative week. During the sixth week, the threaded traction pin is removed and the patient is fitted with the appropriate shoe lift. Since intravenous antibiotic therapy is continued for 4 to 6 weeks for these severe infections, the protracted skeletal traction does not prolong the patient's hospitalization. Sometime between 6 and 7 weeks post-operatively, the patient is discharged home on oral antibiotic therapy which will be continued for a minimum of 12 and ideally 24 months. When the patient is able to bear full weight on the operated limb with comfort, he or she is allowed to go from two crutches to a single crutch. This stage is usually reached somewhere around 9 to 15 months post-operatively. The patient continues to use a crutch until he or she can demonstrate a negative Trendelenburg test with the use of a single cane in the contralateral hand, after which time the cane is used for life. Only the occasional patient will ever walk without support following a Girdlestone; even these patients should use a cane when they leave the protection of their own home. Because this group of patients invariably have a Trendelenburg lurch in gait, it is a tremendous expenditure of energy for them to try to walk without their cane. The average shortening is 2 inches, and the average shoe lift is 1½ inches. The prolonged use of skeletal traction as described above will allow the surgeon to minimize post-operative shortening of the leg.

Since the above-described program and criteria have been instituted in 1976, there have been 28 Girdlestone resections performed at our hospital. Conversion back to a total hip replacement has been requested by only 4 of these 28 patients. The remainder of the patients have been able to adjust to the problems of shortening and instability.

Table 13-10
Major Complications of Triple Antibiotic Therapy

Renal compromise	5
Leukopenia	4
Enterocolitis	2
Renal failure	2
Audiovestibular damage	1
TOTAL	14

Pain has been tolerable in 85 percent of patients in this small group, but all patients have sufficient instability to require support; 25 percent still require two crutches 2 years following surgery.

CONVERSION OF GIRDLESTONE RESECTION ARTHROPLASTY

Evaluation for conversion from a Girdlestone to a total hip replacement is not recommended less than 12 months following the Girdlestone. It is generally preferable to wait a period of 24 months. Ideally, the patient should meet the following criteria:

1. An eager patient who is enthusiastic about the prospect of additional major reconstructive surgery.
2. A patient who has considerable residual pain despite the full-time use of a cane.
3. Healthy bone with stable radiographs and negative radionuclide bone scan for at least 12 months.
4. Lack of any wound drainage for at least 12 months.
5. Sedimentation rate and white blood count normal for at least 12 months.
6. Negative hip aspiration.
7. Realistic patient expectations regarding an end result.

Shea and Nenno have reviewed the success rate in 20 patients who have converted from a Girdlestone to a total hip replacement and they report that only 14 (70 percent) were successful.[69] These authors reported that 6 of 20 patients experienced a poor clinical result due to sepsis, loosening, or to intercurrent medical complications.

Optimum results from conversion of a previously septic Girdlestone resection back to a total hip replacement will be achieved when the seven criteria listed above are met.

ANTIBIOTIC-IMPREGNATED CEMENT

In major reconstructive surgery, and specifically in revision total hip replacement, a scientific rationale for the clinical use of antibiotic-impregnated cement can be formulated. In total hip arthroplasty the femoral head is removed and the medullary canal of the femur is reamed to allow insertion of cement and fitting of the prosthesis. This manuever destroys the endosteal blood supply to the bone immediately adjacent to the cement. Subsequent hematogenous transport of the intravenous antibiotics by the way of periosteal vessels to femoral cortical bone may be compromised. Intravenous and intramuscular antibiotics do not always achieve therapeutic bone levels, even in healthy bone. Therefore, if a means of providing antibiotic directly to the compromised bone-cement interface could be devised, high levels of antimicrobial agents could be achieved both for prophylaxis and treatment.

The clinical use of antibiotic-impregnated surgical cement largely has been pioneered in Europe, where Buchholz has reported successful results both for the prophylaxis and for the treatment of infections.[3-5,7-9] In a series of 1,409 cases using palacos R bone cement without antibiotics, his deep infection rate was 4.1 percent. By incorporating gentamicin with palacos R in a 1.5 percent gentamicin cement mixture, the deep sepsis rate in a subsequent series of 1,095 cases was 0.4 percent.[8] Buchholz, et al have continued to express their satisfaction with the prophylactic use of palacos R cement with gentamicin; their net experience now numbers over 10,000 arthroplasties.[6] The same report provides the largest series of infected hip problems in the literature. Buchholz et al have reported a 77 percent success rate in 583 patients after the first attempt at one-stage revision in the face of documented deep hip infection.[6]

Statistical comparisons of different series are difficult to analyze, especially when technical advances make it impossible to compare new results to old. In addition to the use of antibiotic-impregnated cement, concomitant improvements in operating room cleanliness and air flow, intra-operative aseptic technique, and the prophylactic use of systemic antibiotics have all helped reduce the rate of deep sepsis following total hip arthroplasty.

Nevertheless, information on the leaching of thermostable antibiotics from acrylic cement is available to encourage consideration of the place for this therapeutic combination, in the prophylaxis and treatment of infection.[12,20,24,30,32,35,39,42-45,50,52,59,61,64,73,77]

An antibiotic that creates a successful combination with a surgical cement, such as polymethylmethacrylate, should have the following properties:

1. A broad spectrum of coverage for gram-negative, gram-positive, and anaerobic organisms
2. Little or no evidence of patient sensitivity to the antibiotic or to the cement.
3. Little or no evidence of the emergence of resistant bacterial strains.
4. No significant decrease in the physical properties of the cement consequent to the addition of antibiotic powder.
5. Ability of the antibiotic to leach from the cement in sufficient quantity to saturate the wound hematoma and to obtain a therapeutic bactericidal antibiotic level in the hematoma.
6. Antibiotic thermostability at the polymerization temperature of cement.

Varying combinations of these characterizations have now been demonstrated for tobramycin cloxacillin, oxacillin, methicillin, lincocin, clindamycin, the cephalosporins, colistin, fucidin, neomycin, kanamycin, and ampicillin. In European centers, several antibiotic-cement combinations are available, such as powdered gentamicin in Palacos R cement, an erythromycin-colistin mixture in AKZ* cement, and others.

In the United States, FDA regulations have not permitted manufacturing or marketing of these compounds, but the clinical practice of adding antibiotics to acrylic cement is widespread, although not uniform.

Murray,[49,50] following Buchholz's initial example, has been utilizing erythromycin in acrylic cement since 1971. In 1976, the evidence from Rosenthal, et al[64]

---

*Trademark of Howmedica International, Inc. Professor Kuentscher Str., Kiel, West Germany, DZ301.

demonstrating *in vitro* activity of the combined erythromycin/colistin cement prompted Murray[50] to change to that mixture. Rosenthal, et al[64] showed that the combination of erythromycin and colistin was active against 96 percent of a spectrum of organisms tested, including gram-negative, gram-positive, and anaerobic strains. *In vivo* studies demonstrated leaching of antibiotics over 24 days, with therapeutic blood levels maintained to 48 hours.[64] In addition, Rosenthal demonstrated only a 9 to 18 percent reduction in mechanical properties of the cement, including compressive yield stress, shear stress, flexural stress, and diametral tensile stress. Lautenschlager's studies confirm minimal erosion of the physical properties of cement if the dosage level is kept to 1 gram of antibiotic/40 grams of powdered acrylic cement.[35,36]

Murray has been using erythromycin and colistin in cement since 1976; recently, he reported on 786 total hip replacements with a deep wound infection rate of 0.4 percent (3 of 786).[50] Only four cases of loosening were seen in this series, including three septic cases.

In 1970, Buchholz began work in Europe utilizing gentamicin-impregnated palacos cement, having found its spectrum to be much wider than the initially used erythromycin.[3,4,7] In the U.S., however, powdered gentamicin is unavailable and liquid gentamicin degrades the tensile strength of the cement monomer. Tobramycin, however, is available in a powdered form, which readily mixes with the acrylic polomer.

Miley et al have recently completed a phase II FDA-approved study utilizing tobramycin-impregnated surgical simplex cement.[44] The antimicrobial spectrum and potential toxicity of tobramycin are very similar to gentamicin, with an excellent coverage of both gram-negative and gram-positive organisms. Because of the very low incidence of allergic reactions, tobramycin is an ideal choice for use in major implant surgery.

Miley, et al studied 60 patients who had total hip replacements with follow-up ranging from 8 to 23 months. Twenty-eight patients had primary total hip replacements; 12 patients had revision hip replacements, and 10 patients had surface replacements. Five hundred mg of powdered tobramycin was uniformly mixed with 40 grams of polymethylmethacrylate cement prior to the surgical procedure. Follow-up in the initial 30 patients has now been completed, within a minimum of 12 months and a maximum of 23 months. Figure 13-3 plots the grams of tobramycin cement used against the hematoma concentration of tobramycin at 24 hours in the first group of 30 patients. The mean hematoma levels of tobramycin at 24 hours was 9.5* μg/ml, which is well within the therapeutic range for this drug (3–10 μg/ml). Urinary tobramycin excretion in the initial patient group showed levels in the therapeutic range between 6 and 24 hours postoperatively, with virtually no detectable tobramycin in the urine after 8 days. Serum levels of tobramycin were negligible.

The second group of 30 patients were studied in considerably more detail with hourly hematoma, serum, and urine tobramycin levels being obtained. Data generated by this second group of patients are seen in Figure 13-4, which plots the mean hematoma and urine concentrations against time. This chart demonstrates a biphasic leach-out into the wound hematoma over the initial 40 hours. Study of the

---

* New England Nuclear Radioimmunoassay.

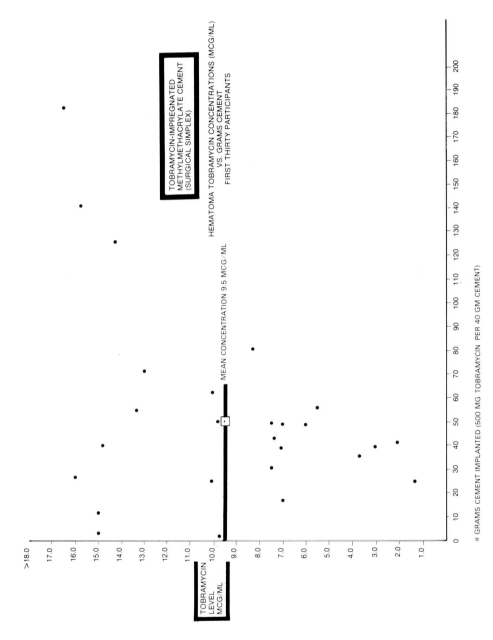

Fig. 13-3. First study group: Grams of tobramycin cement implanted plotted against hematoma concentrations. Mean hematoma concentration was 9.5 µg/ml.

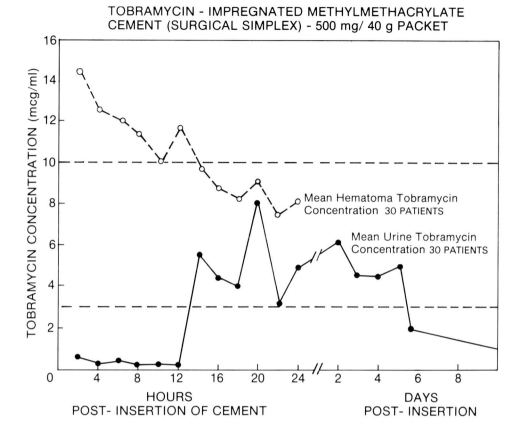

Fig. 13-4. Second study group: Mean hematoma concentration and mean urine concentrations plotted against time.

urinary antibiotic excretion in this patient group confirms the absence of significant urine levels after 8 days, although a few patients demonstrate low levels of urinary excretion for longer periods (Fig. 13-5). Serum levels were detectable in only a few patients, and these were in subtherapeutic ranges. There has been no evidence of either loosening or sepsis in any of these 60 patients, but the follow-up period at this writing is short (8 to 23 months).

Although the literature cited and the data presented are not absolutely conclusive, it appears that antibiotic-impregnated cement may be an adjunct to the prophylaxis of infection in hip replacement surgery. Antibiotic-impregnated cement is recommended for all patients undergoing *revision* total hip surgery. Care should be taken to select a thermostable antibiotic or combination of antibiotics with a broad spectrum of coverage against aerobic and anaerobic organisms.

SUMMARY

The treatment of septic hip joints and revision of septic endoprostheses is complicated and should only be undertaken by a medical and surgical team with

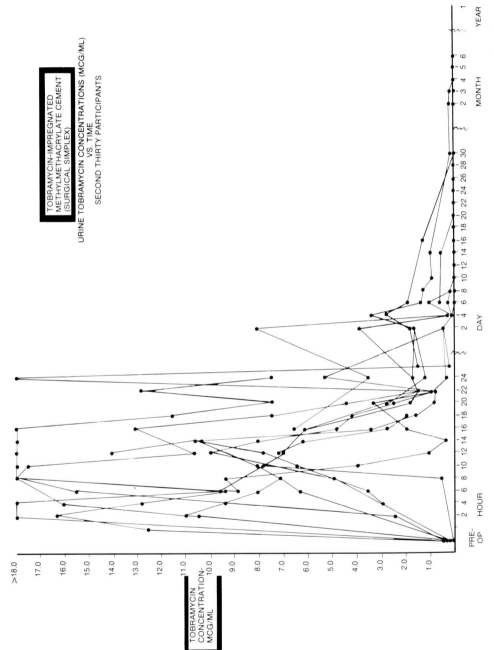

Fig. 13-5. Second study group: Urinary concentrations of tobramycin plotted against time (postinsertion of prosthesis).

310

a commitment to intensive and careful supervision of all aspects of therapy. One-stage revision is an acceptable treatment primarily for gram-positive infections in relatively healthy patients with healthy soft-tissue and good bone structure. Patients with gram-negative infections and those with poor soft tissues or with questionable bone structure are best managed by Girdlestone resection. Medical treatment consisted of intravenous triple drug therapy rather than single antimicrobial therapy. Long-term oral suppressive therapy was continued for 1 to 2 years. Longer term suppressive therapy is indicated in patients on steroid therapy, or in those patients otherwise at increased risk for repeated infection.

The European experience with antibiotic-impregnated cement has indicated that it is useful for both the prophylaxis and treatment of hip infection. The American experience with antibiotic cement combinations is not extensive. Early clinical results and clinical investigative data both support the effectiveness of antibiotic-impregnated cement, both for the prophylaxis as well as for the treatment of hip infections.

BIBLIOGRAPHY

1. Amstutz HC, Kass V: Management of the septic total hip replacement, in *The Hip: Proceedings of the Fifth Open Scientific Meeting of the Hip Society.* St Louis, CV Mosby Co, 1977, pp 152–169.
2. Aufranc OE: *Constructive Surgery of the Hip.* St Louis, CV Mosby Co, 1962, pp 181–190.
3. Buchholz HW: Hip arthroplasty for total replacement, St George model, Hamburg, Germany. Read at the Annual Meeting of The American Academy of Orthopaedic Surgeons, San Francisco, 1971.
4. Buchholz HW: Die operative Behandlung der progressiv chronischen Polyarthritis. *Med Klin* 67:596–602, 1972.
5. Buchholz HW: Klinische Erfahrungen uber die Anwendung von Gentamycin-Poly-methylmethacrylat zur Infektionsprophylaxe in der Huftchirurgie und zur Therapie tiefer Infektionen bei der totalen Endoprothese. In the First International Congress on Prosthetics Techniques and Functional Rehabilitation. Vienna, 1973, pp 119–135.
6. Buchholz HW, Elson RA, Engelbrecht E, et al: Management of deep infection of total hip replacement, *J Bone and Joint Surg* 63(B):342–353, 1981.
7. Buchholz HW, Engelbrecht H: Uber die Depotwirkung einiger Antibiotica bei Vermis-chung mit dem Kunstharz Palacos. *Chirurg* 41:511 515, 1970.
8. Buchholz HW, Gartman HD: Infektionsprophylaxe und operative Behandlung der schleichenden tiefen Infektion bei der totalen Endoprothese. *Chirurg* 43:446–453, 1972.
9. Buchholz HW, Noack G: Results of the total hip prosthesis design St George. *Clin Orth and Rel Res* 95:201–210, 1973.
10. Buck S, Lee AJC, Ling RSM: The effect of antibiotic additions on the mechanical properties of polymethyl methacrylate bone cements. *Med Orth Technik* 181–187, 1976.
11. Carlsson AS, Josefsson G, Lindberg L: Revision with Gentamicin-impregnated cement for deep infections in total hip arthroplasties. *J Bone and Joint Surg* 60(A):1059–1064, 1978.
12. Chapman MW, Hadley WK: The effect of polymethylmethacrylate and antibiotic combinations on bacterial viability, an in vitro and preliminary in vivo study. *J Bone and Joint Surg* 58(A):76–81, 1976.
13. Charnley J: Management of infected cases, in *Acrylic Cement in Orthopaedic Surgery.* London, Churchill Livingstone, 1970, pp 115–118.

14. Charnley J: Post-operative infection after total hip replacement with special reference to air contamination in the operating room. *Clin Orth and Rel Res* 87:167–187, 1972.

15. Charnley J, Eftekhar N: Post-operative infection in total prosthetic replacement arthroplasty of the hip joint with special reference to the bacterial content of the air of the operating room. *Br J Surg* 56:641–649, 1969.

16. Cruess RL, Bickel WS, Von Kessler KLC: Infections in total hips secondary to a primary source elsewhere. *Clin Orth and Rel Res* 106:99–101, 1975.

17. D'Ambrosia RD, Shoji H, Heater R: Secondarily infected total joint replacements by hematogenous spread. *J Bone and Joint Surg* 58(A):450–452, 1976.

18. Downes EM: Late infection after total hip replacement. *J Bone and Joint Surg* 59(B):42–44, 1977.

19. Editorial: L-forms—pathogenic or not? *Lancet* 1:130, 1972.

20. Elson RA, Jephcott AE, McGechie DB, et al: Antibiotic-loaded acrylic cement. *J Bone and Joint Surg* 59(B):200–205, 1977.

21. Fitzgerald RH Jr, Nolan DR, Ilstrup DM, et al: Deep wound sepsis following total hip arthroplasty. *J Bone and Joint Surg* 59(A):847–855, 1977.

22. Fitzgerald RH, Petersen LFA, Washington FA, et al: Bacterial colonization of wounds and sepsis in total hip arthroplasty. *J Bone and Joint Surg* 55(A):1242–1250, 1973.

23. Fremont-Smith P: Sepsis and total hip replacement, in *The Hip. Proceedings of the Second Open Scientific Meeting of the Hip Society.* St Louis, CV Mosby Co, 1974, pp 301–308.

24. Ger E, Dall D, Miles T, et al: Bone cement and antibiotics. *South Africa Med J* pp 276–279, February, 1977.

25. Girdlestone GR: Arthrodesis and other operations for tuberculosis of the hip, in *The Robert Jones Birthday Volume.* London, Oxford Press, 1928, pp 347–374.

26. Girdlestone GR: Acute pyogenic arthritis of the hip. An operation giving free access and effective drainage. *Lancet* 1:419–421, 1943.

27. Gordon SL: Recurrent osteomyelitis. *J Bone and Joint Surg* 53:1150, 1971.

28. Hamblem DL: Girdlestone excision arthroplasty as a salvage procedure for failed total hip replacements. Syllabus of the Second American Orthopedic Association International Hip Symposium, Boston, 1981.

29. Harris WH, Aufranc OE: Mold arthroplasty in the treatment of hip fractures complicated by sepsis. A report on nine cases. *J Bone and Joint Surg* 47(A):31–42, 1965.

30. Hill J, Kelnerman L, Trustey S, et al: Diffusion of antibiotics from acrylic-bone-cement in vitro. *J Bone and Joint Surg* 59(B):197–199, 1977.

31. Hughes PW, Salvati EA, Wilson PD Jr, et al: Treatment of subacute sepsis of the hip by antibiotics and joint replacement. Criteria for diagnosis with evaluation of twenty-six cases. *Clin Orth and Rel Res* 141:143–157, 1979.

32. Hughes S, Field CA, Kennedy MRK, et al: Cephalosporins in bone-cement. Studies in vitro and in vivo. *J Bone and Joint Surg* 61(B):96–100, 1979.

33. Hunter GA, Dandy D: Diagnosis and natural history of the infected total hip replacement, in *The Hip: Proceedings of the Fifth Open Scientific Meeting of The Hip Society.* St Louis, CV Mosby Co, 1977, pp 176–191.

34. Jupiter JB, Karchmer AW, Lowell JD, et al: Total hip arthroplasty in the treatment of adult hips with current or quiescent sepsis. *J Bone and Joint Surg* 63(A):194–200, 1981.

35. Lautenschlager EP, Jacobs JJ, Marshall GW, et al: Mechanical properties of bone cements containing large doses of antibiotic powders. *J Biomed Mater Res* 10:929–938, 1976.

36. Lautenschlager EP, Marshall GW: Mechanical strength of acrylic bone cements impregnated with antibiotics. *J Biomed Mater Res* 10:837–845, 1976.

37. Lazansky MG: Complications revisited. The debit side of total hip replacement. *Clin Orth* 95:96–103, 1973.

38. Leddy JP, Grantham SA, Stinchfield FE: Hip mold arthroplasty and post-operative infection: *J Bone and Joint Surg* 53(A):37–46, 1971.

39. Lindberg L, Carlsson A, Josefsson G: Use of antibiotic-containing cement in total hip arthroplasty done in the presence of or after deep wound infection, in *The Hip: Proceedings of the Fifth Open Scientific Meeting of The Hip Society*, St Louis, CV Mosby Co, 1977, pp 170–175.

40. McDermott W: Microbial persistence. *Yale J Bio Med* 30:257–290, 1958.

41. McDermott W: Microbial persistence. Harvey Lecture, Series 63. New York, Academic Press, 1969, pp 1–31.

42. Marks KE, Nelson CL, Lautenschlager EP: Antibiotic-impregnated acrylic bone cement. *J Bone and Joint Surg* 58(A):358–364, 1976.

43. Medcraft JW, Gardner ADH: The use of an antibiotic bone-cement combination as a different approach to the elimination of infection in total hip replacement. *Med Laboratory Tech* 31:347–353, 1974.

44. Miley GB, Turner RH, Bierbaum BE: *Experimental Studies on Antibiotic-Impregnated Cement.* In press.

45. Moore B: Editorials and annotations, antibiotics in cement. *J Bone and Joint Surg* 59(B):139–142, 1977.

46. Mueller ME: Preservation of septic total hip replacement versus Girdlestone operation, in *The Hip: Proceedings of the Second Open Scientific Meeting of The Hip Society.* St Louis, CV Mosby Co, 1974, pp 308–312.

47. Murray WR: Results in patients with total hip replacement arthroplasty. *Clin Orth* 95:80–90, 1973.

48. Murray WR: Part II, total hip replacement in non-specialized environments, in *The Hip: Proceedings of the Second Open Scientific Meeting of The Hip Society*, St Louis, CV Mosby Co, 1974, pp 271–289.

49. Murray WR: Treatment of deep wound infection after total hip arthroplasty, in *The American Academy of Orthopaedic Surgeons Symposium on Osteoarthritis.* St Louis, CV Mosby Co, 1976, pp 123–131.

50. Murray WR: Prophylactic use of antibiotic cement. *Syllabus of the Second American Orthopedic Association International Hip Symposium*, Boston, 1981.

51. Nelson JP: Operating room environment and its influence on deep wound infection, in *The Hip: Proceedings of the Fifth Open Scientific Meeting of The Hip Society*, St Louis, CV Mosby Co, 1977, pp 129–146.

52. Nelson RC, Hoffman RO, Burton TA: The effect of antibiotic additions on the mechanical properties of acrylic cement, *J Biomed Mater Res* 12:473–490, 1978.

53. Nicholas P, Meyers BR, Levy RW, et al: Concentration of clindamycin in human bone. *Antimicrob Ag Chemother* 8:220–221, 1975.

54. Nolan DR, Fitzgerald RH Jr, Beckenbaugh RD, et al: Complications of total hip arthroplasty treated by reoperation. *J Bone and Joint Surg* 57(A):977–981, 1975.

55. Norden CW: Experimental osteomyelitis IV. Therapeutic trials with rifampin alone and in combination with gentamicin, sisomicin, and cephalothin. *J Inf Dis* 132, No 5:493–499, 1975.

56. Norden CW: Experimental osteomyelitis V. Therapeutic trials with oxacillin and sisomicin alone and in combination. *J Inf Dis* 137, No 2:155–160, 1978.

57. Park JT: in Guze LB (ed): *Microbial Protoplasts, Spheroplasts and L-Forms.* Baltimore, Williams and Wilkins, 1968, pp 52–54.

58. Patterson SP, Brown SC: The McKee-Farrar total hip replacement (preliminary results and complications of 368 operations performed in five general hospitals). *J Bone and Joint Surg* 54(A):257–275, 1972.

59. Picknell B, Mizen L, Sutherland R: Antibacterial activity of antibiotics in acrylic bone cement. *J Bone and Joint Surg* 59(B):302–307, 1977.

60. Poss R, Ewald FC, Thomas WH, et al: Complications of total hip-replacement arthroplasty in patients with rheumatoid arthritis. *J Bone and Joint Surg* 58(A):1130–1133, 1976.

61. Quinlan W, Mehigan C: The release of antibiotics from bone cement. *Irish J Med Sci* 147:425–429, 1978.

62. Rathke FW, Erban WK: Prophylaxis and therapy of infection in joint endoprostheses with antibiotic bone cement (ABC). *Med Orth Technik* 188–191, 1976.

63. Roles NC: Infection in total prosthetic replacement of the hip and knee joints. Proc RSM 64:636–638, 1971.

64. Rosenthal AL, Rovell JM, Girard AE: Polyacrylic bone cement containing erythromycin and colistin I. In vitro bacteriological activity and diffusion properties of erythromycin, colistin and erythromycin/colistin combination. *J Int Med Res* 4:296–304, 1976.

65. Rubin R, Salvati EA, Lewis R: Infected total hip replacement after dental procedures. *So Oral Surg* 41:18–23, 1976.

66. Salvati EA: Infection complicating total hip replacement, in *The Hip: Proceedings of the Fourth Open Scientific Meeting of The Hip Society.* St Louis, CV Mosby Co, 1976, pp 200–218.

67. Sayre LA: *Lectures on Orthopedic Surgery and Diseases of the Joints.* New York, D Appleton and Co, 1876.

68. Schurman DJ, Trindade C, Hirshman HP, et al: Antibiotic-acrylic bone cement composites. *J Bone and Joint Surg* 60(A):978–984, 1978.

69. Shea W, Nenno D: Personal communication, 1979.

70. Smilack JD, Flittie WH, Williams TW: Bone concentrations of antimicrobial agents after parenteral administration. *Antimicrob Ag Chemother* 9:169–171, 1976.

71. Stinchfield FE, Bigliani LU, Neu HC, et al: Late hematogenous infection of total joint replacement. *J Bone and Joint Surg* 62(A):1345–1350, 1980.

72. Turner RH: Revision arthroplasty in the USA, in *Proceedings of the International Revision Arthroplasty Symposium.* Oxford, Elson RA, Caldwell AD (eds): Medical Education Services, 1979, p 85.

73. Wahlig H, Dingeldein E: Antibiotics and bone cements. Experimental and clinical long-term observations. *Acta Orth Scand* 51:49–56, 1980.

74. Wahlig H, Dingeldein E, Bergmann R, et al: The release of gentamicin from polymethyl-methacrylate beads. *J Bone and Joint Surg* 60(B):270–275, 1978.

75. Wahlig H, Hameister W, Grieven A: Release of Gentamicin from polymethylmethacrylate. I. Experimental in vitro tests. *Langenbeck's Arch Chir* 331:169–192, 1972.

76. Waisbren BA: Intensive treatment of bone infections. *Med Counterpoint* 2(Jan.):23–34, 1970.

77. Welch AB: Antibiotics in acrylic bone cement. In vivo studies. *J Biomed Mat Res* 12:843–855, 1978.

78. Wiggins CE, Nelson CL, Clarke R, et al: Concentration of antibiotics in normal bone after intravenous injection. *J Bone and Joint Surg* 60(A): 93–96, 1978.

79. Wilson PD Jr, Aglietti P, Salvati EA: Subacute sepsis of the hip treated by antibiotics and cemented prosthesis. *J Bone and Joint Surg* 56(A)879–898, 1974.

80. Wilson PD Jr, Salvati EA, Aglietti P, et al: The problem of infection in endoprosthetic surgery of the hip joint. *Clin Orth and Rel Res* 96:213–221, 1973.

81. Wilson PD, Salvati EA, Blumenfeld ES: The problem of infection in total prosthetic arthroplasty of the hip. *Surg Clin NA* 55:1431–1437, 1975.

Stephen J. Camer

14

Surgical Complications in Revision Arthroplasty

Revision hip arthroplasty often involves prolonged anesthesia with significant blood loss and replacement. Furthermore, revision hip surgery is often performed on elderly patients who are more susceptible to diseases which can present as acute, nonorthopedic surgical emergencies. The diagnosis of these surgical emergencies can be difficult in the post-revision period unless the orthopedic surgeon has a high index of suspicion. The danger of metastatic infection from a septic focus to the implant must be kept in mind, as has been emphasized in the previous chapter. Further, the proximity of the orthopedic field to other intrapelvic structures (rectum, bladder, and ileofemoral vessels) in hip revision arthroplasty has caused some unique problems that the general surgeon can help solve.

Surgical Abdominal Complications in the Post-Revision Period

Pre-Operative Work-Up

As previously implied, post-operative orthopedic patients are subject to a full range of abdominal surgical catastrophies. To review them all is beyond the scope of this discussion. In many cases, a careful history taken at admission will show symptoms which will alert the examiner to potential causes of acute abdominal disease in the post-revision period. Appropriate pre-operative studies could then be ordered. Thus, patients with diseases such as cholelithiasis, peptic ulcer, or diverticulitis can be identified before they undergo hip surgery. Judgement as to whether the abdominal problem should be treated prior to subjecting the patient to

315

REVISION TOTAL HIP ARTHROPLASTY
ISBN 0-8089-1466-9

revision arthroplasty would properly be rendered at this time. Prophylaxis of abdominal complications is by far the best treatment.

Perforation of Peptic Ulcer

Quiescent peptic ulcers are sometimes reactivated during the stress of major nonabdominal surgery, with perforation or bleeding as the first indication.[14] We have found the first 3 or 4 days after the orthopedic surgery to be the most dangerous for this complication. Steroids have a well-deserved reputation for reactivating dormant ulcer disease or allowing new ulcers to develop.[27] A history of steroid therapy in a rheumatoid patient must be kept in mind when evaluating him or her for abdominal pain in the post-revision period. Aspirin, used in the therapy of arthritis patients, is another ulcerogenic factor. Physical signs and diagnostic features of peritonitis secondary to a perforated duodenal ulcer are well-known.[10]

A few points deserve emphasis: In some cases, perforation can occur; the perforation can then seal with a localized peritonitis, which can be quite evanescent.[5,6] In patients with a known ulcer, this can be misinterpreted as acute exacerbation, and lead the examiner away from the true sequence of events. Hours later, recurrence of the perforation can happen with severe shock and full-blown peritonitis. Thus repeated examinations at short intervals is indicated, to allow early surgery to minimize contamination of the peritoneum. Although the initial efflux from a perforated duodenal ulcer is sterile, as the disease progresses, colonization takes place from oral intestinal tract flora,[2] and the stage is set for intra-abdominal abscess, placing both patient and prosthesis at high risk. Finally, especially in the elderly and patients on high-dose steroid medications, symptoms and signs may be minimal or nonexistent. Abdominal distention may be the only sign and may be confused with post-operative ileus.

If the perforated duodenal ulcer is acute with no previous history of ulcer, simple closure of the perforation is sufficient. If chronic ulcer disease is present, and when the patient's condition allows it, ulcer-curative surgery is the preferred therapy. The decision to embark on a definitive ulcer operation, such as vagotomy and/or resection, as opposed to the speedier alternative of simple closure of the perforation, requires mature surgical judgement and assessment of the abdomen at the time of surgical exploration.[3,5,12,13,16,19,22,28,40]

Acute Cholecystitis Following Joint Replacement Surgery

Since Glenn's report in 1947,[15] acute cholecystitis as a specific entity following surgery in areas remote from the biliary system has received increasing attention in the literature.[16,19,22,28,32,40] Some series since then also implicate severe trauma as an antecedent factor in the development of a particularly fulminating cholecystitis, with a high mortality if it is undiagnosed or inadequately treated.[28,40] An observed increased incidence of such cholecystitis in patients after joint replacement prompted review of our experience at the New England Baptist Hospital (Table 14-1).

This type of acute cholecystitis is most common in the older patient groups, especially in those over 60 years of age. It does not have gender predominance, and

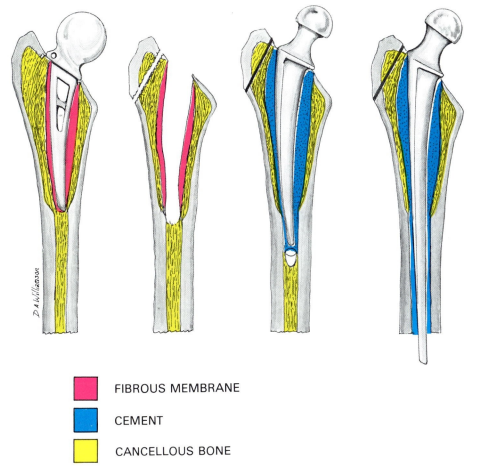

FIBROUS MEMBRANE

CEMENT

CANCELLOUS BONE

Color Plate V. Preparation of proximal femoral canal.

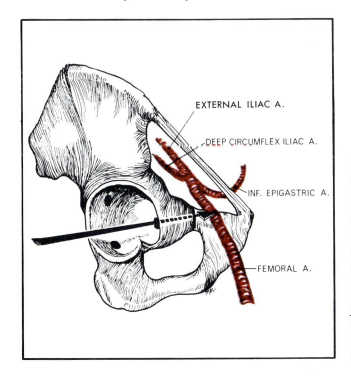

EXTERNAL ILIAC A.

DEEP CIRCUMFLEX ILIAC A.

INF. EPIGASTRIC A.

FEMORAL A.

Color Plate VI.1. Relationship of iliac artery to the acetabulum is illustrated. Mechanical injury or injury by exothermic reaction of cement can occur (indicated by arrow). (Adapted from Aust JC, Bredenberg CE, Murry PG: Mechanisms of arterial injuries associated with total hip replacement. *Arch Surg* 116:345–349, 1981, with permission.)

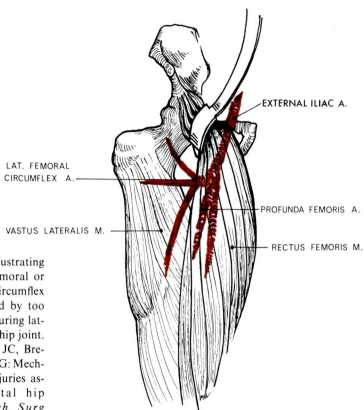

EXTERNAL ILIAC A.

LAT. FEMORAL
CIRCUMFLEX A.

PROFUNDA FEMORIS A.

VASTUS LATERALIS M.

RECTUS FEMORIS M.

Color Plate VI.2. Illustrating how the common femoral or the lateral femoral circumflex artery can be injured by too vigorous retraction during lateral approach to the hip joint. (Adapted from Aust JC, Bredenberg CE, Murry PG: Mechanisms of arterial injuries associated with total hip replacement. *Arch Surg* 116:345–349, 1981, with permission.)

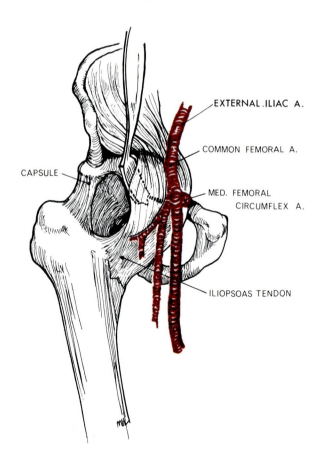

EXTERNAL .ILIAC A.

COMMON FEMORAL A.

CAPSULE

MED. FEMORAL
CIRCUMFLEX A.

ILIOPSOAS TENDON

Color Plate VI.3. The acetabular branch of the medial femoral circumflex artery can also be injured by hip capsule retraction. (Adapted from Aust JC, Bredenberg CE, Murry PG: Mechanisms of arterial injuries associated with total hip replacement. *Arch Surg* 116:345–349, 1981, with permission.)

Table 14-1

Acute Cholecystitis Following Joint Replacement in 25 Patients

Age Range	35–79 years
Sex	15 Females
	10 Males
Orthopedic procedure	23 hip replacements
	2 knee replacements
Treatment	23 emergency surgeries

there is a high incidence of acalculous gallbladders, much higher than would be expected, even in this older age group.[15,16,32,36] We noted 10 cases of acalculous cholecystitis among our 23 surgery patients.

One of the significant features observed both in our patients and in the literature is the onset of symptoms after resumption of intake of food, after a post-operative period of starvation. It has been postulated that during absent or limited oral intake, the gallbladder may fail to empty for 2 or 3 days.[7] Under these circumstances, there is bile stasis, increased viscosity, and sludge formation, causing obstruction of the cystic duct, in patients with and without stones. Acute inflammation then follows. The time interval between resumption of full oral intake and the onset of symptoms appears to be more important than the interval between operation and the attack on cholecystitis.[19,36,40] In our series, the initial episode occurred most commonly between the third and seventh day after revision surgery.

Another possible etiologic factor in these patients is the almost universal use of narcotic drugs. Most narcotics cause increased tonicity of the biliary sphincters, and can also retard gallbladder emptying.[7,16,32]

The diagnosis of cholecystitis can be rendered more difficult by post-operative fever, ileus, and incisional pain. Further, the symptoms are often initially quite mild and rapidly progress, so that repeated clinical examination at short intervals is necessary. Over half of our patients complained of pain in the right upper quadrant, or epigastrium, with associated nausea and vomiting. Fever and abdominal tenderness was present in over 75 percent of the patients. Laboratory studies were not significantly helpful in aiding the diagnosis: The white blood count was elevated in less than half of the patients; liver function tests were abdominal in only a few patients. The serum amylase was elevated in only 3 of the 25 patients. (This test however, should always be performed to rule out pancreatitis, the existence of which may significantly change the management.) The diagnosis of cholecystitis was made on clinical grounds alone in a number of patients. The newer, noninvasive radiologic studies can be of significant benefit in aiding diagnosis. If gallstones are present, ultrasonography can demonstrate them with a high degree of accuracy (Figure 14-1). Radionuclide hepatic iminodiacetic acid (HIDA) scanning can assess the gallbladder and common bile duct obstruction (Figs. 14-2, 14-3). Both of these noninvasive studies can be performed with minimal discomfort to the post-operative hip patient. One must be prepared, however, to undertake surgery on the basis of clinical symptoms and signs alone in some patients, if the radiologic studies are equivocal or negative in the face of severe symptoms and positive signs. In three of our patients with acalculous cholecystitis, the ultrasound and/or HIDA scan were normal.

Once the diagnosis is made, emergent surgery is necessary. Our own experience

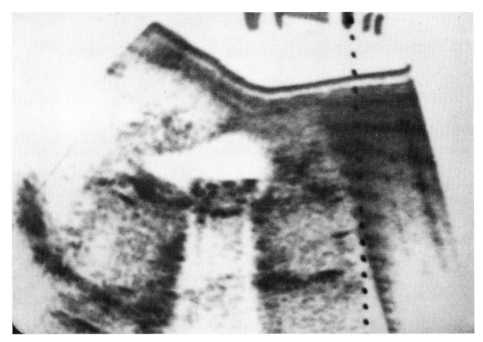

Fig. 14-1 Sonogram showing four medium size gallstones in a patient 4 days after hip replacement with fever, nausea, and right upper quadrant tenderness. At surgery, acute and chronic cholecystitis was noted, in addition to the above-demonstrated cholelithiasis.

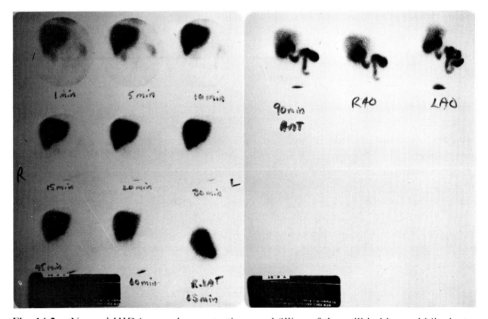

Fig. 14-2. Normal HIDA scan demonstrating good filling of the gallbladder and bile ducts.

318

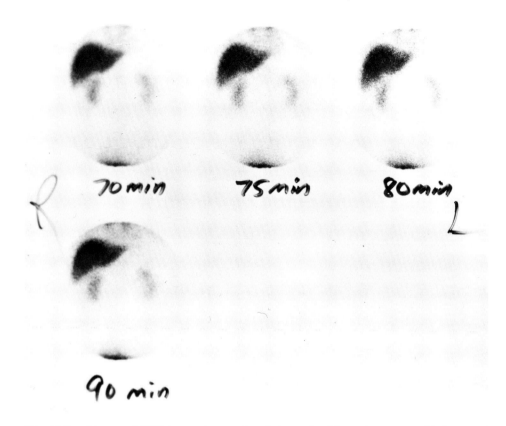

Fig. 14-3. Abnormal HIDA scan in a patient 7 days after hip replacement, with fever and right upper quadrant tenderness. The gallbladder fails to take up the isotope. At surgery, acute inflammation and dilatation of the gallbladder was found, with an impacted stone obstructing the cystic duct.

and that in the literature attest to the unusually fulminant course.[28,40] If the deadly complications of gangrene, empyema, and perforation with biliary peritonitis are to be avoided, cholecystectomy should be performed as soon as the disease is recognized. Simple drainage of the gallbladder without removing it should be avoided, because it has the disadvantage of leaving behind the septic focus with subsequent seeding of the hip prosthesis. Because of the observed increased incidence of this potentially deadly complication in patients undergoing revision arthroplasty, we recommend that cholecystography and/or ultrasonography be performed in all patients who have a history of biliary symptoms, and that the gallbladder be removed prior to the performance of the orthopedic procedure whenever it is in a diseased state. A normal pre-operative cholecystogram or sonogram does not rule out the diagnosis in the post-operative period, because the patient may develop acalculous cholecystitis.[28] Early recognition and treatment can lead to a successful outcome in most cases. All 23 patients operated upon in our series survived. In the two patients who died, the cholecystitis was unrecognized and was confirmed at the autopsy.

Intestinal Obstruction

Mechanical intestinal obstruction of the small or large bowel can occur at any time. The symptoms of abdominal distention, cramps, vomiting, and obstipation are well-known.[35,38] Predisposing factors, such as hernias, previous surgery leading to intra-abdominal adhesions, or a history of intestinal obstruction, should alert one to the possible existence of a mechanical obstruction in the post-replacement period. Small hernias, particularly in the elderly, may be particularly difficult to detect and must be very carefully sought. Irreducible or symptomatic hernias should be repaired prior to arthroplasty. More common problems in the post-revision period are physiologic obstruction (or paralytic ileus), and acute gastric dilatation. Acute gastric dilatation can present quite dramatically with massive vomiting, sometimes amounting to many liters of fluid. In the immobilized patient, such vomiting can lead to severe aspiration and immediate death. Along with this, when the gastric dilatation is truly massive, sudden and profound cardiovascular collapse can occur which can mimic coronary thrombosis, pulmonary embolism, or septic shock. The early warning signs of acute gastric dilatation are an unexplained rise in pulse rate, belching, hiccups, oliguria, and epigastric distension. On observation of these signs, instant aspiration of the stomach will often be rewarded with large volumes of fluid and can be both diagnostic and life-saving.

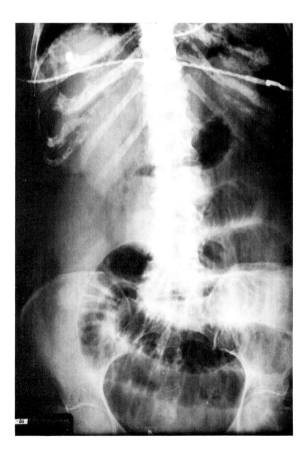

Fig. 14-4. Flat plate of a patient with mechanical obstruction of the small intestine. There is an absence of gas in the large intestine. Note the ladderlike arrangement of distended small bowel. The abnormal distention is confined to the center of the abdomen.

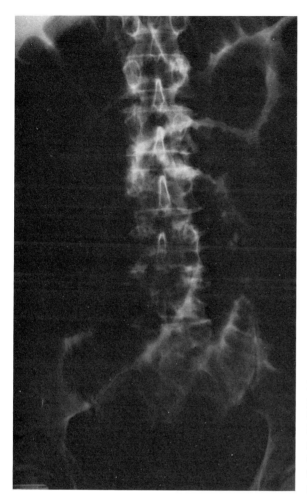

Fig. 14-5. Paralytic ileus was present in both dilated colon and small intestine. The small-bowel loops are more randomly arranged than in mechanical obstruction, and the abnormal loops are scattered throughout the abdomen.

Patients with known sliding hiatus hernia are particularly prone to regurgitation and aspiration in the recumbent position. The post-operative hip patient with hiatus hernia, narcotized and in traction, is at high risk for the development of these complications. In patients with known sliding hiatus hernia, nasogastric decompression with levin tube and intermittent suction should be instituted during the operation and continued during the immediate post-operative period, until the patient is alert and can be elevated in bed.

Paralytic ileus refers to a physiologic small bowel obstruction without a mechanical component. It occurs in the post-operative period and can be initiated by retroperitoneal bleeding, such as is often present in revision arthroplasty. Anesthesia may also contribute to the development of paralytic ileus. The differentiation between paralytic ileus and mechanical obstruction may be quite difficult, and becomes more so as the ileus is of long standing.[37] The degree of distention may be greater in paralytic ileus; and the distention is usually painless. The most helpful immediate study is a flat film of the abdomen, which will show diffuse dilatation of the entire small and large intestines in paralytic ileus and distal collapse of the intestines in mechanical obstruction (see Figs. 14-4, 14-5). Once the diagnosis of paralytic ileus is established, nasogastric aspiration and careful attention to fluid and electrolyte balance, particularly potassium replacement, is mandatory if the ileus is to resolve. One must guard against premature removal of the nasogastric tube and institution of oral intake, as this may lead to vomiting and aspiration in the recumbent position.

COMPLICATIONS OF ANTICOAGULANT THERAPY

In patients on anticoagulant therapy, bleeding and hematoma formation may mimic acute surgical conditions. Bleeding into the mesentery of the small bowel can cause hematoma with small bowel obstruction. Retroperitoneal hemorrhage can lead to paralytic ileus. A hematoma may form in the rectus abdominus sheath secondary to straining and coughing, and can resemble a strangulated inguinal hernia or lead to signs of tenderness, mimicking peritonitis. A patient history of anticoagulant therapy, along with a drop in the hematocrit, should alert one to the possible presence of these complications. Administration of vitamin K and cessation

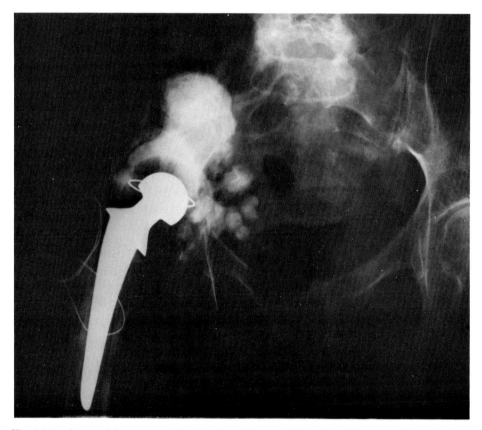

Fig. 14-6. Intrapelvic cement collection in a 53-year-old female with groin pain and edema of right lower extremity. The cement was easily palpable rectally and vaginally.

of the anticoagulant medication is the obvious treatment. However, in some cases, surgical exploration may be necessary to relieve obstruction, to rule out peritonitis, or to drain a compressing hematoma. In such cases, if anticoagulant therapy is indicated but undesirable, alternate modes of treatment (such as insertion of a vena caval filter or partial vena cava interruption with vena cava clip) should be considered to protect the patient from pulmonary embolus.

TECHNICAL COMPLICATIONS OF HIP SURGERY

Injury to Vessels

In the course of the performance of hip arthroplasty, damage to the external iliac artery or to the common femoral artery and its branches may result. These injuries may present as hemorrhage, ischemia, or the development of false aneurysm. Previous authors have emphasized the anatomic proximity of the external iliac and common femoral arteries to the hip joint.[1,8,9]

Injury to the external iliac artery can be caused by direct instrumental trauma during preparation of the acetabulum, or subsequently, by exothermic reaction of extruded methymethacrylate cement (see Color Plate VI).[1]

Injury to the common femoral artery and its branches can be caused by too-vigorous retraction of the hip capsule, as well as by exothermic reaction from extruded cement. Disruption, false aneurysm formation, and rupture of atherosclerotic plaque with immediate occlusion and ischemia have all been described (see Color Plate VI).[1]

Careful clinical assessment of pre-operative vascular status should be part of the routine work-up of every patient in whom hip revision arthroplasty is planned, in order to assess post-operative changes. Knowledge of the anatomic relationship of the vessels to the hip joint is of extreme importance. Patients who are known to have intrapelvic cement protrusions should have a routine pre-operative venogram to ascertain the exact location of the external iliac vessels in relationship to the cement (see Fig. 14-7). Any compression of the iliac vein may contribute to venous stasis and increase the possibility of thromboembolic complications (discussed in Chapter 15). The venogram also provides a "road map" for the revision surgeon and forewarns him or her of the possibility of intra-operative laceration of the iliac vessels during cement removal. Cement removal by a retroperitoneal approach may be more satisfactory than a transacetabular removal; this will also be discussed in a later chapter.

The proximity of the iliac artery to the acetabulum must also be kept in mind during the operative preparation of this structure. Gouging of the acetabulum can cause direct trauma to the iliac vessels; they can also be damaged by the exothermic reaction of extruded cement, especially in patients with major medical acetabular defects (see Color Plate VI).[1,8,33]

The course of the common femoral artery and its branches must always be kept in mind when placing retractors in the region of the rectus femoris and vastus lateralis muscles. The atherosclerotic vessels of the elderly patient undergoing hip arthroplasty are particularly prone to injury (see Color Plate VI).[1,9,11,30]

If vascular injury is suspected because of massive intra-operative or post-operative hemmorhage or ischemia, the assistance of a vascular surgeon should be immediately obtained. Angiography may be of value in delineation of an arterial injury.[1]

Cement Extrusion

Extrusion of cement from the acetabular defect into the pelvic retroperitoneal space can cause impingement on other structures in addition to the arteries. We have seen chronic erosion into the urinary bladder with arthrovesical fistula in two cases. We have also seen impingement on the rectum and vagina with a palpable mass on ditigal examination. During the orthopedic procedure, repair of acetabular defects, care in placement of the cement, and protection of the soft tissue from exothermic reaction should minimize extrusion and damage to intrapelvic structures. If the extruded intrapelvic cement is causing symptoms, or if one fears possible gradual erosion, removal of the cement is indicated. We have used a retroperitoneal approach with careful identification of the ureter and vessels. The cement mass was invariably surrounded by a pseudocapsule. Incision of the iliacus muscle allows the extruded cement to be exposed. It can then be freed laterally by drill and osteotome, and gently "levered" out without harming adjacent structures.

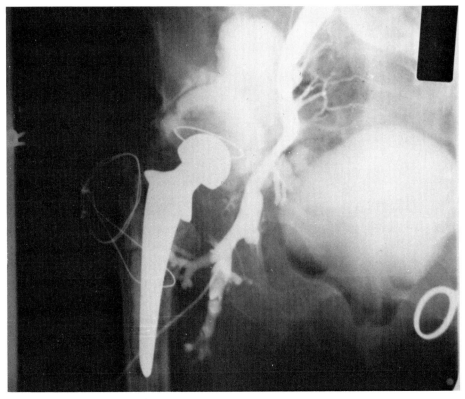

Fig. 14-7. Venogram in the same patient illustrated in Fig. 14-6. The cement is partially surrounding and narrowing the iliac vein.

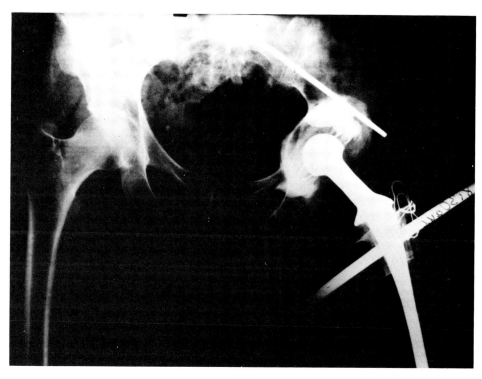

Fig. 14-8. A Kirschner wire has penetrated the pelvic wall and was found to be lying partially within the abdominal cavity. Removal was made through a lower midline laparotomy. No vascular or intestinal injury was noted in this patient after careful exploration. Removal of the wire by attempting to withdraw it through the hip joint should not be done, since this may infect the orthopedic field if the wire has penetrated the intestinal tract or the bladder.

Instrument Perforation

Instrument perforation of the pelvis and into the abdominal cavity and urinary bladder has also been noted (see Fig. 14-8). Immediate and thorough exploration of the abdomen with identification and repair of any urologic, intestinal, or vascular injury is mandatory. We do not recommend a policy of "watchful waiting," since the grave consequences of infection of the prosthesis, should an intestinal or bladder perforation be present, must be avoided.

SUMMARY

The prevention, diagnosis, and management of general surgical complications are an important part of the complete management of the revision hip arthroplasty patient. Only by maintaining a high index of suspicion and an acute awareness of these complications may they be detected and promptly treated.

BIBLIOGRAPHY

1. Aust JC, Bredenberg CE, Murry PG: Mechanisms of arterial injuries associated with total hip replacement. *Arch Surg* 116:345–349, 1981.
2. Bach NP, Amdrup E: Pre-operative bacteriologic examination of the stomach and duodenum. *Acta Chir Scand* 129:521–523, 1965.
3. Berne CJ, Mikkelsen WP: Management of perforated peptic ulcer. *Surgery* 44:591–598, 1958.
4. Booth RAD, Williams JA: Mortality of perforated duodenal ulcer treated by simple suture. *Br J Surg* 58:421–424, 1971.
5. Cohen MM: Treatment and mortality of perforated peptic ulcer: A survey of 852 cases. *Can Med Assoc J* 105:263–266, 1971.
6. Cope O, Wight A: Metabolic derangements imperiling the perforated ulcer patient. VI. The Plan of Therapy. *Arch Surg* 72:571–578, 1956.
7. Copher, GH, Illingworth CFW: Mechanism of emptying of the gallbladder and common duct. *Surg Gynec Obstet* 46:459–462, 1928.
8. Coventry MB, Beckenbaugh RD, Holan DR, et al: 2012 total hip arthroplasties. A study of post-operative course and early complications. *J Bone and Joint Surg* 56:273–284, 1974.
9. Dameron TB: False aneurysm of femoral profundus artery resulting from fixation device. *J Bone and Joint Surg* 46:577–580, 1964.
10. DeBakey M: Acute perforated gastroduodenal ulceration. *Surgery* 8:852–860, 1940.
11. Dorr LD, Covaty JP, Kahne R, et al: False aneurysm of the femoral artery following total hip surgery. *J Bone and Joint Surg* 56:1059–1062, 1974.
12. Eisenberg MM: Physiological approach to the surgical management of duodenal ulcer. *Curr Probl Surg* January, 1977.
13. Emmett JM, Williams HL: Gastric resection: A definitive treatment for perforated peptic ulcer. *Am Surgeon* 23:993–996, 1957.
14. Fletcher DG, Harkins HN: Acute peptic ulcer as a complication of major surgery, stress or trauma. *Surgery* 36:212–215, 1954.
15. Glenn F: Acute cholecystitis following the surgical treatment of unrelated disease. *Ann Surg* 126:477–483, 1947.
16. Glenn F, Wartz GE: Acute cholecystitis following the surgical treatment of unrelated disease. *Surg Gynec Obstet* 102:145–153, 1956.
17. Gray JG, Roberts AK: Definitive emergency treatment of perforated duodenal ulcer. *Surg Gynecol Obstet* 143–146:1, 1976.
18. Green DL: Complications of total hip replacement. *South Med J* 69:1559–1564, 1976.
19. Hoffman E: Acute gangrenous cholecystitis secondary to trauma. *Amer J Surg* 91:288–292, 1956.
20. Jordan GL Jr, Angel RT, DeBakey ME: Acute gastroduodenal perforation: comparative study of treatment with simple closure, subtotal gastrectomy and hemi-gastrectomy and vagotomy. *Arch Surg* 92:449–456, 1966.
21. Kirkpatrick JR: The role of definitive surgery in the management of perforated duodenal ulcer disease. *Arch Surg* 110:1016–1020, 1975.
22. Knudson RJ, Zuber WF: Acute cholecystitis in the post-operative period. *N Engl J Med* 269:289–291, 1963.
23. Mikal S, Morrison WR: Acute perforated peptic ulcer: Criteria for operation and analysis of 500 Cases. *N Engl J Med* 247:119–125, 1952.
24. Müller ME. Total hip prostheses. *Clin Orthop* 72:46–68, 1970.
25. Patterson FP, Brown CS: The McKee-Farrar total hip replacement: Preliminary results and complications of 368 operations performed in five general hospitals. *J Bone and Joint Surg* 54:257–275, 1972.

26. Rees JR, Shan KG, Thorbjarnson B: Perforated duodenal ulcer. *Am J Surg* 120:775–779, 1970.

27. ReMine WH, McIlrath DC: Bowel perforation in steroid-treated patients. *Am Surg* 192:581–583, 1980.

28. Robertson RD: Noncalculous acute cholecystitis following surgery, trauma, and illness. *Am Surgeon* 36:610–614, 1970.

29. Roseman PL, Econmav SG: Treatment of complications of gastroduodenal "steroid ulcers." *Arch Surg* 90:488–492, 1965.

30. Salama R, Stavorosky MM, Itellin A: Femoral artery injury complicating total hip replacement. *Clin Orthop* 85:143–144, 1972.

31. Sawyers JL, Herrington JL, Mulkerin JL, et al: Acute perforated duodenal ulcer. *Arch Surg* 110:527–534, 1975.

32. Schwegman CW, DeMuth WE: Acute cholecystitis following operation for unrelated disease. *Surg Gynec Obstet* 97:167–171, 1953.

33. Scullin JP, Nelson CL, Bever GB: False aneurysm of the left external iliac artery following total hip arthroplasty. *CLin Orthop* 113:145–149, 1975.

34. Singer HA, Vaughan RT: Treatment of the forne fruste type of perforated peptic ulcer. *Surg Gynec Obstet* 54:945–948, 1932.

35. Smith GA, Perry TE, Yoehero EG: Mechanical intestinal obstruction: A study of 1252 cases. *Surg Gynec Obstet* 100:651–654, 1955.

36. Thompson JW, Ferris PO, Baggenstoss AA: Acute cholecystitis complicating operation for other diseases. *Ann Surg* 155:489–492, 1962.

37. Torgerson WR: Three-year experience with total hip replacement. *Clin Orthop* 95:151–157, 1973.

38. Waldron GW, Hampton JM: Intestinal obstruction: A half-century comparative analysis. *Ann Surg* 153:839–846, 1961.

39. Welch CE: *Intestinal Obstruction.* Chicago, Year Book Publishers, 1958.

40. Winegarner FG, Jackson GF: Post-traumatic acalculous cholecystitis. A highly lethal complication. *J Trauma* 116:567–569, 1971.

Michael Hume

15

Thromboembolic Complications in Revision Arthroplasty

ORGANIZATION AND FACILITIES

Thromboembolic complications after revision hip surgery can be anticipated and prevented. The resources which are absolutely essential for success of this type of surgery are similar to those desirable for any major joint replacement. Effective organization ultimately begins with the orthopedic surgeon; he or she must be assured of the cooperation of an experienced vascular surgeon. Familiarity with the routine major arterial reconstruction is often less required than in-depth experience with the complications of thromboembolic disease, chronic venous insufficiency, and arteriolitis. Facilities must include high-quality angiography, nuclear medicine, and physiologic vascular testing. Diagnosis will be discussed in the sequence on the work-up of the patient undergoing revision hip surgery. Necessary equipment includes at least the following:

1. A bedside plethysmographic method (impedance plethysmography, or IPG).
2. An ultrasound technique for peripheral vascular testing and supraorbital examination of the carotid arterial system.
3. Scanning instruments for isotope localization (the ^{125}I fibrinogen uptake test).
4. Trained technologists to perform these tests.
5. A pneumatic calf-compression apparatus.
6. A coordinated arrangement, permitting sterile technique and fluoroscopy for placement of the inferior vena cava umbrella filter.[16]

329

REVISION TOTAL HIP ARTHROPLASTY
ISBN 0-8089-1466-9

OUTPATIENT WORK-UP

An informal specialist can determine by careful history and detailed physical examination the likelihood of most vascular complications that may befall the revision total hip replacement patient. Signal elements in the history and physical suggest consultation before the patient is admitted to the hospital. The following should be noted:

1. The dates and details of all prior surgical operations on the lower extremities, giving particular attention to whether swelling of the limb persisted after surgery.
2. Details of the duration and effectiveness of measures necessary for control of swelling.
3. Documentation of any episodes of embolism or thrombosis for which treatment was given.
4. The timing of the appearance of skin changes characteristic of chronic venous insufficiency, including the location of ulceration and its response to therapy.
5. The duration of steroid therapy for inflammatory joint disease.
6. The requirement for aspirin, or gastric intolerance to aspirin.
7. Episodes of bleeding from any source, such as the gastrointestinal or genitourinary tract.
8. Transient focal neurologic events such as transient ischemic attacks (TIA).
9. The quality and character of pain resembling claudication in the legs with exercise.
10. A history of coldness of the operated leg exacerbated by chilly weather, suggesting reflex dystrophy.

Physical examination should confirm the following routine findings regarding the arteries:

1. Pedal pulses should be palpable.
2. The abdominal aorta pulse should not be dilated to an extent suggesting aneurysm.
3. No bruit should be present in the carotid arteries.

The skin of the lower extremities should be inspected for changes suggesting chronic venous insufficiency, such as edema, obvious swelling, pigmentation, induration, ulceration, and dermatitis. In addition, it should be noted whether there is atrophy of the skin, characteristic of chronic steroid therapy. The location of ulceration of the legs is important. Stasis ulcers occur on the medial aspect of the leg; the ulceration of arteriolitis related to inflammatory joint disease is more common the lateral aspect of the legs (Fig. 15-1). Other differences between these types of ulcer should be familiar to the experienced vascular specialist.

Referral of the patient to a vascular specialist is indicated by the finding of ulceration or other abnormalities during the initial work-up. Additionally, any circumstances that would increase the risk of bleeding in the post-operative period when drug prophylaxis against thromboembolism is required must be evaluated. Gastrointestinal (GI) or genitourinary (GU) ulceration with history of bleeding should be investigated by the appropriate specialist; any known defect of hemostasis requires referral for work-up by a hematologist.

Conditions that can be evaluated on an outpatient basis by the vascular consultant include a noninvasive work-up of carotid bruit and measurement of the abdominal aorta to determine the presence of an aneurysm. Both are done by ultrasonic techniques, which are noninvasive. Some assessment of occlusive arterial disease is possible in the office with a Doppler probe. If chronic venous insufficiency is revealed (e.g., typical skin changes) it is appropriate to arrange for fitting of elastic stockings to control edema. Prior to hospitalization, it is also possible to determine by Doppler examination whether incompetent perforator veins are present.

The timing of admission for revision hip surgery depends on complete healing of any leg ulcers due to chronic venous insufficiency or arteriolitis. The technique of the Unna-type compound dressing is demonstrated in the accompanying illustration (Fig. 15-2). In the hands of an experienced practitioner, virtually every instance of small- or medium-sized areas of ulceration due to chronic venous insufficiency can be induced to heal without hospitalization. The challenge is distinctly more complex if there is a notable degree of skin atrophy due to steroid therapy. Hospitalization for skin grafting of large ulcers may be required to save time, or if the compound Unna-type dressing is not effective.

After healing, the patient can either be immediately admitted to the hospital for hip surgery, or conservative measures can be employed to prevent recurrence

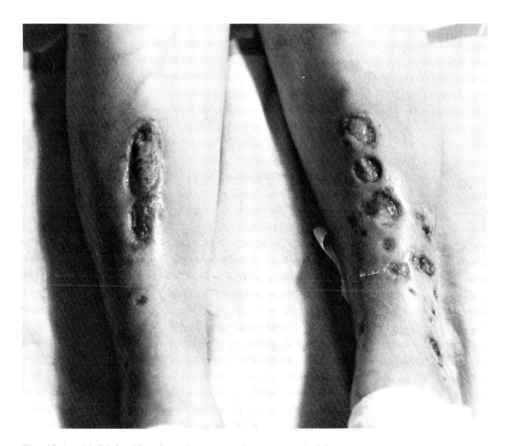

Fig. 15-1. Multiple skin ulcerations secondary to arteriolitis.

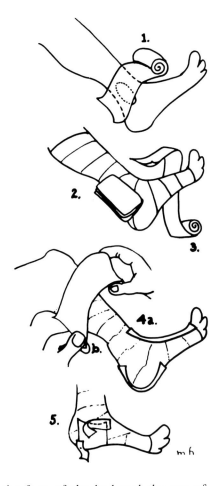

Fig. 15-2. Technique for Unna-type compound dressing. (1) unna bandage, 3 inches wide. Begin over ulcer and cover from base of toes to tibial tubercule. Caution: for mild dermatitis use cortisone lotion (¼ percent) on skin; for severe dermatitis use aluminum acetate soaks (½ strength) instead of boot. (2) Absorbent gauze pad, enough to absorb all exudate until next application. Put outside Unna dressing opposite ulcer. Caution: in presence of occlusive arterial disease add lambswool as extra padding over bony prominences. Priority in treatment should be given to ischemia, if sever, rather than venous insufficiency. (3) Conforming gauze bandage, one layer to hold all in place. (4) Elastic adhesive plaster, 4 inch roll. (a) Cut strips ½ width of roll; put front and back of ankle for protection from pressure. (b) Hold roll by edges; overlap ½ width; apply with increasing pressure going down. (5) Adhesive plaster, 1 inch wide. Secur ends of elastic adhesive with short, noncircumferential pieces of 1 inch tape. (From Hume M, Sevitt S, Thomas DP: *Venous Thrombosis and Pulmonary Embolism.* Cambridge, Mass, Harvard University Press, 1970. Reprinted by permission.)

until hip surgery is performed. Elevation of the foot of the bed and the use of pressure-gradient elastic stockings are fundamental, but these methods are difficult for patients disabled by arthritis. Admission to the hospital should therefore promptly follow healing of the skin ulcers. It would be a serious error to undertake major joint revision while an ulcer remains unhealed; the potential for infection of the prosthesis is great.

There are several reasons why the patient with crippling arthritis may not be able to comply with a good plan for management of venous insufficiency, including knew-length elastic stockings and elevation of the foot of the bed. Arthritis of the hands may make it too difficult for the patient to handle stockings which have adequate compression. Joint disease of the hip or knee may interfere with tying shoe laces. In such cases, slippers may be worn instead of conventional footwear. It is always necessary to prevent swelling due to valvular venous insufficiency. Shoes must be worn, and pressure-gradient stockings fitted. The help of family members (or even of neighbors) may be required. By elevating the foot of the bed, gravity will quickly remove edema when the patient is recumbent. Cement blocks under the bed osts are practical, sturdy, and exactly the correct height (Fig. 15-3). A lesser degree of elevation may be necessary in the presence of chronic obstructive pulmonary disease, congestive heart failure, or hiatus hernia.

EVALUATION IN HOSPITAL

If noninvasive imaging of the carotid artery reveals or suggests a significant stenosis, it is prudent to obtain a carotid arteriogram before scheduling hip surgery. This procedure is required in order to decide whether carotid endarterectomy should take precedence. After the patient is admitted to the hospital, laboratory work-up is related in part to the prevention of thrombosis and embolism. To arrange for all of the work-up to take place on the day the patient is admitted is difficult. The presumption by third-party insurance carriers that the work-up can be done on an outpatient basis or in a single day pre-operatively is fallacious; an adequate work-up routinely takes 2 pre-operative days in the hospital.

If x-rays reveal protrusio acetabulae, it is necessary to obtain a phlebogram (Fig. 15-4), in order to determine the relation of the iliac vein to the acetabular component and the intrapelvic cement. An IPG test should be performed pre-operatively, if possible. If the results are abnormal, it is necessary to consider monitoring for thrombosis with ^{125}I fibrinogen. Saturated solution potassium iodide (SSKI) must be given to block thyroid uptake of the isotope. All patients should have a partial thromboplastin time, but a prothrombin time is necessary only if the patient has been receiving oral anticoagulant therapy. If the patient has been on aspirin or the number of platelets is reduced on the blood smear, a bleeding time is performed. Any history of GI bleeding requires a stool guaiac.

PROPHYLAXIS

The choice of prophylaxis for the prevention of post-operative thromboembolism is made after considering the risk of bleeding and the outcome of prophylaxis at any previous surgery. The risk is statistically greater early post-operatively and in overweight and elderly patients. For most patients, the preferred prophylaxis is aspirin (10 grains twice a day). For reasons which remain unclear, it appears that protection against thrombophlebitis by aspirin may not extend to women undergoing total hip replacement[2,7] although this is not confirmed by the New England Baptist Hospital experience.[11] The incidence of pulmonary embolism, however, has been reported to be extremely low in both men and women receiving prophylactic aspirin following total hip replacement.[2,7,11,14,15] Among all patients undergoing total hip replacement at the New England Baptist Hospital who are given aspirin, the

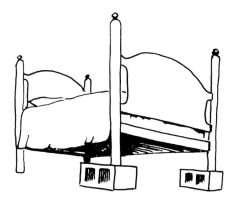

Fig. 15-3. Standard size construction cement blocks are practical and provide sturdy elevation of the foot of the bed to the correct height.

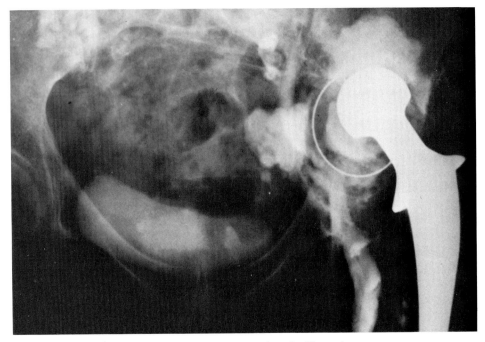

Fig 15-4.   Iliac venogram shows cement compressing the iliac vein.

occurrence of pulmonary embolism is 0.87 percent (4 of 462). This incidence is significantly lower than was found in a carefully studied group of 140 patients during the period before aspirin was used prophylactically.[14] During that time there were six incidents of embolism, a rate of 4.3 percent.

It should be noted that the mechanism by which aspirin protects against thromboembolism after hip replacement is not fully understood, although it has been suggested that an endothelial injury is characteristic of this operation.[2,4,20] Decreased levels of the clotting factor antithrombin III found in postoperative hip arthroplasty patients has been reported by Gitel et al.[4] The evidence for protection by aspirin after other types of surgery is far less convincing and, indeed, it may be unwarranted to assume that aspirin is an effective prophylaxis for any type of surgery other than total hip replacement.

There are exceptions to the general preference for aspirin prophylaxis; alternatives should be selected for the following types of patients (Fig. 15-5):

Some patients know that they cannot tolerate aspirin by mouth, usually because of gastritis and occasionally because of bowel irritability. It is a serious mistake to substitute enteric-coated aspirin for such individuals. The absorption of aspirin is unpredictable in the post-operative period; enteric-coated aspirin may not be absorbed at all. We know of one instance of fatal embolism that occurred because this was not appreciated. Enteric-coated aspirin is not an acceptable substitute prophylaxis if GI intolerance of buffered aspirin must be taken into account.

Some subjects undergoing revision hip surgery have had thromboembolic complications after previous operations on the hip, in spite of aspirin prophylaxis. We feel that it is better to consider such cases as failures of aspirin and to select an alternative plan of prevention rather than to assume that this was a unique experience which will not be repeated. The principal drug alternatives to aspirin are warfarin and dextran.[1,5,12] There has been extensive experience in the United States with warfarin, but dextran has been used on a much more limited basis in the U.S. than in Europe. If dextran is selected, a recommended dosage, based on the experience of Berqvist et al,[1] is 500 ml of dextran 70 during surgery, followed by 50 ml in the recovery room, and another 500 ml on the first and third post-operative days. Warfarin should be given orally in a dosage of 10 mg the night before surgery and daily thereafter. The same dose is repeated until the prothrombin time approximates one-and-one-half times to twice the control.

Patients with recent active bleeding probably should not be selected for elective revision of the hip joint. Surgery should be postponed until the risk of bleeding is no longer a reason for not using the standard drug prophylaxis. If it is not possible to postpone surgery, pneumatic calf compression may be considered as an alternative.[6,9] In an early comparison of pneumatic calf compression with warfarin, the two methods seemed approximately equally effective.[6] Since that report, a technical modification of pneumatic compression has been reported by Hull et al.[9] Patient acceptance of alternate compression of the legs during the long period of prophylaxis is quite good. Until there are reports that pneumatic calf compression is an effective prophylaxis after hip surgery, its use as an alternative to drug prophylaxis must be undertaken circumspectly. However, pneumatic compression seems better than no protection at all if coupled with prospective monitoring for venous thrombosis with IPG. We previously suggested that it may be possible to avoid the problem of bleeding if monitoring is substituted for drug prophylaxis under special circumstances.[14] When impedance plethysmography is combined with ^{125}I fibrinogen scanning, the presence and extent of vein thrombi can be monitored with reassuring accuracy in those patients who cannot be given aspirin.[14]

Investigators have found low-dose heparin to be ineffective in prophylactic anticoagulation of patients underoing total hip surgery.[3] Others have found that, at the dosage required to provide adequate protection, the rate and severity of hemorrhagic complications are unacceptable.[5,13,17] Heparin therefore does not appear to be a useful alternative to aspirin in routine prophylactic anticoagulation of the total hip patient.

Revision THR

Selection of Prophylaxis

---

1. Aspirin unless (a) GI intolerance to ASA
                    (b) Prior ASA failure
                    (c) Risk major bleeding
2. Warfarin (or dextran) for (a), (b).
3. For (c): Postpone THR, treat bleeding risk or monitor by ^{125}I-Fg & IPG, use pneumatic calf compression

Fig. 15-5.   Alternative selections for prophylaxis against thromboembolic complications.

POST-OPERATIVE MANAGEMENT

Post-operative complications may occur in spite of appropriately chosen prophylaxis; they should be anticipated. Noninvasive bedside testing is mandatory, if there are symptoms. It is difficult to obtain good plethysmographic tracings in post-operative patients during the first 5 to 6 days, encumbered as they are by balanced suspension and other devices, beset by incisional pain and limited in regard to positioning in bed by arthritic involvement of multiple joints. Early post-operatively, there may be multiple symptoms in muscle groups that have been roughly handled during strenuous manipulations under general anesthesia. Technical problems in obtaining a reliable plethysmographic test in these patients early post-operatively may surpass the ability of a well-trained technologist. Experience in frequent testing of the post-operative patient is required for the test to be reliable. There are alternate monitoring methods which should be available if the plethysmographic tests are not feasible. At the discretion of the vascular surgeon, alternative diagnostic measures which may be helpful include: Doppler vein examination; determination of fibrin degradation products in the blood; and ^{125}I fibrinogen uptake.[12]

It is helpful for the orthopedic surgeon to have some understanding of the causes of false-positives of any of these tests in the post-operative state. For instance, plethysmography requires the knee to be flexed between 10° and 25° to achieve the maximum venous outflow. After the leg can be removed from balanced suspension any plethysmographic test is easier to perform. The likelihood of venous thrombosis after hip replacement reaches a peak at about the same time that technical problems with IPG become simpler to resolve. For that reason, we believe that monitoring by plethysmographic techniques is of limited use early post-operatively, but should be done if symptoms arise, or after the fourth or fifth post-operative day. A pre-operative IPG for comparison is invaluable. Those patients who are abnormal pre-operatively should be monitored post-operatively by ^{125}I fibrinogen leg scan. One hundred μC of ^{125}I fibrinogen are given intravenously after confirming that SSKI had been administered pre-operatively.[14]

Hemorrhage, particularly wound hematoma, is a significant post-operative complication. This occurs in about 6 percent of patients, regardless of the prophylactic treatment. Wound hematoma occurs in about 7 percent of patients given aspirin; twice as often if warfarin is used. As noted, subcutaneous heparin given three times a day has been found to induce an unacceptably high occurrence of wound bleeding.[3,5,17] The wound should be examined daily and the bleeding time is checked if a large or painful hematoma develops. Consideration is then given to alternative prophylaxis. When it is necessary to discontinue aspirin or warfarin, two choices remain. If the noninvasive monitoring techniques indicate no evident active thrombosis, one can then consider substituting pneumatic calf compression. The calf compression option should not be undertaken if the monitoring suggests that venous thrombosis is present, because this would increase the risk of converting thrombosis to embolism. In such circumstances, interruption of the inferior vena cava with an umbrella filter is the only acceptable alternative.[16]

The other major vascular complication is venous thrombosis, with or without pulmonary embolism. We have demonstrated, using IPG and ^{125}I fibrinogen uptake scanning with selective phlebograms, that: (1) minor calf vein thrombi, demonstrated only as "hot spots" by the fibrinogen uptake test, often spontaneously resolve, even without treatment; (2) major venous thrombosis, demonstrated by a positive IPG, is uncommon during the first week; and (3) symptomatic embolism, proven by a lung scan, occurs somewhat later, around the end of the second post-operative week.[14] However, many patients have leg symptoms soon after major joint replacement. It is necessary to explain these symptoms if noninvasive monitoring techniques are normal. Manipulation of the limb during anesthesia provokes considerable muscle soreness away from the operative field; this is often associated with a positive "Homans sign," or tenderness in the calf muscles. A normal IPG is reassuring under such circumstances but, as previously noted, the IPG occasionally is technically uneatisfactory in the early post-operative period. A Doppler examination may reveal normal venous flow sounds at the location of the posterior tibial veins. Spontaneous and augmented flow sounds characteristic of a patent main venous outflow can be recognized by an observer who is experienced with the Doppler probe. This reassurance may permit one to defer phlebography, or to avoid it, if the IPG subsequently returns to normal. The phlebogram should be obtained if the noninvasive tests remain abnormal for 2 successive days. Fibrin degradation products are elevated during the first 10 to 14 days after hip surgery. The diagnostic value of these "split products" tests is limited when they may be most needed. However, if normal, the test can be interpreted as evidence against the diagnosis of extensive venous thrombosis.

Pulmonary embolism should immediately be suspected if pleuritic chest pain occurs post-operatively, particularly in the second week or later. Embolism rarely is the cause of chest symptoms during the first week. During this early period arterial pO2 is often below the normal range; this test adds little to the diagnosis of embolism after hip replacement. Ventilation-perfusion lung scans should be compared with the best obtainable chest x-ray if symptoms suggest pulmonary embolism. The finding of a pleural friction rub and tachypnea are confirmatory. Heparin can provisionally be started intravenously pending the result of the lung scan, after the bleeding time is determined. The risk of a wound hematoma is high for a patient receiving aspirin if the bleeding time is already prolonged. Clinical diagnosis should be substituted for lung scanning; the complications of anticoagulant management of pulmonary embolism are complex. Too often heparin can result in hemorrhage; it should be used only for positive indications and not merely for clinical suspicion. A more detailed discussion of the diagnosis and treatment of pulmonary embolism has been presented by Hume, Sevitt, and Thomas.[10]

ANTICOAGULANT THERAPY

Heparin is to be administered intravenously by pump at an hourly unit dose related to body size, age, and sex. Elderly women are more susceptible to bleeding complications.[21] The following factors are also considered in determining the primary dose of heparin, given as a bolus: (1) What is the likelihood of bleeding on heparin? To answer this the bleeding time must be determined, particularly if the patient has been receiving aspirin. We found that only 8 of 23 subjects given aspirin had a prolonged bleeding time 1 week post-operatively. (2) Is there a hematoma present in the wound and, if so, how extensive is it? (3) How extensive is the thrombosis revealed by phlebography, or how extensive is the embolism based on the perfusion defects present on the lung scan? In general, a loading dose is used for extensive involvement or severe symptoms. If thrombosis is asymptomatic, having been detected only by monitoring, it is not necessary to give any loading dose. Pulmonary embolism should generally be treated by larger doses of heparin than thrombosis in the leg. A loading dose, if there has been an embolism, should equal at least 100 units/kg of body weight.

The duration of anticoagulant therapy for demonstrated venous thrombosis should be approximately 12 to 14 weeks. The treatment of pulmonary embolism should extend for a similar period of time, although some recommend a period of up to 6 months. Heparin should be given for at least 1 week; warfarin is added after a stable hourly dosage of heparin has been established. A continuous-infusion pump is used. Fewer hemorrhagic complications of heparin have been encountered with this technique than with the previous routine of bolus injections of heparin every 4 hours.[18] Laboratory control of heparin therapy is simplified by continuous perfusion because it is not necessary to maintain a precise time interval between the last dose of heparin and the collection of blood for partial thromboplastin time (PTT). However, mistakes in interpreting the effects of heparin can be made if blood is collected for PTT too soon after a change is made in the hourly infusion dose of heparin. We therefore prefer to collect routine PTTs each morning and to make no adjustments in heparin dosage after midnight. The desired range for laboratory control is 50 to 80 seconds, as determined by the activated PTT. When a response in this range has been achieved, heparin is continued at constant dosage while warfarin, 10 mg daily, is orally administered. Heparin is discontinued when the prothrombin time is between one-and-one-half and two times the control value. Thereafter, daily dosage of warfarin is adjusted according to the prothrombin time. Figure 15-6 is a schematic representation of the phased transition from heparin to warfarin during anticoagulation therapy. Arrangements are made for laboratory control after the patient is discharged from the hospital.

Physical therapy appropriate to the stage of post-operative rehabilitation may not need to be interrupted because of venous thrombosis. Leg symptoms which are due to venous thrombosis, if made worse by out-of-bed activity, require such activities to be postponed. Similarly, for pulmonary embolism, the accompanying pleuritic pain may limit movement in bed or ambulatory exercises; until the pain subsides, physical therapy is curtailed. Although there is a tendency to fear that a thrombus may dislodge and thus become an embolus, such an accident is extraordinarily uncommon after full heparin therapy is established.

Rehabilitation following venous thrombosis depends on the establishment of venous collaterals, for the main venous drainage is obstructed by the presence of thrombi. The Trendelenburg bed position is extremely important in the acute phase of management, and is continued for as many months thereafter as swelling persists. The patient is advised that the position actually accelerates the recovery from thrombosis. At meal times the head of the bed may be elevated. At all other times it should be down and the shoulders should rest on the mattress. Extra pillows are allowed under the head for reading or television viewing. A 4-inch ace bandage is wrapped from the base of the toes to the level of the knee and rewrapped every 8 hours, or more often if it becomes loose. As soon as the edema is under control, a knee-length pressure-gradient stocking should be fitted. The patient is required to wear this stocking for as long as any edema can be demonstrated.

Besides the physical measures described above, the symptomatic treatment of venous thrombosis is relatively simple. Pain is not usually severe if the physical

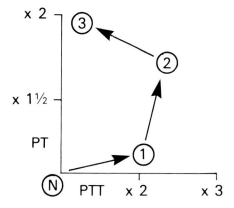

PHASE	DOSE	DRUG	LAB CONTROL
1.	Heparin I.V.	1000 + u./hr*	PTT Q. a.m.
2.	Warfarin p.o. & Heparin I.V.	10 mg/day steady dose	Daily PT, PTT
3.	Warfarin p.o.	5 + mg/day*	Daily PT

* Dosage adjusted per lab test to desired therapeutic range.

Fig. 15-6. A schematic representation of the phased transition from heparin to warfarin during anticoagulation therapy.

measures are duly applied. Moist heat makes the leg comfortable. Analgesics should not contain aspirin. After the patient is on the anticoagulant treatment, anti-inflammatory drugs add very little further symptomatic relief. Because they may interfere with platelet function, the use of anti-inflammatory medications is discouraged.

The follow-up management of venous thrombosis requires understanding and commitment by the patient, and cooperation with the referring physician. Orientation begins several days before the patient leaves the hospital. (We supply an informational booklet, prepared with the assistance of the nursing service.[8]) The nurse reviews with the patient various measures, such as elevation of the bed at home on cement blocks, the use of elastic compression to control edema, regulation of anticoagulants, and other home instructions.

HEMORRHAGIC COMPLICATIONS OF ANTICOAGULANT THERAPY

Major hemorrhagic complications of anticoagulant therapy undertaken for proven venous thrombosis or embolism must be seriously considered in the post-operative period following revision hip surgery. Because it may be necessary to interrupt the inferior vena cava, one must require firm proof of thrombosis and/or embolism and the presence of a serious hematoma. The phlebogram should be reviewed to determine that all the evidence for venous thrombosis is accounted for by recent, acute venous thrombosis. It is possible that the phlebogram may show a small amount of fresh thrombus and extensive abnormality due to an old thrombus, present for perhaps many months. The utility of a baseline IPG and a carefully done history becomes obvious when such decisions have to be made. Similarly, the lung scan must be examined to determine the extent of the perfusion defects. If more than a few days elapse after these determinations are made, it may be appropriate to repeat the lung scan in order to discover if there has been some resolution or new emboli. By such comparison, and by other means, it may be possible to exclude nonembolic causes for the perfusion defects. A painful expanding hematoma will require termination of anticoagulant therapy. A normal IPG may result if anticoagulants were given because of embolism. Under such circumstances, it seems appropriate to substitute pneumatic calf compression for the anticoagulant prophylaxis. Such treatment has, in some cases, obviated the need for interruption of the vena cava. However, if one of these options is available, caval interruption should be expeditiously carried out. This operation is done under local anesthesia with fluoroscopic control in the radiology department and has presented few technical difficulties. The umbrella filter, placed permanently, serves well as protection against major embolism.[16]

SUMMARY

A rational plan has been outlined for the protection of post-operative revision hip arthroplasty patients from thromboembolic complications following major hip surgery. If prophylaxis fails, the orthopedic surgeon and the vascular surgical consultant must be prepared to swiftly and logically move to limit the extent and severity of venous thrombosis. Pulmonary embolism is a dreaded and potentially fatal complication. All of our preventive and therapeutic programs are directed towards reducing the chance of a major pulmonary embolism. If medical measures fail, or if systemic treatment is complicated by major hematoma formation, implantation of a vena cava umbrella filter should be seriously considered.

REFERENCES

1. Bergqvist D, Efsing HO, Hallbook T, et al: Thromboembolism after elective and post-traumatic hip surgery—A controlled prophylactic trial with dextran 70 and low-dose heparin. *Acta Chir Scand* 145:213–218, 1979.
2. DeLee JC, Rockwood CA: Current concepts review: The use of aspirin in thromboembolic disease. *J Bone and Joint Surg* 62(A):149–152, 1980.
3. Evarts CM, Alfidi RJ: Thromboembolism after total hip reconstruction: Failure of low doses of heparin in prevention. *JAMA* 515–516, 1973
4. Gitel SN, Salvati EA, Wessler S, et al: The effect of total hip replacement and general surgery on anti-thrombin III in relation to venous thrombosis. *J Bone and Joint Surg* 61(A):653–656, 1979.
5. Harris WH, Salzman EW, Athanasoulis C, et al: Comparison of warfarin, low-molecular-weight dextran, aspirin, and subcutaneous heparin in prevention of venous thromboembolism following total hip replacement. *J Bone and Joint Surg* 56(A):1552–1562, 1974.

6. Harris WH, Raines JK, Athanasoulis C, et al: External pneumatic compression versus warfarin in reducing thrombosis in high-risk hip patients, in Madden JL, Hume M (eds): *Venous Thromboembolism—Prevention and Treatment.* New York, Appleton Century Crofts, 1976, pp 51–60.

7. Harris WH, Salzman EW, Athanasoulis CA, et al: Aspirin prophylaxis of venous thromboembolism after total hip replacement. *N Engl J Med* 297:1246–1248, 1977.

8. Hume M: *Your Veins.* Privately printed, 1979.

9. Hull R, Delmore TJ, Hirsh J, et al: Effectiveness of intermittent pulsatile elastic stockings for the prevention of calf and thigh vein thrombosis in patients undergoing elective knee surgery. *Thrombosis Res.* 16:37–45, 1979.

10. Hume M, Sevitt S, Thomas DP: *Venous Thrombosis and Pulmonary Embolism.* Cambridge, Mass, Harvard University Press, 1970.

11. Hume M, Donaldson WR, Surprenant J: Sex, aspirin, and venous thrombosis. *Ortho Clin North Amer* 9:761–767, 1978.

12. Hume M, Kuriakose TX, Jamieson J, et al: Extent of leg vein thrombosis determined by impedance and ^{125}I fibrinogen. *Am J Surg* 129:455–458, 1975.

13. Hume M, Kuriakose TX, Zuch L, et al: ^{125}I fibrinogen and the prevention of venous thrombosis. *Arch Surg* 107:803–806, 1973.

14. Hume M, Turner RH, Kuriakose Tx, et al: Venous thrombosis after total hip replacement. *J Bone and Joint Surg* 38(A):933–939, 1976.

15. Jennings JJ, Harris WH, Sarmiento A: A clinical evluation of aspirin prophylaxis of thromboembolic disease after total hip arthroplasty. *J Bone and Joint Surg* 58(A):926–928, 1976.

16. Mobin-Uddin K, Callard GM, Bolooki H, et al: Transvenous caval interruption with umbrella filter. *N Engl J Med* 286:55–58, 1972.

17. Moskovitz PA, Ellenberg SS, Feffer HL, et al: Low-dose heparin for prevention of venous thromboembolism in total hip arthroplasty and surgical repair of hip fractures. *J Bone and Joint Surg* 60(A):1065–1069, 1978.

18. Salzman EW, Deykin D, Shapiro RM, et al: Management of heparin therapy. Controlled prospective trial. *N Engl J Med* 292:1046–1050, 1975.

19. Salzman EW, Harris WH, DeSanctis RW: Reduction in venous thromboembolism by agents affecting platelet function. *N Engl J Med* 284:1287–1292, 1971.

20. Stamatakis JD, Kakkar VV, Sagar S, et al: Femoral vein thrombosis and total hip replacement. *Brit Med J* 2:223–225, 1977.

21. Walter AM, Jick H: Predictors of bleeding during heparin therapy. *JAMA* 244:1209, 1980.

Kenneth Moller, Henry M. Steady,
Klaus W. Korten, and Roderick H. Turner

16

Blood Conservation in Revision Arthroplasty

Difficult orthopedic surgery often results in significant blood loss. In procedures such as scoliosis fusion and revision hip surgery, involving extensive soft-tissue dissection and large cancellous bone surfaces, the estimated blood loss will commonly range from 1,000 to 3,000 ml,[32] sometimes as high as 5,000 ml. Such prodigious bleeding taxes not only the patient, as pointed out by Pasteyer et al, who documented electrolyte, coagulation, cardiodynamic, thermoregulatory, and pulmonary problems in such patients, but also puts great demands on the blood bank.[30] Further, there are significant risks incurred with transfusion of homologous blood products. We will explore four options available for conserving a patient's own blood: pre-operative autologous blood banking; acute pre-operative hemodilution; induced hypotensive anesthesia and epidural analgesia; and intra-operative red-cell salvage and autologous transfusion.

BLOOD BANKING: RISKS AND COSTS

In the United States alone, nearly 11.8 million units of blood are transfused each year.[26] Supplementation of the volunteer donations with paid donors or imported blood is required to meet increasing demand. The risks of using homologous blood include isosensitization; hemolytic reactions; transmission of malaria,

343

syphilis, or bacterial contaminants; mismatch due to clerical error; and post-transfusion serum hepatitis.[24] The risk of hepatitis has been 20 to 46 percent with paid donors; 8 to 13 percent with volunteer donors. These cases are difficult to detect without routine post-transfusion liver function studies and antigen screening, since only 25 to 35 percent of the patients become clinically icteric.[7] Myhre has pointed out that fatalities related to transmission do occur;[26] 113 deaths were reported to the Food and Drug Administration from April 1976 to January 1980. Forty-one percent of these were related to clerical error, another 29 percent due to hepatitis, 7 percent due to laboratory errors, and 23 percent related to miscellaneous causes.

The processing and crossmatching costs of a unit of homologous blood are high, currently amounting to about $100 at New England Baptist Hospital in Boston. Six to eight units may typically be required in the operative period. Blood which has been stored frozen has a 3-year shelf life and costs approximately twice as much as liquid-stored blood. Certainly not all the shortages, risks, and costs apparent in homologous transfusions can be avoided with autologous blood, but they can be significantly reduced.

PREOPERATIVE AUTOLOGOUS BLOOD BANKING

Autologous transfusion on an elective basis was reported in 1921 by Grant,[11] and gained popularity after a report by Milles.[25] The success of autologous transfusion in orthopedic patients was demonstrated in 1968 by Turner,[35] while Cowell and Swichard, in 1974, published an account of a series of pediatric orthopedic patients in which this method of blood conservation was effectively used.[4]

Better understanding of the hemodynamics of phlebotomy for blood banking began in 1941, when Ebert showed that the plasma volume would increase over 72 hours to compensate for lost red blood cells.[6] Finch proved in 1950 that after blood donation the limiting factor in effective hematopoiesis was the body's iron stores.[8] Later, McCurdy showed that iron could be supplied as effectively by mouth as parenterally, and more safely.[23] Hamstra and Block pointed out in 1969 that phlebotomy itself could stimulate erythropoiesis.[12]

Three separate series involving patients undergoing total hip arthroplasty with preoperative blood banking have been published (see Table 16-1). Mallory in 1976,[21] Marmor in 1977,[22] and Eckardt in 1978,[7] using slightly different protocols, had similar results. The guidelines for donations were that, prior to any single phlebotomy, patients be in good general health, weigh over 100 pounds, and have hematocrits greater than 38 percent in Mallory's series and greater than 34 percent in Mallory's and Eckardt's series. Mallory and Marmor used only liquid-stored blood, while Eckardt used both liquid and frozen storage. Liquid blood was citrated and stored at 4°C, while frozen blood was kept at −87°C with glycerol as a cryoprotective agent. In Mallory's group, 60 percent of transfusion requirements (average four units/patient) were supplied by autologous blood. In Eckardt's study, 49 percent of the patients required no homologous blood, while 22 percent required only one additional homologous unit. In Marmor's patients, 62 percent received their own blood only; he used no pre-operative antibiotics, pointing out, as had the

Table 16-1

Published Reports of Total Hip Arthroplasty with Pre-Operative
Autologous Blood Banking

Author	Total no. of cases	Average no. of units donated	Donation intervals	Average admission hematocrit	Average post-op hematocrit
Mallory (1976)	50	2.5	7 days	38	32*
Marmor (1977)	61	2.7	5 days	35	28†
Eckardt (1978)	50	2.7	3–4 days	35	—§

* 60% of transfused units were autologous blood.

† 62% of patients received *no* homologous blood.

§ 49% of patients received *no* homologous blood; post-operative hematocrits not reported.

others, that lower average pre-operative hematocrits do not increase the incidence of sepsis nor adversely affect the rate of wound healing.

Pre-operative autologous blood banking has been shown to be safe for the patient undergoing elective orthopedic surgery. With supplemental iron the patient/donor hematocrit may be as low as 34 percent, and there are virtually no contraindications to such blood donation. The logistics and cost of an autologous predeposit blood bank program may limit this technique to larger centers, and clerical mishaps are still possible. However, the need for added anesthesia expertise and the high equipment costs of some of the other methods are avoided.

ACUTE ISOVOLEMIC HEMODILUTION

Acute isovolemic hemodilution has been recognized as a safe method of conserving whole blood. It developed as an outgrowth of techniques devised to facilitate surgery involving large blood losses with Jehovah's Witness patients.[36,37] These patients will usually accept acute isovolemic hemodilution as long as the blood is not entirely separated from their circulation.

The ideal patient for acute hemodilution is in good general health with a hematocrit greater than 40 percent. Immediately preceding the incision and the shedding of blood, up to 50 percent of the patient's red cell mass can be safely removed, as long as the circulating blood volume is kept constant. While blood is sequestered via a large-bore peripheral arterial cannula and stored in a citrate-phosphate-dextrose bag, isovolemia is maintained by simultaneously infusing plasma protein solution (except in Jehovah's Witness patients), plasma expanders, or balanced salt solutions in a ratio of three volumes of crystalloid solution (or one volume of crystalloid and one volume of colloid solution) to one volume of blood removed. The patient's hematocrit is decreased, thereby reducing the intra-operative red cell loss. After reinfusion of the sequestered blood during the later stages of the operation, the hematocrit usually rises to about 28 percent, at the time of surgical closure.[31] Laks has shown the feasibility of acute isovolemic hemodilution in total hip surgery.[14,15] This work proved that the body can compensate for the decreased oxygen-carrying capacity of low hematocrit blood, when insovolemia is maintained, by increasing cardiac output. For each patient in this series, the arteriovenous oxygen difference, 2,3-diphosphoglycerate level, lactate:pyruvate ratio, and skeletal muscle surface pH all remained essentially unchanged. With a mean volume of 1,618 ml of blood removed, only 1.5 units of homologous blood were required on average in the intra-operative and post-operative periods. Mean hematocrits obtained were 42 percent preoperatively, 22 percent post-operatively, and, finally, 33 percent at the time of discharge.[16]

Isovolemic hemodilution is safe and can be useful when surgical blood loss greater than 500 ml is anticipated. An experienced anesthesia team is essential to the careful monitoring and control of this technique. A urinary catheter and arterial monitoring cannula are required, but the equipment costs are relatively low. This procedure is probably contraindicated in patients with congestive heart failure, or generalized artherosclerotic cardiovascular disease, due to the large dynamic fluid shifts.

INDUCED HYPOTENSIVE ANESTHESIA AND EPIDURAL ANALGESIA

While not "true" forms of autotransfusion, induced hypotensive anesthesia and epidural analgesia can be regarded as intracorporeal methods of sequestering part of a patient's blood volume and returning it to the circulation at a later time. Induced hypotension during surgery was first reported by Gardner in 1946,[10] using simple arteriotomy and reinfusion, while in the 1950s, high-spinal, epidural analgesia, and ganglion-blocking agents were used; Linacre in 1962 reported 1,000 cases of hypotensive anesthesia successfully used in major gynecologic surgery.[18] Complications of cerebral thrombosis and anoxia have been reported by Little.[19] In a review of several papers covering 13,264 operative procedures, there were 113 deaths;[16] however, Bodman pointed out that these deaths were due to technical errors and were not inherent to hypotensive anesthesia as a method.[3]

Epidural analgesia, first advocated in 1948, has been reported for total hip surgery in the anesthesia literature. Keith divided 27 patients scheduled for total hip replacement into three groups, epidural analgesia in the first, halothane anesthesia in the second, and a modified neuroleptic anesthetic in the third, and used a colorimetric technique to measure blood loss.[13] The mean blood loss for the three groups was 340 ml, 648 ml, and 744 ml respectively, with no significant differences in the post-operative period. Though the number of patients in each group was small, the results were encouraging, and 60 percent of those under epidural analgesia required no blood transfusion. Deliberate hypotension was not employed. Sculco has reported on 224 total hip arthroplasties comparing spinal anesthesthesia and general anesthesia in a carefully controlled study.[32] The average blood loss was reduced by 600 ml with spinal anesthesia; post-operative complications were also less in this group.

Amaranath examined 167 cases to ascertain the variables responsible for differences in blood loss.[1] Revision surgery, neoplasms, and bilaterality had increased losses, but the strongest correlation was with blood pressure. In a prospective study of 58 of these patients, through lowering the systolic pressure by 20 to 30 percent of the pre-operative level (using trimethopan or nitroprusside), the blood loss, operative time, and hypotensive and hypoxic response to the acrylic decreased. The amount of blood transfusion required was also reduced by 2 to 3 units, compared with patients whose systolic pressure was not lowered.

Hypotensive anesthesia was advocated by Charnley for use in orthopedic surgery, and there is now a wealth of experience with this technique (see Table 16-2). It has been shown to decrease blood loss and operative time, as well as to facilitate surgery. Improved cement techniques result from a drier operative field. Hypotensive anesthesia, however, should not be used in patients with coronary artery disease, general arteriosclerosis, or renal disease. Patients on antihypertensive medications that depress catecholamines should also be excluded, as well as those with severe chronic obstructive pulmonary disease,[5] liver disease, or compensatory hypertension.[27]

Mallory reported a 25 percent decrease in operating time, 55 percent decrease in expected blood loss (40 percent decrease in revision hip arthroplasty), and 50 percent decrease in post-operative transfusion requirements.[20] In a study by Davis,[5] using halothane and pentolinium as anesthetic agents in 253 patients undergoing total hip replacement, there were no complications with respect to renal, coronary, or cerebral circulation. The mean blood replacement was reduced from 2,965 ml in revision arthroplasty to 1,730 ml (a 41 percent reduction); and from 2,250 ml in primary arthroplasty to 1,150 ml (a 51 percent decrease), with systolic blood pressure kept at 60 to 75 mm Hg. Thompson, in a smaller series (30 total hip arthroplasties (21 hypotensive and 9 normotensive controls)), showed a decrease in the average estimated intra-operative blood loss, from 1,183 ml in the normotensive group to 406 ml with halothane-induced hypotension, and to 326 ml with nitro-prusside-induced hypotension.[33] Using more extensive and detailed testing (including psychological batteries, neurological examinations, serial electrocardiograms, and multiple clinical laboratory tests), Thompson found no evidence of cerebral, hepatic, renal, or myocardial toxicity.[33] All patients in this series showed no increase in post-operative hemorrhage.

Table 16-2
Published Reports of Total Hip Arthroplasty Performed Under Hypotensive Anesthesia

Author	Total no. of cases		Anesthetic agent	Intra-op Ebl*	Operative time*	Total transfusion*
Mallory (1975)	40		Pentolinium	55%	25%	—
Davis (1974)	253		Pentolinium	—	—	51%
Thompson (1978)	30	(9)	Halothane	65%	25%	62%
		(12)	Nitroprusside	72%	45%	82%
Nelson (1980)	119		Nitroprusside	39%	32%	100%

*Given as % decrease from normotensive controls

Nelson, in a study of 119 patients (37 of whom had undergone prior hip surgery), performed total hip arthroplasty under hypotensive conditions using general anesthesia with halothane and nitroprusside.[27] The mean arterial pressure was approximately 65 mm Hg, a decrease of 35 percent from a matched group of controls. The response was so consistent that a dosage nomogram was developed for the use of the nitroprusside.[17] In this group of patients, utilizing meticulous hemostasis and an Ace spica, as well as the hypotensive anesthesia, he was able to perform surgery without any transfusions. Operating time was decreased approximately 30 percent, estimated operative blood loss was decreased approximately 40 percent, and average hemoglobin at the time of discharge was 10.5 g/dl versus 12.2 g/dl in the control group. Two complications were encountered: acute tubular necrosis and excessive post-operative bleeding; both of these responded to appropriate management.

It appears that hypotensive anesthesia, and epidural or spinal analgesia, can be effective in reducing blood-bank requirements as well as facilitating surgery. A skilled anesthesia team and careful monitoring are required. However, with proper patient selection and control, these techniques are safe and can be used without increased complications.

INTRA-OPERATIVE AUTOLOGOUS TRANSFUSION

Intra-operative salvage of blood with subsequent reinfusion was first reported in 1818 by Blundell who used it in 10 cases of post partum hemorrhage.[2] As currently used, the technique involves suctioning blood with accompanying irrigating fluid and debris from the surgical wound into a double-lumen tube, through which anticoagulant is delivered close to the suction tip.[34] The suction pressure is maintained at less than -100 mm Hg to minimize damage to the salvaged red blood cells, even though this can result in slightly slower clearing of blood and irrigation fluid from the operative field. The sanguineous aspirate is passed into a reservoir with a 170 micron screen which serves as a coarse filter to remove fat, soft tissue, bone, and any surgical debris resulting from use of power instruments, such as tiny fragments of metal or plastic. Using a roller pump, the filtrate is transferred to a centrifuge bowl where it is washed with 1 liter of 0.9 percent sodium chloride solution (approximately seven times the volume of the red cells present). Plasma, with activated clotting factors, heparin, red cell stroma, free hemoglobin, and myoglobin, are removed by dilution and flotation. The supernatant wash solution is removed to a waste collection bag and the salvaged, washed red cells, suspended in saline are pumped into a reinfusion bag and returned to the patient through a 40-micron in-line microaggregate filter.

Use of the Cell Saver®

The foregoing account describes the workings of the Haemonetics Cell Saver® (see Fig. 16-1). The anticoagulant can be either heparinized saline (40,000–60,000 units of heparin/liter of 0.9 percent sodium chloride) or standard acid citrate dextrose (ACD) used in blood banking. The IBM Blood Cell Processor can also be effective in providing washed salvaged red blood cells intra-operatively, though

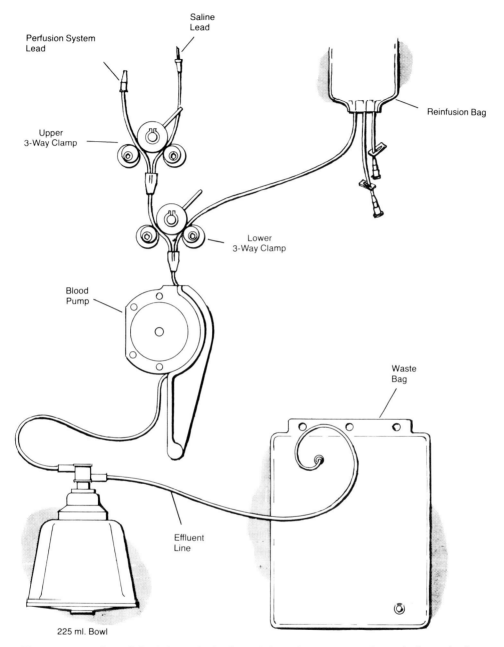

Fig. 16-1. Outline of the fluid paths in the Cell Saver® system (not shown is the aspiration-anticoagulation assembly).

there is less continuity in the processing. Basic research with the Cell Saver® by Orr has shown that during processing there is essentially no significant damage to blood components.[29] Use of this kind of system is best indicated for intra-operative autologous transfusion when the expected blood loss is greater than 1500 ml, in order to be cost-effective when compared with the costs of homologous transfusions.

Reinfusion and washed, salvaged autologous red blood cells suspended in saline carries no risk of hepatitis or transfusion reaction. It seems acceptable to Jehovah's Witness patients. This method of blood conservation should not be used in cases of gross bacterial contamination or malignancy involving the operative site. Red-cell salvage shares with the other methods of autologous transfusion previously discussed obvious advantages for patients who have multiple antibodies or previous unexplained reactions to homologous blood transfusions. It is unique among the methods of blood conservation considered in that it can also be used in the immediate post-operative period simply by connecting the suction tubing to the sterile wound drainage tube.

Flynn and Metzger of Orlando, Florida, have reported a 2-year experience with 99 cases, mostly spinal fusions, using the Haemonetics Cell Saver® (see Fig. 16-2). Their salvage of blood shed from the surgical wound averaged 54 percent; this was obtained by computations of red cell mass based on the patient's preoperative hematocrit and an assigned hematocrit of 60 percent for the Cell Saver units. Turner and Steady, also using the Haemonetics Cell Saver®, at New England Baptist Hospital, over a 2½-year period compiled 328 cases, (217 were included in an earlier report).[9] Ninety percent of these were total hip arthroplasties, of which two-thirds were cases of revision total hip replacement. The Baptist Hospital Cell Saver experience is considered in three periods. In Period A (the first 18 months) with 106 patients, the results were analyzed in a manner similar to the Florida cases, and yielded a red cell salvage of 53 percent. During Period B (the next 6 months), there were 111 cases. Of these, a select group of 61 patients was reviewed, because hematocrit data on the individual Cell Saver units recovered were also available. The more accurate calculations from this group showed a mean salvage rate of 61 percent for blood shed and returned to the patient. In some cases where particular attention was paid to diligent use of suction, keeping the tissue moist, and minimizing the use of sponges and wound towels, the salvage rate was close to 90 percent. The Cell Saver® was also taken to the recovery room in a few cases, when significant blood loss continued post-operatively.

No patient complications referable to the Cell Saver® system were encountered during the Baptist Hospital study. However, Flynn had two cases of excessive bleeding after the initial 2-year study; both were controlled by transfusing fresh frozen plasma.[9] Currently, based on studies by Orr, Flynn recommends transfusing 1 unit of fresh frozen plasma for every 4 or 5 units of red cells salvaged, and 8 to 10 units of platelet concentrate after 10 units of red cells salvaged.[9] Using such a regimen, excessive bleeding due to depletion of coagulation factors can be avoided. Some do not advocate this "rule-of-thumb" approach, but favor tailoring coagulation therapy to each patient's actual needs, based on determinations of the usual coagulation parameters.

From Period C (the next 6 months), 32 revision total hip arthroplasties were reviewed. In these, the proportion of red cells salvaged varied from 33 to 89 percent. The amount of red cells saved/case ranged from 2 to 11 units. Overall, 138 units were saved, an average of 4.3 units of autologous red blood cells/operation. Computing the red cell mass of the shed blood as a function of the patient's preoperative and intra-operative hematocrits, and the red cell mass of the individual 225-ml Cell Saver® units, an average of 578 ml of red blood cells were saved and reinfused, yielding a mean salvage rate of 61 percent. Homologous blood transfused ranged from 5 to 10 units, a mean of 3.6 units of banked blood/case. Without intra-operative salvage, the usual amount of banked blood crossmatched for revision hip arthroplasty was 6 to 10 units. Thus the use of banked blood is considerably reduced with the red-cell salvage system, which answers more than half of the intra-operative red-blood-cell requirement.

The Cell Saver technique provides an adjunct to autologous blood banking and an alternative to acute hemodilution and hypotensive anesthesia. It requires the attendance of a perfusionist or technician. Operators can be trained to assemble and operate the instrument in about a week and can, with experience, simultaneously attend one or two Cell Saver® Systems, if the surgeries are in adjacent rooms. To lessen the need for the constant attention of a skilled operator, there have been developments in the automation of red cell recovery systems. The Haemonetics Cell Saver® II is a semiautomated system, which provides a choice of a programmed processing cycle or complete manual operation. The shortcomings of that system were pointed out,[34] particularly the failure of the photoelectric sensor to distinguish between saline/plasma with a high concentration of free hemoglobin and intact erythrocytes in suspension. This and other minor problems of design have been overcome in the Haemonetics Cell Saver® III, billed by the manufacturer as an "automated autologous blood recovery system." This instrument provides automation for the standard Cell Saver functions outlined earlier.

The Cell Saver® III, after assembly, permits blood collection from the wound by the operating surgeon as usual; after a reasonable amount of blood and irrigation fluid has been collected—usually about 1 liter—the rest of the processing proceeds with minimal operator involvement. The volume of wash solution desired can also be programmed; and we have found that 1 liter of saline wash is best for our purposes, given the amount of debris generated in revision hip surgery. The

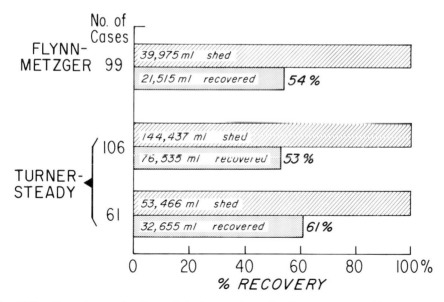

Fig. 16-2. Percentages of estimated shed operative red cell mass recovered by autotransfusion using Cell Saver®.

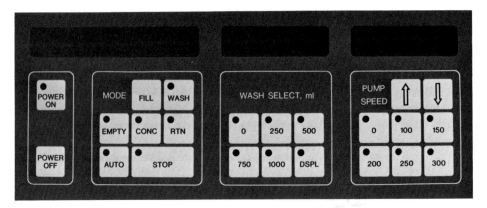

Fig. 16-3.   The touch-sensitive control panel of the Cell Saver® III.

automated processing cycle (fill, wash, and transfer to reinfusion pack) is initiated by pressing a single button on a control panel (see Fig. 16-3). Sensors detect when erythrocytes reach a predetermined level in the centrifuge bowl, or when air enters the system, at given points, and the next phase of the cycle is then automatically initiated. Thus the system detects when the saline wash is empty and displays "out of saline," reminding the operator to replace the empty bag. In this regard, it should be possible to use larger volumes of 0.9 percent sodium chloride than the 1-liter bags currently available as sterile injectable saline. However, this might require additional approval, since the 3-liter bags of sterile 0.9 percent sodium chloride solution are not yet FDA-approved for intravenous injection. However, as new technology allows larger volumes to be safely handled without increasing the risks of fluid overload to the patient, such approval will no doubt be forthcoming. Use of a 3-liter bag of sterile saline as the reservoir for wash solution will allow 3 to 4 units of salvaged red cells to be processed before the saline supply needs to be replenished.

Another significant advantage of the Cell Saver® III is the display panel which, at the touch of a button, indicates, in addition to the phase of the cycle in operation, the volume of sanguineous fluid processed, and the volume of red cells already salvaged. In revision hip arthroplasty with extensive soft-tissue dissection, breach of the nutrient artery of the femur, and almost-continuous irrigation for cleansing and cooling during the use of power instruments, the volumes of blood and other fluids processed are considerable. The cumulative recording of the volumes processed and salvaged facilitates computation of the blood shed and autologous red

Fig. 16-4.   Radiographs of a Jehovah's Witness patient before (top) and after (bottom) bilateral total hip replacement using intra-operative autologous blood transfusion. (AC, a 31-year-old Jehovah's Witness with bilateral congenital dysplastic hips underwent removal of hardware after an osteotomy in 1974. It was accompanied by a large blood loss; a planned reconstruction was therefore aborted. With the use of the Cell Saver® in 1980, both hips underwent reconstruction as shown, at separate procedures; estimated blood losses were 2,660 ml and 1,640 ml respectively, with respective salvage rates of 55% and 87%, and postoperative hematocrits of 34% and 19%, at their lowest. Hypotensive anesthesia was used with the first procedure.)

cells replaced, and thus should be a boon to anesthesiologists who strive to keep up with the patient's "estimated blood loss" and replacement transfusions.

The automatic functions can be varied to suit the operator or the prevailing conditions. They may even be set aside and the instrument manually operated, with the operator in full control. Whether automated or manual, an intra-operative red

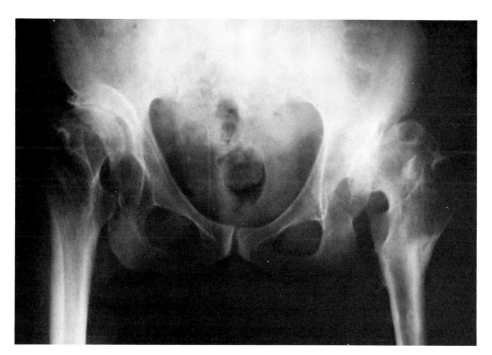

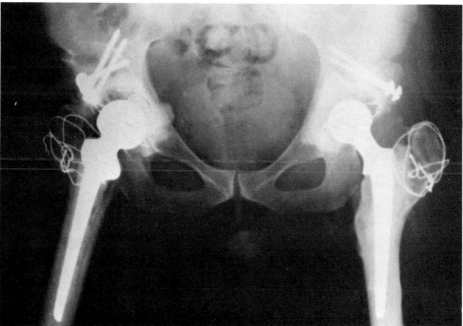

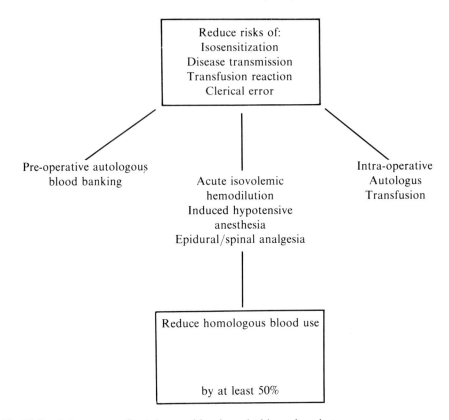

Fig.16-5.   Advantages of autologous blood use in hip arthroplasty.

cell salvage system can be used in those patients who, for general health reasons, do not meet the criteria for the other methods discussed.

COMBINED TECHNIQUES

Little has been written about combining the techniques described here. North, in a series of 20 patients undergoing total hip arthroplasty, combined intra-operative autotransfusion and nitroprusside-induced hypotensive anesthesia.[28] With a mean blood pressure of 64 mm Hg, blood loss was reduced to 460 ml, or one third of that expected. In addition, he achieved a 32 percent salvage of blood actually shed using a Bentley ATS-100® Autotransfuser. Therefore, approximately 77 percent of the expected net blood loss was avoided by the combination of these two techniques. It is hoped that further improvement on these results can be obtained by combining the techniques of pre-operative autologous blood banking, acute isovolemic hemodilution, induced hypotensive anesthesia or epidural/spinal analgesia, and intra-operative autotransfusion, and tailoring them to the specific needs of each patient, we should be able to reduce, by at least 50 percent, the amount of blood lost during major orthopedic surgery (see Fig. 16-5). Thus, both the demand for and the risks of replacement by banked homologous blood are decreased. A combination of these techniques is successfully employed during surgery on Jehovah's Witness patients who refuse transfusion of any banked blood or blood components. A combination of these techniques with a potential risk is the use of both isovolemic hemodilution and hypotensive anesthesia or epidural/spinal analgesia in the same patient. Such combinations have not been reported in a large series, though we have used them in a few of our patients.

SUMMARY

Difficult orthopedic surgery results in significant blood loss. In this chapter, we discuss ways to lessen the requirement for the over 11,000,000 units of homologous blood transfused each year in this country, thereby decreasing the risks involved, which include isosensitization, transmission of viral and bacterial disease, and mismatch due to clerical error. Pre-operative autologous blood banking has been shown in series involving total hip arthroplasty to afford some 50 to 60 percent of patients the possibility of not requiring any homologous blood in the operative period. Acute isovolemic hemodilution can be used to obtain 2 to 3 units of blood before the initial surgical incision, to be reinfused near the end of the operation, and in the immediate post-operative period. Induced hypotensive anesthesia during total hip arthroplasty can provide for a reduction in blood replacement requirements as well as a shorter operating time. Intra-operative autotransfusion using a device such as the Cell Saver® can salvage blood shed at the wound, and return to the patient slightly over 50 percent of the red cells (during scoliosis surgery), and approximately 60 percent to those patients undergoing arthroplasty of the hip. All of these techniques are currently used and have been proven safe in the series reported.

REFERENCES

1. Amaranath L, Cascorbi HF, Singh-Amaranath AV, et al: Relation of anesthesia to total hip replacement and control of operative blood loss. *Anesth Analg* 54:641–648, 1975.
2. Blundell J: Experiments on the transfusion of blood by the syringe. *Medico Chir Trans* 9:56–92, 1818.
3. Bodman RI: Controlled hypotension: Recent advances in anesthesia. *Int Anesthesiol Clin* 5.90–117, 1968.
4. Cowell HR, Swichard KW: Autotransfusion in children's orthopaedics. *J Bone and Joint Surg* 56(A):908–912, 1974.
5. Davis NJ, Jennings JJ, Harris WH: Induced hypotensive anesthesia for total hip replacement. *Clin Orthop* 101:93–98, 1979.
6. Ebert RV, Stead EA, Gibson JG: Response of normal subjects to acute blood loss. *Arch Intern Med* 68:578–590, 1941.
7. Eckardt JJ, Gossett TC, Amstutz HC: Autologous transfusion and total hip arthroplasty. *Clin Orthop* 132:39–45, 1978.
8. Finch S, Haskins D, Finch CA: Iron metabolism hematopoiesis following phlebotomy: Iron as a limiting factor. *J Clin Invest* 29:1078–1086, 1950.
9. Flynn JC, Metzger CR, Steady HM, et al: Intra-operative autotransfusion (IAT) in elective orthopaedic surgery. Presented at the American Academy of Orthopaedic Surgeons, Las Vegas, Nevada, 1981.

10. Gardner WJ: Control of bleeding during operation by induced hypotension. *JAMA* 132:572–574, 1946.

11. Grant FC: Autotransfusion. *Ann Surg* 74:253–254, 1921.

12. Hamstra RD, Block MH: Erythropoiesis in response to blood loss in man. *J Appl Physiol* 27:503-507, 1969.

13. Keith I: Anesthesia and blood loss in total hip replacement. *Anesthesia* 32:444–450, 1977.

14. Laks H, Handin RI, Martin J, et al: The effects of acute normovolemic hemodilution on coagulation and blood utilization in major surgery. *J Surg* 20:225–230, 1976.

15. Laks H, Pilon RN, Klovekorn WP, et al: Acute hemodilution: Its effect on hemodynamics and oxygen transport in anesthetized man. *Ann Surg* 180:103–109, 1974.

16. Larson AG: Deliberate hypotension. *Anesthesiol* 25:682–706, 1964.

17. Lawson NW, Thompson DS, Nelson CL, et al: A dosage nomogram for sodium nitroprusside-induced hypotension under anesthesia. *Anesth Analg* 55:574–580, 1976.

18. Linacre JL: Induced hypotension in gynecological surgery, a review of 1,000 major cases. *Br J Anaesth* 33:45–50, 1961.

19. Little DM: Induced hypotension during anesthesia and surgery. *Anesthesiol* 16:320–332, 1955.

20. Mallory TH: Hypotensive anesthesia in total hip replacement. *JAMA* 224:248, 1973.

21. Mallory TH, Kennedy M: The use of banked autologous blood in total hip replacement surgery. *Clin Orthop* 117:254–257, 1976.

22. Marmor L, Berkus D, Robertson JD, et al: Banked autologous blood in total hip replacement. *Surg Gynecol Obstet* 145:63, 1977.

23. McCurdy PR: Oral and parenteral iron therapy. *JAMA* 191:859–862, 1965.

24. McKittrick JE: Banked autologous blood in elective surgery. *Am J Surg* 128:137–141, 1974.

25. Milles G, Langston H, Dalessandro W: Experience with autotransfusions. *Surg Gynecol Obstet* 115:689–694, 1962.

26. Myhre BA: Fatalities from blood transfusion. *JAMA* 244:1333–1335, 1980.

27. Nelson CL, Martin K, Lawson NW, et al: Total hip replacement without transfusion. *Contemp Orthop* 2:655–658, 1980.

28. North ER, Nelson CL, Lawson NW: Prevention of blood loss in total hip replacement surgery by hypotensive anesthesia and intra-operative autotransfusion. *Surg Forum* 25:517–518, 1975.

29. Orr MD, Blenko JW: Autotransfusion of concentrated selected washed red cells from the surgical field: A biochemical and physiological comparison with homologous cell transfusion. Proceedings of the Blood Conservation Institute, 1978.

30. Pasteyer J, Jean N, Shebabou C: Massive hemorrhage during major orthopedic surgery. Metabolic consequences. *Rev Chir Orthop* 62:585–593, 1976.

31. Pilon RN, in Continuing Education Course on Fluid and Electrolyte Therapy. Lecture given at Harvard Medical School, 1978.

32. Sculco TP, Ranawat C: The use of spinal anesthesia for total hip replacement arthroplasty. *J Bone and Joint Surg* 57(A):173–177, 1975.

33. Thompson GE, Miller RD, Stevens WC, et al: Hypotensive anesthesia for total hip arthroplasty: A study of blood loss and organ function (brain, heart, liver, and kidney). *Anesthesiol* 48:91–96, 1978.

34. Turner RH, Steady HM: Cell washing in orthopedic surgery, in Hauer JM, Thurer RL, Dawson RB (eds): *Autotransfusion, Proceedings of the First International Autotransfusion Symposium.* New York, Elsevier/North Holland, 1981, pp 43–50.

35. Turner RS: Autologous blood for surgical autotransfusions. *J Bone and Joint Surg* 50(A):834, 1968.

36. AR _____: *Blood, Medicine, and the Law of God.* Watchtower Bible and Tract Society of New York Inc., International Bible Students Association, Brooklyn, 1961.
37. AR_____: *Jehovah's Witnesses and the Question of Blood.* Watchtower Bible and Tract Society of New York Inc., International Bible Students Association, Brooklyn, NY, 1977.

J. Drennan Lowell

17

Heterotopic Ossification in Revision Arthroplasty

Eighty thousand total hip arthroplasties are annually performed in the United States.[10] The end result of a significant number of these arthroplasties is adversely affected by the development of heterotopic ossification during the post-operative period. The exact mechanism that triggers this untoward event is unknown, but it is apparent that in affected patients, pluripotential mesenchymal cells lay down an osteoid matrix in which there is calcium deposition with ultimate ossification.[11]

In some patients heterotopic ossification is seen only as a few isolated islands of bone visible on post-operation radiographs but in no way compromising hip motion or the ultimate functional result. In others, large masses develop which ultimately coalesce and lead to complete joint ankylosis.

Over the years, a population at risk for heterotopic ossification has been identified. The largest group are males with either hypertrophic osteoarthritis or post-traumatic arthritis with a limited arc of motion (70° or less), and extensive osteophyte formation.[13,18] The risk is maximum in patients who have developed heterotopic ossification following surgery on one side, and present for surgery on the opposite. When revision hip surgery is performed on a hip already involved with ossification, recurrence is the rule rather than the exception. Another group of patients at high risk for heterotopic ossification in the convalescent period are those with ankylosing spondylitis, particularly if the disease is in an active phase at the time of operation.

The incidence of heterotopic ossification varies widely, from a low of 2 to 4 percent of patients following total hip arthroplasty, as reported by Reigler and Harris, to a high of 53 percent, as reported by Nollen and Slooff.[2,3,11,14,16,20]

Complete ankylosis following total hip arthroplasty reportedly occurs in 2 to 7 percent of patients.[2,11,14,16,20] The frequency of occurrence of this complication, as

359

REVISION TOTAL HIP ARTHROPLASTY
ISBN 0-8089-1466-9

it exists in the literature, deals almost exclusively with a random patient population as it presents for total hip arthroplasty in major clinics.

When high-risk patients are selected from the general population, for example, those males with osteoarthritis, the incidence of heterotopic ossification will rise to 65 percent, with the condition being severe in one third of these.[13] There is to date no sizeable series dealing with the limited issue of heterotopic ossification and its occurrence in patients undergoing revision surgery in whom heterotopic ossification was already present. It can be presumed to be at least as likely an occurrence as in any of the recognized high-risk groups.

GENERAL PREVENTIVE MEASURES

Several general preventive measures are currently considered useful in reducing the likelihood of heterotopic ossification, and are practiced by the great majority of reconstructive hip surgeons. These measures are as follows:

1. Use a lateral or a posterolateral surgical approach, rather than an anterior approach.
2. Minimize periosteal stripping if an anterior approach is indicated, or preferred for any reason.
3. Avoid detaching the greater trochanter in most cases of primary hip surgery, as discussed in Chapter 11.
4. Use gentleness in the handling of tissues.
5. Cauterize and/or bone wax raw bone surfaces.
6. Carefully institute hemostasis; meticulously debride any devitalized tissues.
7. Use pulsating jet irrigation to remove fragments of bone and other particulate debris.
8. Use soft-tissue compression with wound suction drainage for 24 to 48 hours, to reduce both dead space and the likelihood of hematoma formation.

Prophylactic cortisone administration during convalescence has not seemed to be useful. The usefulness of oral diazepam is debated, but the use of indomethacin during convalescence shows some promise.[17]

SPECIFIC MEASURES

There exist two therapeutic regimes with established effectiveness in reducing the incidence of heterotopic ossification in the patient convalescing from primary or revision total hip replacement arthroplasty. These are the oral administration of diaphosphonate (EHDP), and radiation therapy.[4-6,11] EHDP inhibits the growth of hydroxyapatite crystals in vitro, and thus may be responsible for the prevention of pathologic calcification and, ultimately, heterotopic ossification in vivo.[7-9,11] There is no evidence offered that EHDP inhibits the formation of osteoid matrix.[15]

Local radiation of the operated area during early convalescence appears to have the potential to prevent mesenchymal cells from laying down osteoid matrix, which ultimately would calcify and ossify.[4,11] It is a regime which must be approached with caution, particularly in younger patients, since the long-term effects of radiation are not known.

EHDP (DIPHOSPHENATE) STUDY

To more precisely determine the benefits of EHDP in the prevention of heterotopic ossification in a group of patients at risk for this complication, a multicenter double-blind study,* in which the Peter Bent Brigham Hospital participated, has recently been completed. It is with this investigation that the next portion of this chapter is concerned.

Materials and Methods

The study was a double-blind placebo-controlled study carried out in seven different orthopedic centers, with written informed consent obtained from all participants. The youngest patient was age 18; the oldest, 83. An attempt was made to select those in the highest risk group for this complication: patients with hypertrophic osteoarthritis with less than a 70° arc of flexion, patients wih rheumatoid arthritis or ankylosing spondylitis, or those who had developed heterotopic ossification following previous hip surgery (Tables 17-1 and 7-2).

All patients in the study were scheduled to undergo total hip arthroplasty. They were divided into two groups, based on the presence or absence of heterotopic ossification, established by radiographs of the hip to be replaced taken at the time of entry into the study (Table 17-3). By computer-generated random numbers, the

Table 17-1
Primary Diagnoses

Primary diagnosis	Number of patients
Osteoarthritis	104
Traumatic arthritis	29
Rheumatoid arthritis	19
Ankylosing spondylitis	12
Congenital hip dysplasia	11
Osteonecrosis	5
Legg-Calvé-Perthes disease	2
Osteomyelitis	1
Paget's disease	1
Paraplegia	1
Acetabular protrusion	1
Septic arthritis	1
Nonspecific diagnoses	4
TOTAL	191

*The material relating to the EHDP experience was developed as part of a multicenter study, funded and tabulated by the Procter and Gamble Company of Cincinnati, Ohio. The chief investigator was Gerald A. Finerman, M.D. Other participants were Jack W. Bowerman, M.D., Richard H. Gold, M.D., Walter F. Krengel, M.D., J. Drennan Lowell, M.D., William R. Murray, M.D., and Robert G. Volz, M.D.

Table 17-2
Reasons Patients Failed to Complete the Study

	Number of patients	
Reason	Placebo	EHDP
Death	1[a]	1[b]
Fractures	1[c]	1[d]
Side effects	2[e]	14[f]
Intercurrent illness	5	3
Patient request	2	3
Investigator decision	1	4
Lost to follow-up	3	0
Surgery cancelled	1	1
TOTAL	16	27

[a] Myocardial infarction—on placebo 7 weeks.
[b] Cardiopulmonary arrest—on EHDP 4 weeks.
[c] Fracture of femur and hip—on placebo 4 weeks.
[d] Supracondylar comminuted fracture, traumatic—on EHDP 8 weeks.
[e] One report each of diarrhea and flatulence, and headaches and dizziness.
[f] Thirteen reports of gastrointestinal complaints; one report of rash.

patients were assigned to receive either a placebo or EHDP. All investigators were "blind" as to the patient's treatment assignment. Patients received identically appearing tablets, either a placebo or 200 mg of EHDP/tablet. Placebo or 20 mg/kg/day of EHDP was administered for 4 weeks before hip surgery, and for 3 months afterwards. No corticosteroids, fluorides, estrogens, calcitronin, calcium supplements, or vitamin-D medications were administered during the study period. The patients were evaluated 4 weeks prior to surgery, at surgery, then at 2, 6, 12, and 18 weeks post-surgery, and at 6, 9, and 12 months post-surgery. Walking ability, hip pain and function, and range of motion ratings were made at all examinations (except, obviously, 2 weeks post-surgery).[1] Radiographs of the pelvis and affected hip were obtained prior to surgery and at 3, 6, and 12 months post-surgery in all patients, and at more frequent intervals, if medically indicated. Radiographic findings were assessed by each patient's operating surgeon and by two independent radiologists, blinded to the patient's assigned treatment as well as the sequence of the radiographs. The extent of heterotopic ossification on a scale of 0 to 5 (0 indicates no evidence of heterotopic ossification; 5 indicates severe bone formation with apparent ankylosis) were used.[5] The same radiographs were assessed by the radiologists who, in addition, traced the area of heterotopic ossification on the anterior-posterior projection. The result represented area rather than volume, but provided an approximation of the degree of heterotopic ossification.

For the radiologic assessment of heterotopic ossification, the data were based on the observations made 4 weeks prior to surgery, at 12 weeks post-surgery (which corresponded to the end of the EHDP or placebo treatment regime), and at 12 months post-surgery. If the 12-week visit was missed, the 6-week measurement was used, because there was a plateau in response profiles for both treatment groups from week 6 to week 12. If the 12-month visit was missed, then the previous visit was used for assessment, provided it corresponded to a period of at least 6 or 9 months post-surgery.

Table 17-3

Characteristics of Patients Evaluated for Efficacy

	Treatment	
	Placebo	EHDP
Characteristics	(n = 76)	(n = 72)
Sex		
Male	53	45
Female	23	27
Age (in years)		
Range	18–79	18–83
Mean	56	55
Pretreatment HO* Grade		
HO = 0	53	52
HO > 0	23	20

*HO = Heterotopic ossification.

Results

Both end-of-treatment and last-visit data were not available for all patients. End-of-treatment data were available for 74 of 76 placebo-treated patients and 68 of 72 EHDP-treated patients. Twelve-week data were available for 68 patients in each treatment group. Twelve-month data were used for the majority of patients. (The difference in the number of patients for whom end-of-treatment and last-visit data were available explain why, in Figures 17-1 through 17-5, and in Tables 17-4 and 17-5, the number of patients is not constant.)

In patients with no evidence of heterotopic ossification prior to treatment, the incidence of heterotopic ossification was found to be lower in EHDP-treated patients than in placebo-treated patients. At the end of treatment, heterotopic ossification was present in 17 percent of EHDP-treated patients and 37 percent of placebo-treated patients. At the last visit, heterotopic ossification was present in 40 percent of EHDP-treated patients and 54 percent of placebo-treated patients.

Table 17-4

Prevalence of Clinically Significant Heterotopic Ossification
(Grade ≥ 3)

		Evaluation At	
		End of treatment	Last visit
Treatment group	Grade	(No. reporting/no. eval.)	(No. reporting/no. eval.)
EHDP	3	0	1
	4	0	2
	5	0	1
		(0/48)*	(4/50)
Placebo	3	4	4
	4	3	3
	5	0	1
		(7/51)*	(8/48)

*Statistically significant difference favoring EHDP ($P < 0.05$).

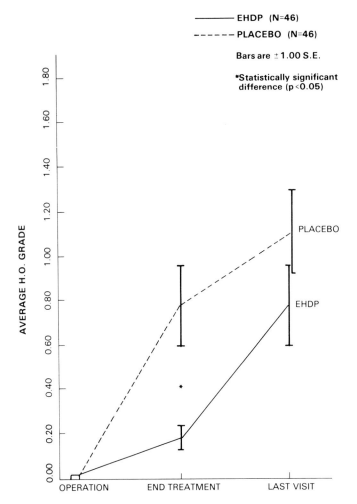

Fig. 17-1. Average heterotopic ossification (HO) grades among patients with zero pretreatment HO (operating surgeons' evaluations).

If the grade of heterotopic ossification was assessed, there was significantly more heterotopic bone in placebo-treated patients than patients treated with EHDP at the end of the treatment period. EHDP-treated patients continued to have a lower grade of heterotopic ossification than placebo-treated patients at the final visit (Fig. 17-1).

Looking at the area of heterotopic ossification revealed highly significant differences in measurement between the EHDP- and placebo-treated patients, both at the end of treatment and at the last visit (Fig. 17-2).

Clinically significant heterotopic ossification, defined as Grade 3 or greater, was 0 percent at the end of treatment in the EHDP-treated patients, and 14 percent in the placebo-treated patients. At the time of the last visit, it was 8 percent in the EHDP-treated patients and 17 percent in the placebo-treated patients (Table 17-4).

In summary, a review of all patients in whom no heterotopic ossification existed prior to surgery, with respect to incidence, grade, area, and clinically significant heterotopic ossification, showed that the amount of heterotopic ossification subsequently observed was less in the EHDP-treated patients than the placebo-treated patients, both at the end of treatment and at the last visit. Statistically different degrees ($P < 0.05$) were present at the end of treatment, with respect to incidence, grade, and area, and at the last visit, with respect to area.

In patients with osteoarthritis or traumatic arthritis without pre-existing heterotopic ossification, the placebo-treated patients again showed a greater incidence of heterotopic ossification than those given EHDP. At the end of treatment, it was 40 percent in the former and 18 percent in the latter. At the last visit, it was 67 percent in the former and 42 percent in the latter.

With respect to the average grade, there was a statistically significant difference

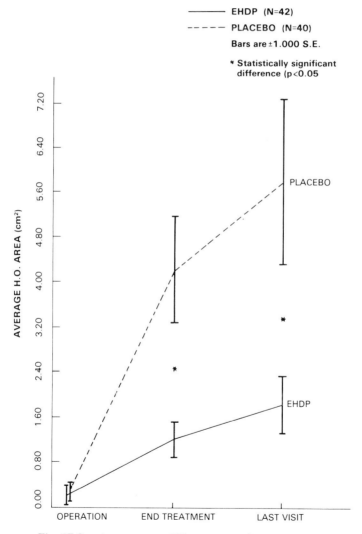

Fig. 17-2.   Average area HO among patients with zero pre-treatment HO (radiologists' evaluation).

both at the end of treatment and at the last visit ($P < 0.05$) (Fig. 17-3). The difference was even more striking when the average area was assessed. At the final visit, this was 4.8 times greater in the placebo-treated patients than in the EHDP-treated patients (Fig. 17-4). Clinically significant heterotopic ossification was found at final visit in 8 percent of EHDP-treated patients and in 24 percent of patients receiving the placebo.

In those patients exhibiting heterotopic ossification prior to treatment, the change in grade and area was assessed both at the end of treatment and at the time of the last visit. The difference was statistically significant ($P < 0.05$) at the end of treatment, but no longer statistically significant at the time of final visit, although an apparent benefit continued to be present (Fig. 17-5).

When the ultimate range of motion was assessed at the time of the final visit,

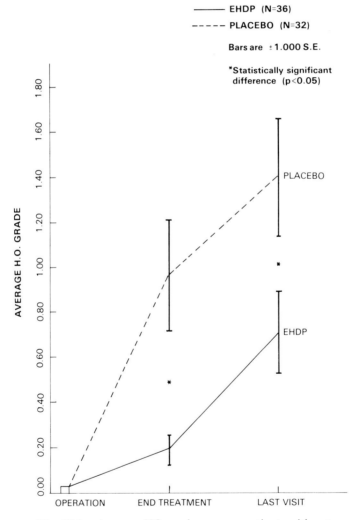

Fig. 17-3. Average HO grades among patients with osteo-arthritis or traumatic arthritis and zero pretreatment HO (operating surgeons' evaluations).

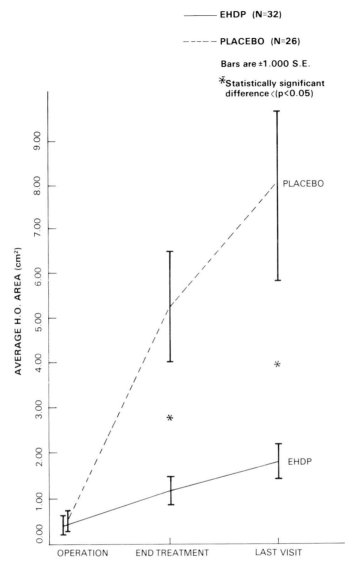

Fig. 17-4. Average area of HO among patients with osteoarthritis or traumatic arthritis and zero pretreatment HO
(radiologists' evaluation).

there was no statistical difference in the figures obtained between the two treatment
groups. However, there appeared to be a greater increase in the range of motion in
the EHDP-treated patients when pre-operative and last visit observations were
compared. In looking at one of the study sites, however, there appeared to be
satisfactorily better motion in those patients treated with EHDP than those who
received a placebo.

When the parameters of pain, walking ability, and activity rating were assessed,
the known beneficial effects of total hip arthroplasty were evident, but there was no
clear difference between the two treatment groups (Table 17-5).

The safety and tolerance of EHDP and the placebo were assessed throughout the trial. The side effects were similar, with the exception of gastrointestinal effects. Although nausea, vomiting, and upset stomach were seen with equal frequency in both treatment groups, the incidence of diarrhea and flatulence was clearly higher in the EHDP-treated patients (Table 17-6). It was necessary for 13 of 99 EHDP-treated patients to discontinue the study because of this complication. In 20 other patients exhibiting this complication, control was obtained by modifying the dosage schedule. The original schedule called for all of the medication to be taken an hour before breakfast; the modified schedule called for half the dose being taken an hour before breakfast and the other half an hour before the noon meal.

One patient in each group experienced a traumatic fracture (Table 17-2). The medication was discontinued in both patients at the time their fractures occurred; no undesirable side effects were evident.

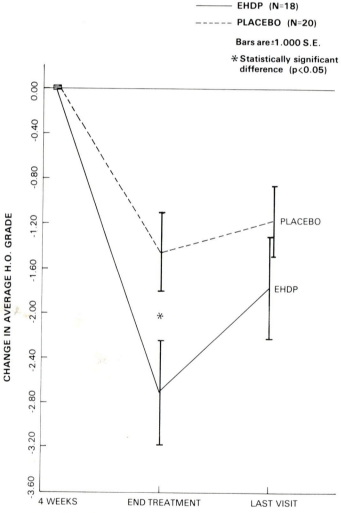

Fig. 17-5. Change in average HO grades among patients with evidence of HO pretreatment (operating surgeons' evaluations).

Table 17-5

Pain, Walking Ability, and Function

	Treatment group		
	EHDP	Placebo	
Subjective evaluation	Mean rating (n)	Mean rating (n)	
Pain[a]			
Pre-surgery	4.2±0.3 (69)	4.0±0.2 (71)	
End of treatment	8.3±0.3 (45)	8.6±0.2 (49)	
Last visit	8.8±0.2 (62)	9.0±0.2 (60)	
Walking ability[b]			
Pre-surgery	5.7±0.2 (71)	5.8±0.2 (73)	
End of treatment	6.6±0.4 (45)	7.1±0.3 (48)	
Last visit	8.6±0.2 (63)	8.6±0.2 (60)	
Function[c]			
Pre-surgery	4.9±0.3 (66)	4.9±0.3 (68)	
End of treatment	6.2±0.4 (41)	6.0±0.4 (43)	
Last visit	8.2±0.3 (58)	8.1±0.3 (58)	

[a] Rated from 1 (unbearable) to 10 (no pain).
[b] Rated from 1 (bedridden) to 10 (unrestricted).
[c] Rated from 1 (confined) to 10 (normal).

Complications of reattachment of the greater trochanter were seen in both groups. A total of 14 migrations occurred in 10 placebo-treated patients and 8 trochanter migrations in 7 EHDP-treated patients. There was no evidence of increased radiolucency at the cement-bone interface in the EHDP-treated patients.

The only laboratory abnormality observed was hyperphosphatemia in the patients receiving EHDP therapy (Table 17-7). The mean serum phosphorus levels were significantly higher after 4 weeks of treatment ($P < 0.05$) than in the placebo-treated patients, but did not persist 4 weeks after cessation of therapy.[19] Serum calcium levels did not significantly differ in either treatment group, during or after therapy.

Discussion

EHDP in a dosage schedule of 20 mg/kg/day, 1 month before and 3 months after total hip arthroplasty decreases the incidence and severity of heterotopic

Table 17-6

Summary of Gastrointestinal Side Effects

	Patients reporting/Patients discontinuing therapy	
Symptoms[a]	EHDP (n = 99)	Placebo (n = 92)
Upper gastrointestinal tract (nausea, vomiting, upset stomach)	11/3	9/0
Lower gastrointestinal tract (diarrhea, flatulence)	33/10[b]	8/1

[a] Some patients had both upper and lower gastrointestinal complaints
[b] Statistically significant difference, $x^2 = 15.74$, $P < 0.001$

Table 17-7

Effects of Treatment on Serum Calcium and Phosphorus

Time in relation to surgery	Mean value ± standard error			
	Serum phosphorus[a]		Serum calcium[a]	
	EHDP (n)	Placebo (n)	EHDP (n)	Placebo (n)
–4 wks	3.538±0.148 (91)	3.588±0.193 (82)	9.744±0.053 (91)	9.626±0.127 (82)
0 wk	5.305±0.114[b] (66)	3.354±0.080 (57)	9.662±0.058 (66)	9.446±0.084 (57)
6 wks	5.205±0.136[b] (57)	3.946±0.331 (46)	9.732±0.079 (57)	9.794±0.086 (46)
12 wks	5.987±0.697[b] (45)	3.667±0.216 (39)	9.858±0.094 (45)	9.785±0.105 (39)
18 wks	3.791±0.146 (35)	3.477±0.081 (30)	9.451±0.298 (35)	9.573±0.230 (30)
12 mo	3.427±0.245 (48)	3.878±0.387	9.804±0.113 (48)	9.735±0.094 (48)

[a] Normal ranges: Calcium, 9.0–11.0 mg/dl
Phosphorus, 2.5–3.5 mg/dl
[b] Statistically significant difference $p < 0.05$

ossification. Patients receiving the placebo experienced a 17 percent incidence of clinically significant heterotopic ossification, a finding similar to that appearing in other published studies. By contrast, those receiving EHDP developed an 8 percent incidence of clinically significant heterotopic ossification. In the subset of patients with osteoarthritis or traumatic arthritis, the incidence of clinically significant heterotopic ossification was again 8 percent in the EHDP-treated patients, but 24 percent in those receiving the placebo. In those patients who had developed heterotopic ossification following previous surgery and were undergoing revision arthroplasty, although EHDP prevented formation of bone during the treatment period, at the time of the last visit, the incidence of heterotopic bone formation was not statistically different in the EHDP-treated and placebo-treated patients. However, the delay of onset of the ossification may have had a beneficial effect in allowing patients to develop better motion during their early convalescence than otherwise might have been possible.

Following this study, the possibility of further enhancing the inhibition of heterotopic ossification with a 10 mg/kg/day dose of EHDP given over 6 months (instead of the 20 mg/kg/day over 3 months dose schedule) was assessed. This dosage level was not found to be efficacious; consequently, the current recommended dosage of EHDP is 20 mgm/kg/day given for 2 weeks to 1 month prior to surgery, and for 3 months after surgery.[5,12]

The medication is generally well-tolerated, with patients only occasionally requiring discontinuance due to gastrointestinal symptoms. Hyperphosphatemia will be a constant finding during EHDP administration, but appears to have no adverse effect; it does provide a method of assessing compliance.

The medication appears to be particularly helpful in high-risk patients, namely those with osteoarthritis or traumatic arthritis, and especially in male patients with decreased range of motion, abundant osteophyte formation, and without pre-existing heterotopic ossification.

RADIATION STUDY

Materials and Methods

A study to assess the effectiveness of post-operative radiation to prevent heterotopic ossification in high-risk patients and in patients in whom this complication had previously occurred was undertaken at the Mayo Clinic.[4,11] Their patient population was 42 in number (31 males and 11 females); 48 hips were treated. The patients' age ranged from the third to the eighth decade, with a mean age of 62. 2000 Rads, divided into 10 daily doses, was given to the operated hip. Optimum effects were noted if the treatment regime was begun within 5 or 6 days of surgery. If treatment was delayed until heterotopic ossification was visible on post-operative radiographs, no beneficial effect was achieved; the effect was only moderate if treatment began as late as the 10th day.

The patients were divided into five groups: (1) those with massive bone excised after previous total hip arthroplasty; (2) those with rheumatoid spondylitis with pre-operative ankylosis; (3) those with ectopic bone following previous surgery, leading to total hip arthroplasty; (4) those with ectopic bone following surgery on the opposite hip; and (5) those with ectopic bone present early in the post-operative treatment.

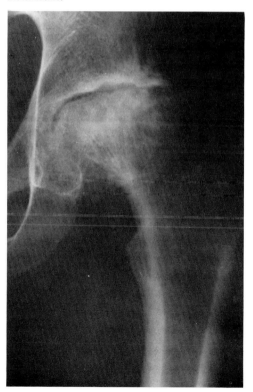

Fig. 17-6. A 39-year-old male presented with progressive hip pain and stiffness over a 5 year period. At the age of 15, he had had a slipped capital femoral epiphysis treated by open reduction and internal fixation. Radiographs showed marked degenerative changes.

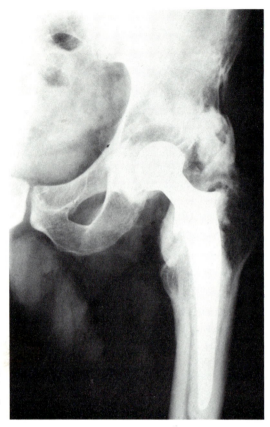

Fig. 17-7. At 1 year after total hip arthroplasty, the hip exhibited a 10° flexion-extension arc; the radiograph revealed severe heterotopic ossification.

Results

The greatest benefit appeared to occur in the first and third patient groups; those with ectopic bone following previous total hip arthroplasty, and those with ectopic bone following other previous surgery. In the first group of 12 hips, all had severe involvement prior to surgery. After surgery, four hips developed no further heterotopic ossification; one developed it mildly; and seven showed moderate involvement. There were 13 hips in the group with previous surgery other than total hip arthroplasty in whom heterotopic ossification was present. Heterotopic ossification pre-operatively was severe in 11; moderate in 1; mild in 1. Post-operatively, of those with severe pre-operative involvement, ossification was none in two hips; mild in four; moderate in two; severe in three. The patient with moderate pre-operative heterotopic ossification developed mild changes post-revision surgery; the patient with mild involvement pre-surgery developed none post-operatively.

Of three hips with solid ankylosis secondary to rheumatoid spondylitis pre-surgery, two developed no heterotopic ossification during their convalescence; one developed it mildly. Of seven hips with bone in the hip opposite to the one operated, two developed none, four developed mild involvement, and one moderate involvement post-surgery. No effect was apparent in those patients in whom radiation treatment was started after heterotopic ossification had already appeared.

Discussion

If we summarize their data, the following additional useful information becomes apparent. In 23 hips with severe involvement due to heterotopic bone prior to surgery, 6 showed no bone post-radiation treatment, 5 mild involvement, 9 moderate involvement, and 3 severe involvement. There were no complications of delayed wound healing; no subjective or objective symptoms; hospitalization time was slightly increased due to the treatment regime; six trochanters did not unite after osteotomy, but there seemed to be technical reasons present in each instance.

The method then appears to be useful; it is not a panacea and, on the best information currently available, referred to within the paper, it is sufficiently safe to justify employment in these extreme situations.

EHDP–RADIATION COMBINED THERAPY

Our own experience with the radiation technique has been limited to four hips in three patients; it has been effective in each instance. It has been employed in conjunction with EHDP, as now suggested by the Mayo Clinic group. The first patient developed complete ankylosis of his hip after initial total hip arthroplasty, had gone on to re-ankylosis after excision of the heterotopic bone on two occasions, under cover of EHDP given 1 month before surgery and for 3 and 6 months after

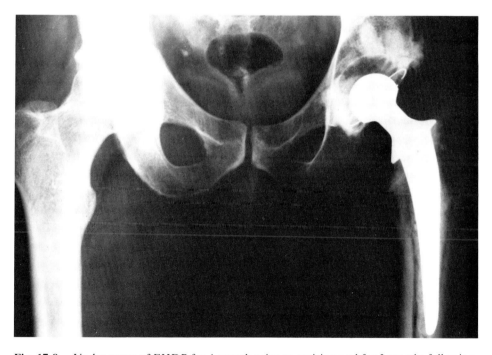

Fig. 17-8. Under cover of EHDP for 1 month prior to excision and for 3 months following, the heterotopic ossification was removed. The radiograph at the time of discontinuing EHDP shows a few patches of heterotopic ossification; the flexion-extension arc was 70°.

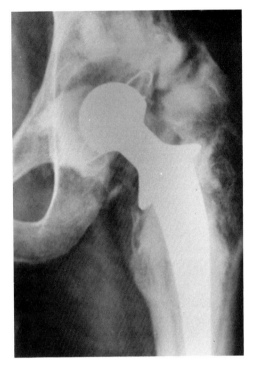

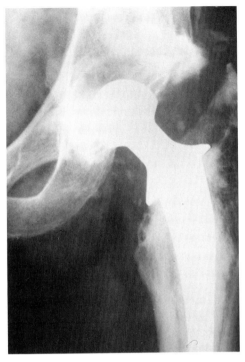

Fig. 17-9. Radiograph 2 years after initial excision of heterotopic ossification. There is almost complete bony bridging and the flexion-extension arc was now 15°. Heterotopic ossification had recurred promptly after discontinuation of EHDP. Clinically, the hip had stiffened within 2 weeks.

Fig. 17-10. Radiographs 6 months after re-excision of heterotopic ossification under cover of EHDP for 1 month prior and 6 months after operation. EHDP was discontinued at this time. There was a 30° flexion-extension arc. There had been no significant reossification since the surgery.

the operations. After discontinuation of the EHDP, re-ankylosis occurred each time. After a third excision, both EHDP and local radiation were used; only moderate ossification has occurred and a satisfactory arc of motion has been maintained (Figs. 17-6–17-12).

A second patient developed incomplete fibrous and bony ankylosis of each hip after total hip arthroplasty. On separate admissions, the bone from each hip was excised. Treatment with EHDP alone for the first hip and EHDP and radiation for the second hip followed. The greatest improvement occurred when the two regimes were used in combination.

In a third patient, almost complete bony ankylosis developed following total hip arthroplasty complicated by dislocation and open reduction during the immediate post-operative period (Figs. 17-13, 17-14). Nine years later, the bone was excised because of the development of progressive back pain. Both EHDP and radiation therapy were employed. Six months after bone removal, there has been minimal recurrence; there is a 90° flexion-extension arc and good function (Fig. 17-15).

SUMMARY

The problem of heterotopic ossification remains incompletely resolved. Three high-risk groups can be identified: (1) males who have not had previous hip surgery and who present with osteoarthritis and a limited range of hip motion; (2) males or females who have had previous hip surgery, developed heterotopic ossification during convalescence, and for whom revision surgery is planned; and (3) patients with ankylosing spondylitis in an active phase.

Beyond the technical aspects of the operative procedure itself, there exist two treatment modalities that appear to be effective in reducing the frequency of reformation of heterotopic ossification. These are the oral administration of EHDP at a dose range of 20 mg/kg/day, beginning 2 weeks to 1 month prior to surgery and continuing for 3 months after surgery, and the use of post-operative radiation at a dosage level of 2000 Rads in 10 divided doses, starting within the first week after operation. Both methods of treatment appear to be independently effective. They each address the biology of the problem at different phases of its development; it would thus appear that the suggestion of the Mayo Clinic group, that EHDP therapy be considered as a supplement to radiation treatment in the particularly high-risk patient, is worthy of serious consideration.

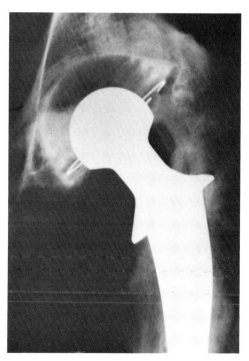

Fig. 17-11. Radiograph 2½ years after second excision of heterotopic ossification. A solid bridge of bone crosses the joint and there is no motion. Heterotopic ossification had recurred again shortly after discontinuation of the EHDP, and clinical stiffening, though more slowly, also returned.

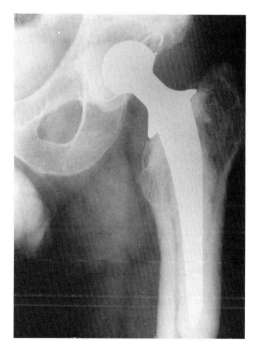

Fig. 17-12. Radiograph 6 months after third excision of heterotopic ossification under cover of EHDP 1 month prior and 6 months post-operation. 2000 Rads of radiation were given over a 10-day period, starting on the fifth post-operative day. At 9 months, he has a 70° flexion-extension arc of moion, and "feels fine."

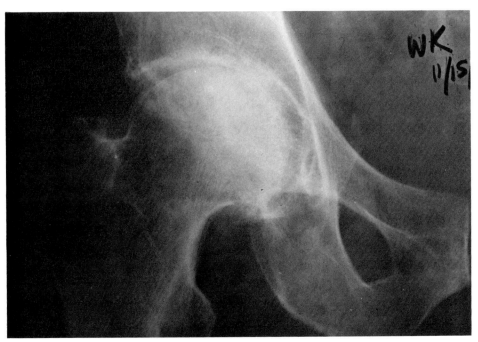

Fig. 17-13. Original radiograph of a 71-year-old male who underwent total hip arthroplasty for progressive pain and disability secondary to degenerative osteoarthritis.

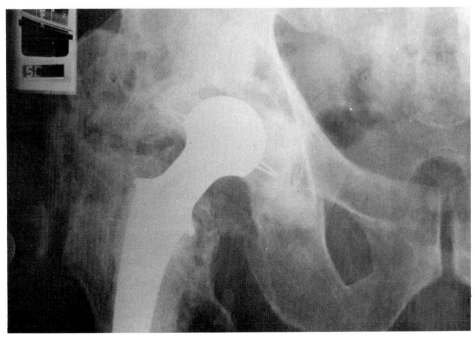

Fig. 17-14. Heterotopic ossification developed post-operatively with restriction of motion. The radiograph 9 years later shows nearly complete ankylosis. There was a 20° flexion-extension arc of motion; the patient had developed incapacitating back pain.

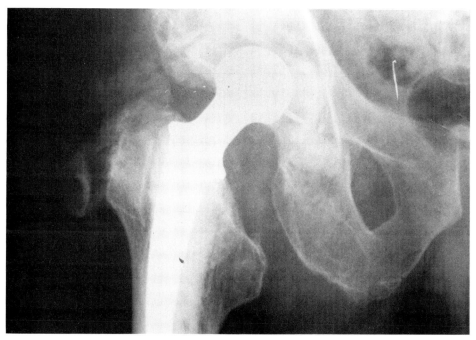

Fig. 17-15. The heterotopic ossification was excised and the prosthesis retained. EHDP was given for 1 month prior and 3 months post-excision. 2000 Rads of radiation were given in 10 divided doses, beginning 6 days after operation. Three months after the operation, when this radiograph was taken, there was a 90° flexion-extension arc of motion and the back pain had largely disappeared.

REFERENCES

1. Amstutz HD: Trapezoidal-28 total hip replacement. *Clin Orthop* 95:158–167, 1973.

2. Brooker AB, Bowerman JW, Robinson RA, et al: Ectopic ossification following total hip replacement: Incidence and a method of classification. *J Bone and Joint Surg* 55(A):1629–1632, 1973.

3. Charnley J: The long-term results of low-friction arthroplasty of the hip performed as a primary intervention. *J Bone and Joint Surg* 54(B):61–76, 1972.

4. Coventry MB, Scanlon PW: The use of radiation to discourage ectopic bone. *J Bone and Joint Surg* 63(A):201–208, 1981.

5. Finerman GAM, Krengel WF Jr, Lowell JD, et al: Role of diphosphonate (EHDP) in the prevention of heterotopic ossification after total hip arthroplasty: A preliminary report, in *The Hip, Proceedings of the Fifth Open Scientific Meeting of the Hip Society.* St Louis, CV Mosby, 1977, pp 222–234.

6. Fleisch H, Russell RGG, Bisaz S, et al: The inhibitory effect of phosphonates on the formation of calcium phosphate crystals in vitro and on aortic and kidney calcification in vivo. *Europ J Clin Invest* 1:12–18, 1970.

7. Flora L: Comparative anti-inflammatory and bone protective effects of two diphosphonates in adjuvant arthritis. *Arthritis Rheum* 22:340–346, 1979.

8. Francis MD: The inhibition of calcium hydroxyapatite crystal growth by polyphosphonates and polyphosphates. *Calcif Tissue Res* 3:151–162, 1969.

9. Francis MD, Russell RGG, Fleisch H: Diphosphonates inhibit formation of calcium

phosphate crystals in vitro and pathological calcification in vivo. *Science* 165:1264–1266, 1969.

10. Hori RY, Lewis JL, Zimmerman JR, et al: The number of total joint replacements in the United States. *Clin Orthop* 132:46–52, 1978.

11. Jowsey J, Coventry MB, Robins PR: Heterotopic ossification: Theoretical consideration, possible etiologic factors, and a clinical review of total hip arthroplasty patients exhibiting this phenomenon, in *The Hip, Proceedings of the Fifth Open Scientific Meeting of the Hip Society.* St Louis, CV Mosby, 1977, pp 210–221.

12. Mack HP: Personal communication, (Proctor and Gamble Company, Miami Valley Laboratories, Cincinnati, Ohio 45247.), 1979.

13. Matos M, Amstutz HC, Finerman G: Myositis ossificans following total hip replacement. *J Bone and Joint Surg* 57(A):137, 1975.

14. Nollen AJG, Slooff TJJH: Para-articular ossifications after total hip replacement. *Acta Orthop Scand* 44:230–241, 1973.

15. Plasmans CMT, Kuypers W, Slooff TJJH: The effect of ethane-1-hydroxy-1, 1-diphosphonic acid (EHDP) on matrix-induced ectopic bone formation. *Clin Orthop* 132:233–243, 1978.

16. Riegler HF, Harris CM: Heterotopic bone formation after total hip arthroplasty. *Clin Orthop* 117:209–216, 1976.

17. Ritter MA: Personal communication, 1981.

18. Ritter MA, Vaughan RB: Ectopic ossification after total hip arthroplasty. *J Bone and Joint Surg* 59(A):345–351, 1977.

19. Russell RGG, Fleisch H: Pyrophosphate and diphosphonates in skeletal metabolism. *Clin Orthop* 108:241–263, 1975.

20. Slatis P, Kiviluoto O, Santavirta S: Ectopic ossification after hip arthroplasty. *Ann Chirurg Gynaecol* 67:89–93, 1978.

Otto E. Aufranc, John McA. Harris, III,
Sandra J. McKay, and Donna M. Dinardo

18

Rehabilitation in Hip Arthroplasty

No volume on the art of revision arthroplasty would be complete without some comment on the rehabilitation of patients who have undergone the procedure. In the past, the few articles that have spoken of the rehabilitation of the hip arthroplasty patient have focused on the primary arthroplasty patients.[1-8]

Experience at the New England Baptist Hospital and at the Boston Veterans Administration Medical Center has shown that, if abuse of a total hip arthroplasty is one of the causes for its painful loosening, abuse of a revision total hip arthroplasty will almost certainly lead to similar failure. It is doubly important, therefore, that a program of rehabilitation be established for revision arthroplasty patients that is directed not only at the restoration of function in the immediate post-operative period, but also at establishing a life-long set of habits that protect the hip. The program that is outlined below begins in the pre-operative period, and continues during hospitalization and the post-discharge months, when the patient should follow a specific home program. The pre operative evaluation and education are almost as important as the various exercises and activities utilized during the post-operative period. For that reason, we recommend the following approach as a guide, even if specific activities or exercises do not seem to apply in the case of every revision arthroplasty patient.

PRE-OPERATIVE EVALUATION

During the pre-operative evaluation of the revision total hip replacement candidate, an extensive physical and social history is necessary. Only if the clinician

379

is familiar with the physical and emotional environment of the home to which the patient will return will the patient and therapist be able to jointly determine realistic goals for post-operative treatment.

It is important to know the specifics about the patient's home, as a barrier-free physical layout is an important goal. This includes such things as removal of scatter rugs and other movable hazards about the house. The patient should plan to either live on the main floor of the house, so as to eliminate stair-climbing, or to organize his or her life to minimize stair-climbing.

A person living alone who undergoes revision hip surgery is encouraged to arrange and to accept outside assistance for most activities, including basic activities of daily living. This help can be a friend, family member, or service provider from an outside agency coming into the home. Alternatively, the patient may convalesce at the home of a family member or friend upon hospital discharge. This emphasizes the importance of strict adherence to partial weight-bearing with crutches, and to allow the patient sufficient time and energy to complete a post-operative exercise program.

The patient should be made to understand that the time spent recovering from revision hip surgery is not merely an inconvenience, but is a vital contribution to the success and long-term survival of the revision arthroplasty. He or she should be discouraged from feeling "free" to use or abuse the affected hip, on the assumption that repeated revision hip surgery is always available. The patient is encouraged to examine his or her life-style, and to make necessary adjustments to a specific set of guidelines, including the use of external support, first in the form of crutches, and ultimately, a cane. The patient is encouraged to understand that the prosthesis is an artificial device, and that both muscle and bone are weakened through multiple surgical procedures. The rehabilitative course is longer, therefore; the cane is a permanent reminder to treat the hip with respect.

Weight control is essential to revision arthroplasty success, when obese patients undergo revision hip surgery. Necessary weight reduction should begin while the patient is in the hospital, not only by reducing calories, but also by establishing appropriate protein intake for adequate healing. Educating the patient must include consultation with the dietitian, for both patient and family, in order to establish an effective weight-reduction regime following discharge.

The patient is encouraged to ask questions and to express feelings concerning this and prior hospitalizations. The patient is reminded that communication is a two-way street. During the initial 3-week post-operative phase, his or her world will be limited to arm's reach, so the patient must make his or her needs known. A good understanding of the patient's reaction to hospitalization will help in the planning of the pre-operative instruction, in gaining the patient's cooperation, and in anticipating the patient's reaction to a post-operative course that will probably differ from that which followed previous hip surgery.

The patient who has undergone many hospitalizations and operative procedures often expresses financial concerns. If the patient is the family provider, this can become a major concern and stress factor. If the patient has incomplete insurance coverage, he or she will express worry over accumulated hospital and physician fees. Another concern of the patient will be his or her ability to return to a previous occupation. Revision hip surgery entails extended periods of crutch-walking, usually incompatible with even partial employment. At this point, additional input is needed from the physician, perhaps in the form of a letter suggesting job modifi-cation, or in the exploration of job training programs.

A pre-operative physical assessment of the patient is performed, with emphasis upon the involved hip. Specific ranges of hip motion are recorded, as are any fixed contractures. The degree of involvement of other joints is noted, as is the muscle strength of all extremities. This data provides a baseline for re-evaluation during the post-operative course, as well as the basis for the planning of post-operative exercise and mobilization. The patient's gait pattern and leg lengths are noted; abnormalities are recorded. If an abnormality is present, it is important to determine that it is specifically due to the painful hip, rather than other causes such as leg-length discrepancy or pathology in the contralateral limb. Thorough knowledge of these factors facilitates post-operative ambulation training when the goal is a normal gait pattern.

PRE-OPERATIVE TEACHING

The patient usually has had crutch-walking experience, but the basic three-point partial weight-bearing gait is reviewed. Emphasis is again placed upon the long-term use of crutches, and the eventual use of a cane. The importance of protecting the hip, hip muscles, and the osteotomized greater trochanter will be repeatedly stressed, with each activity planned for the recovery period.

The hospital bed should be equipped with a balkan frame, and side handles or a trapeze. The patient is instructed in bed mobility activities, particularly lifting himself (or herself), for such activities as for bedmaking (Fig. 18-1). The patient is encouraged to use the electric bed control to obtain positions of comfort while on a program of bedrest, and is instructed to use the overhead frame to help achieve maximum hip flexion (Figure 18-2) and the bed controls for equal amounts of "flat time," to decrease or prevent a flexion contracture. If the balanced suspension is not yet on the bed, the patient is oriented to it by pictures in a pre-operative teaching manual or by observing a post-operative patient.

Succession of the specific activities to expect in the post-operative phase are discussed with the patient in detail. The patient is reminded that a pillow will be placed between his or her knees, and that the abducted position must be maintained, especially when sitting down in, or when rising from a chair, bed, or toilet. The bed exercise and activity program is reviewed with the patient, who must give an independent demonstration of the exercises at this time.

The patient will first be encouraged to do deep breathing and coughing. This begins in the recovery room and continues on the nursing unit. The patient may also have an incentive spirometer or respiratory therapy treatments at bedside to help raise secretions and clear the lungs. Use of this equipment should be reviewed pre-operatively.

Ankle dorsi and plantar flexion will be performed so as to simulate the heel-toe action of walking and, therefore, promote good circulation. At the same time, the patient is instructed in post-operative use of knee-length surgical elastic stockings.

Quadriceps, gluteal, hamstring, and abdominal exercises will be taught to maintain and to improve muscle tone, as well as to prevent the pooling of blood in

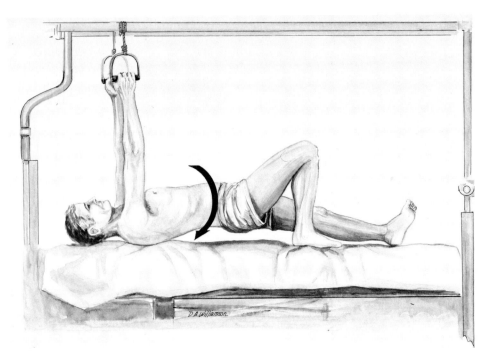

Fig. 18-1. The patient is instructed in bed mobility activities, particularly lifting himself, for such activities as bed-making.

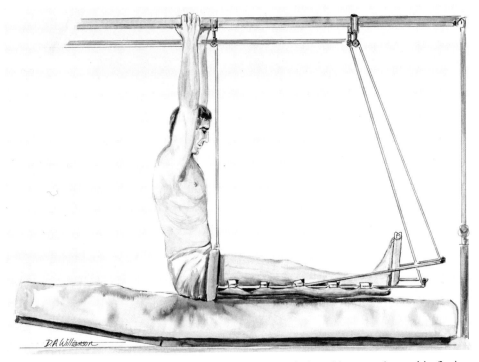

Fig. 18-2. Use of the overhead frame is encouraged to help achieve maximum hip flexion.

382

the lower extremities and lower abdomen. The patient will be instructed in internal and external rotation exercises, done bilaterally, supine alternating hip-hiking, and pelvic tilting exercises. These exercises will provide initiation of gentle stretching of hip muscles, within the patient's comfort limit. If a flexion deformity is noted, the patient is instructed in the Thomas stretch test. Since the hip muscles are often sore and sensitive, the patient is instructed in the use of the overhead frame to begin gaining early passive hip motion.

Pre-operative assessment and teaching is valuable to the patient and to all members of the health care team. During this time, principles concerning revision hip surgery as established during the office visit are reinforced to the patient and the family. Another goal of the pre-operative period is to establish trusting patient and therapist relationships. This is important, so as to create a psychologically positive atmosphere necessary for the success of the rehabilitation program. The ultimate goal is to impress upon the patient a realization that with acceptance of, and strict adherence to, imposed limitations, he or she can return to relatively independent living.

IMMEDIATE POST-OPERATIVE PERIOD

The use of balanced suspension is strongly advocated in the post-operative phase of revision hip surgery. This apparatus not only maintains an abducted position and facilitates nursing care, but also provides a dynamic system which allows active assisted range of motion to the hip and knee. The patient should be transferred directly from the operating table to a bed equipped with balanced suspension to minimize both discomfort and the chance of dislocation (Fig. 18-3).

For the safety and monitoring of these patients, they remain in the recovery room overnight, after being placed in balanced suspension and Buck's traction. When the patient is returned to the nursing unit the following morning, a check of

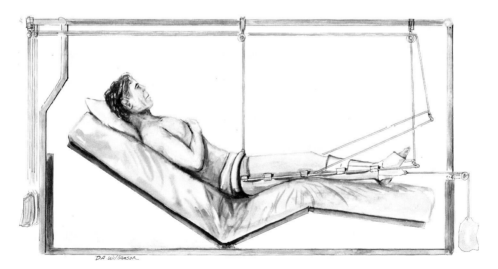

Fig. 18-3. Transferring the patient directly from the operating table to a bed equipped with balanced suspension can minimize discomfort and the chance of dislocation.

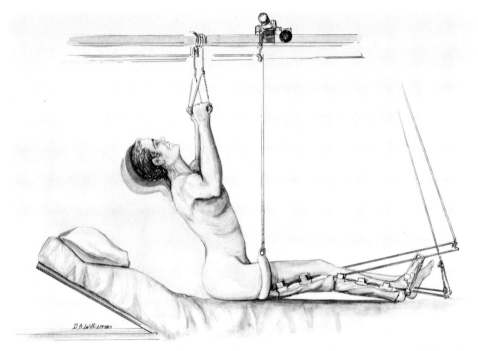

Fig. 18-4. To relieve low back pain, the patient rises to a seated position using side handles and returns to the bed by arching the back into a "C" shape, shown here.

the suspension apparatus is carried out. It is important to readjust weights, center the limb in the splint, and do a neurovascular check. Frequent checks of this type are necessary while the patient is in balanced suspension, for the patient's comfort and to avoid skin and neurologic problems associated with improper position. As the patient regains active muscular control of the limb, the weights must be adjusted to keep the limb balanced as the patient moves about in bed.

Elevation of the head and foot of the bed will lessen spasm in the hip. To encourage the patient to maintain an abducted position and to discourage extremes in passive rotation of the limb, the bedside table and other items of interest to the patient (eg, the television) are moved to the operative side of the bed, within arm's reach.

The stability of the trochanteric fixation dictates the length of time the patient is confined to suspension bedrest. In general for revision arthroplasty, this time is 10 to 21 days. This allows not only for decrease of swelling and initial healing, but further reinforces the importance of patient participation in assuring a durable and lasting hip replacement.

During the supine bedrest, passive handling of the patient's hip should be gentle. One should never touch the post-operative patient without first explaining exactly what is planned. The patient should initiate any movement with support supplied by the surgeon, nurse, or therapist, to reduce the load on his or her muscles. This will decrease antagonistic muscle contraction and spasm, increase patient comfort and, therefore, cooperation.

Any person confined to the supine position for an extended period of time may complain of low back pain. A simple technique for patient comfort is to have

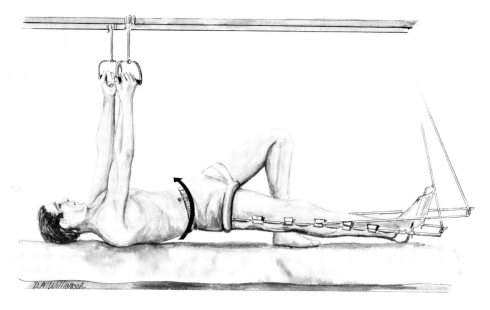

Fig. 18-5. Another mobilization technique involves planting the unaffected foot with knee bent and using that leg and both hands on side handles, lifting up off the bed.

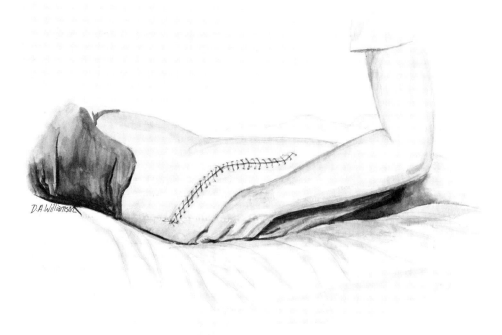

Fig. 18-6. An additional comfort is to have a nurse gently pull the flesh of the proximal thigh and buttock outwards, while the patient has lifted up, using the trapeze or side handles and the unoperated lower limb.

the patient mobilize his spine by using the trapeze or side handles to come to a seated position and then to return to the bed by arching the back into a "C" shape (Fig. 18-4). The head is lowered first, followed by the shoulders, and lastly the buttocks. Another mobilization technique involves having the patient plant the unoperated-side foot, with the knee bent and, using that leg and both hands (on the trapeze or side handles), lifting off the bed (Fig. 18-5). In order for the patient to do this, the suspension must be properly balanced and should move freely to lift the weight of the leg. These activities, as well as pelvic tilts, can prevent or reduce back discomfort and the generalized aching associated with prolonged reduced mobility at bedrest. Another comfort measure is to have the nurse gently pull the flesh of the proximal thigh and buttock outwards from the midline starting at the gluteal folds, while the patient has lifted up, using the trapeze or side handles and the unoperated lower limb (Fig. 18-6). The patient then lowers back down to the bed with the soft tissues thus replaced in a position that both enhances comfort and avoids fixed external rotation contracture.

The bed exercise program at this time consists of ankle dorsi and plantar flexion, quadriceps and gluteal sets, alternating hip-hiking (Fig. 18-7), and active internal and external rotation, all of which have been rehearsed in the pre-operative period. Since hip flexion contracture is often present, the patient is instructed in the Thomas test as an exercise. To achieve further hip extension, "flat time" is spent three times a day for 20 to 30 minutes, as tolerated. The patient is encouraged to do quad, gluteal, and abdominal sets simultaneously in the balanced suspension. Mobilization of the hip and knee is begun in balanced suspension by the patient's use of appropriate ropes to flex and extend the Thomas splint and the Pierson attachment of the suspension (Fig. 18-8).

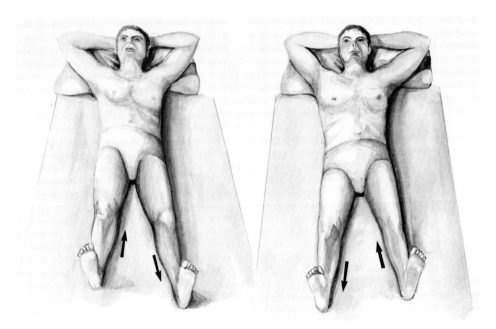

Fig. 18-7. Alternative hip-hiking, one component of the immediate post-operative bed exercise program.

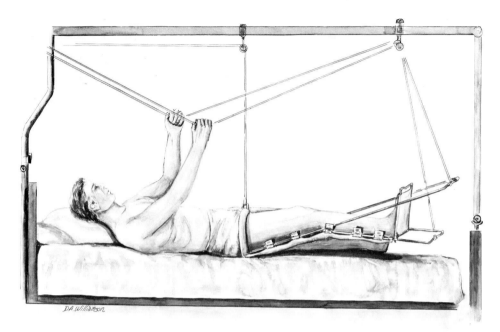

Fig. 18-8. Mobilization of the hip and knee is begun in balanced suspension through the patient's use of appropriate ropes to flex and extend the Thomas splint and the Pierson attachment of the suspension.

When the balanced suspension is removed, maximum hip extension can be achieved by prone lying. Care must be taken to maintain relative abduction of the operated hip at all times while turning to the prone position (Fig. 18-9).

During the patient's confinement, a close relationship develops with the health team, which helps to reinforce the necessity in life-style changes and also provides the patient with further understanding of the complexity of his or her hip problem.

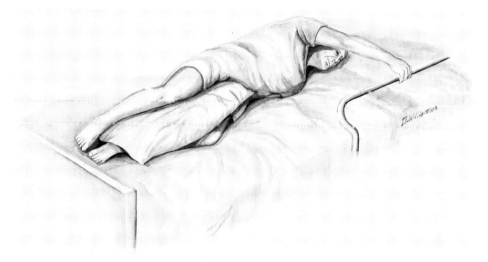

Fig. 18-9. Care must be taken to maintain relative abduction of the operated hip at all times while turning to the prone position, once balanced suspension is removed.

POST-OPERATIVE AMBULATION

Balanced suspension is usually continued for 10 to 21 days post-operatively, to allow sufficient soft-tissue healing to protect trochanteric repair. Time in suspension varies, as discussed in Chapters 4 and 11. Once the suspension is removed, a knee sling is applied, and the patient is taught further active assisted range of motion (Fig. 18-10). It is important to stress that the knee sling remain in place whenever the patient is in bed. The sling also lifts the leg slightly up off the bed to make active abduction exercises easier to perform.

After removal of the suspension, the patient is allowed to sit on the side of the bed, usually on the same day, as comfort and tolerance allows. It is preferable to

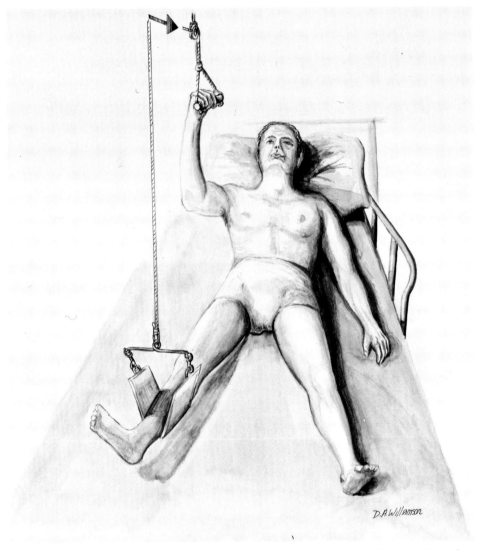

Fig. 18-10. After balanced suspension is removed, a knee sling is applied and the patient is taught further active, assisted range of motion. Sling must be in place whenever the patient is in bed.

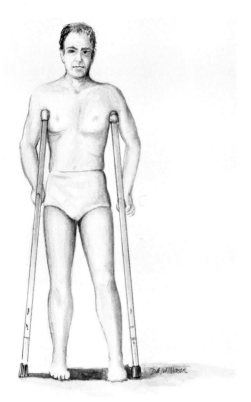

Fig. 18-13. The feeling (on the part of the patient) that the operated leg is too long may be due to temporary abduction contracture and/or distal advancement of the greater trochanter.

Premature initiation of flexion in gait is another common early gait error. The patient is instructed to make strides of equal length, to stand erect, and keep the knee in full extension with the heel flat on the floor in the stance phase of gait. A full-length mirror is a very useful teaching tool for the patient to visualize gait and correct faults.

Stair-climbing instruction follows the achievement of satisfactory level gait. The instruction is standard: going up unaffected leg first, then affected leg, then both crutches; going down crutches first, then affected leg, then, finally, unaffected leg. This permits the patient to raise and lower body weight with both crutches and the unaffected leg (Fig. 18-14).

Seated activities should begin only when 70° of hip flexion have been obtained and the patient has good muscular control of the operated limb. Selection of proper chairs is dependent on the patient's height and degree of disability. In general, an armchair with a straight back and a seat that is 18 to 21 inches from the floor is satisfactory for the unilateral hip revision patient of average height. Patients with greater disabilities (eg, bilateral arthroplasties, limited hip flexion, generalized debility, and weakness of specific muscle groups, such as the knee extensors or upper extremity motors), may need special consideration, as will taller patients. In these cases, chair height will have to be raised by cushions or blocks to a level that does not require rising from a position of 90° of hip and knee flexion, but permits the patient to slide into a semi-erect position before lifting the body weight from the chair (Fig. 18-15). The same basic criteria applies to toilet-seat height. Short

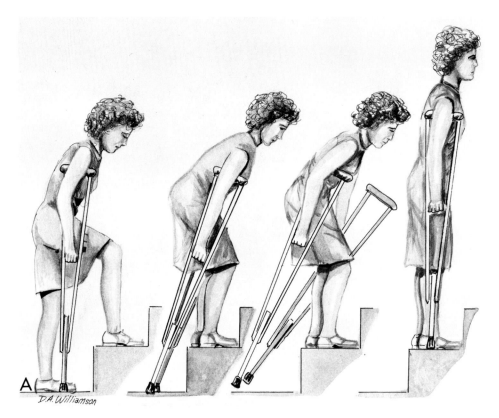

D.A. Williamson

Fig. 18-14. Stair-climbing with crutches. (**A**) *Upstairs:* unaffected leg first, then affected leg, and lastly crutches. (**B**) *Downstairs:* crutches first, then affected leg, and finally unaffected leg.

people with good hip flexion do not need an elevated toilet seat. When arising from the seated position, the patient relies mainly on the unaffected leg, however, the operated leg should "help," within the limits of comfort.

Tub and shower techniques are taught after suture removal. A stable stool placed inside the tub or shower stall is recommended for safety and protection from standing fatigue. A good-quality stable rubber mat is advised for both tub and shower.

DISCHARGE PLANNING

Criteria for discharge include a good understanding of the precautions imposed by revision hip surgery. The patient must demonstrate exercises independently and be stable with crutches on level surfaces and on stairs. He or she should be afebrile for at least 48 hours prior to discharge, and the wound should show signs of primary healing. The patient should also have a good understanding of any prescribed medications and diet for home use. The patient should understand follow-up arrangements including return visits to the physician.

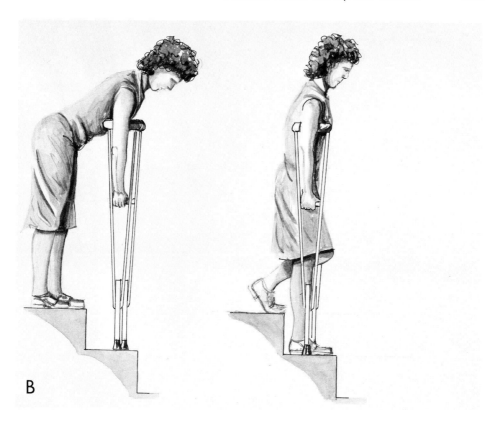

B

Whether the patient returns home independently, with assistance, or requires temporary placement, a written home activity guideline is provided. This includes specific exercises and frequency of performance. It is advisable to review this program with a responsible individual who will be involved in the patient's care to avoid any conflicts over the level of activity.

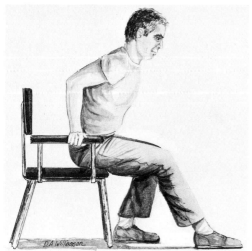

Fig. 18-15. Chairs used must not require rising from a position of 90° of hip and knee flexion, but must permit the patient to slide into a semi-erect position before lifting the body weight from the chair.

Proper positioning in bed including use of a pillow between the knees when lying, turning, or side lying, must be reinforced. Low chairs are to be avoided, and appropriate equipment, such as a "hip chair" and raised toilet seat, must be available prior to discharge. With physician's approval, patients may be allowed pool swimming, provided that the pool has steps with a handrail that permits the patient to descend into the pool with crutches until buoyancy unloads the hip. Patients are instructed to perform as many activities as possible, such as showering, while using a chair or stool to avoid any unsupported weight-bearing. Unnecessary bending and lifting are discouraged. Patients are advised to rearrange their kitchen, for example, to allow easy access to frequently used articles. Patients may resume sexual activity as indicated by hip comfort and mobility. The patient is advised to be the less active partner.

Patients having sedentary jobs may return to work while still on crutches. All patients, however, are cautioned against sitting for longer than 45 minutes without getting up and walking around with the crutches. Extended periods of sitting will cause stiffness of hip muscles and may lead to permanent, fixed-flexion deformity. Sitting with legs in the dependent position for long periods may lead to stasis edema.

Following revision surgery of the left hip, the patient is able to resume driving when comfortable getting behind the wheel, provided that the car has an automatic transmission and the left leg is not used. Patients having right hip revision who drive are advised to avoid driving until the first post-operative physician visit. However, many patients having chronic pain and disability with the right hip will be adept at using the left leg for braking. In this case, the physician may permit driving within 2 to 3 months after hospital discharge.

Finally, upon hospital discharge, it is ascertained that the patient has the telephone numbers of the physician and of a member of the health care team at the hospital. The patient is encouraged to telephone, should questions or problems arise. This assures the patient of the continued concern for his or her needs on the part of the team, and may serve to reinforce in the patient the need to care for himself or herself.

OUT-PATIENT THERAPY

During the first 2 months following surgery, the revision hip patient will bear up to one third of body weight on the operated extremity. To better visualize this concept, simulated weight-bearing on a foot scale may be necessary. Into the third and fourth post-operative months, progressive weight-bearing, up to one half body weight, is permitted. During the fifth month, the patient is allowed up to two thirds body weight-bearing through the operated hip. The patient is allowed to progress to full weight-bearing during the sixth month following surgery, still using crutches. Weight-bearing instructions will be altered depending on trochanteric fixation and on the recovery of the musculature about the operated hip, particularly the abductors. Increased weight-bearing should not be permitted until the patient can support an increasing percentage of the lower-extremity weight against gravity in the side-lying position. As abductor strength increases, weight-bearing with crutches can be increased.

When the patient comes from a distant location where close follow-up by the health team is not possible, good communication with a local physical therapist is necessary to monitor progress and assure compliance with the previously established program.

At approximately 3 months post-operatively, use of an exercise bicycle can be added, to gain some additional motion as well as endurance. Initial tension should be little or none, and should be very slowly increased as endurance increases. The seat height should start sufficiently high to have the knee in full extension when the pedal is in its lowest position. The seat can be lowered half an inch each week, as permitted by comfort and range of hip flexion, provided that the patient has sufficient knee flexion to pedal through a full cycle.

When the patient has complete control of the limb and demonstrates a negative Trendelenburg test to static testing, he or she may progress to walking with a single crutch under the opposite arm, *provided that muscle strength is the only limiting consideration.* The average revision patient is kept on two crutches for 6 months. Patients with major acetabular reconstruction or other major body deficits may have to be on crutches for as long as a year, and a cane may always be necessary.

SUMMARY

This chapter has outlined in detail a comprehensive rehabilitation program to be planned for, and followed by, patients undergoing revision total hip arthroplasty. It is no coincidence that this program resembles in many ways the program developed for patients recovering from vitallium mold arthroplasty.[1] Patience is required on the part of all members of the health team. Following this extensive program, the rewards for the patient will be an enduring and successful hip replacement arthroplasty.

REFERENCES

1. Aufranc OE:*Constructive Surgery of the Hip.* Saint Louis, CV Mosby Co, 1962.
2. Charnley J: *Low-Friction Arthroplasty of the Hip: Theory and Practice.* New York, Springer-Verlag, 1979, pp 302-307.
3. Charnley J: Total hip replacement by low-friction arthroplasty. *Clin Orthop Rel Res* 72.7–21, 1970.
4. Demopoulos JT, Selman L: Rehabilitation following total hip replacement. *Arch Phys Med and Rehabil* 53;51–59, 1972.
5. Frankel VH, Burstein AH: *Orthopedic Biomechanics.* Philadelphia, Lea and Febiger, 1970, pp 21–27.
6. McCann VH, Philips CA, Quigley TR: Pre-operative and post-operative management. The role of allied health professionals, In Millender LH, Sledge CB (Eds): Symposium on Rheumatoid Arthritis. *Orthop Clin North Amer* 6:881, 1975.
7. Opitz JL: Total joint arthroplasty: Principles and guidelines for post-operative physiatric management. *Mayo Clin Proc* 54:602–612, 1979.
8. Yoslow W, Simeone J, Heustis D: Hip replacement rehabilitation. *Arch Phys Med and Rehabil* 57:275–278, 1976.

Index